Clinical Nursing Diagnosis Series

# A GUIDE TO THE
# NURSING OF CHILDREN

Clinical Nursing Diagnosis Series

# A GUIDE TO THE
# NURSING OF CHILDREN

**Susan B. Dickey, MSN, RNC**

*Assistant Professor, Department of Nursing*
*Temple University, Philadelphia, Pennsylvania*
*Doctoral Student, University of Pennsylvania*

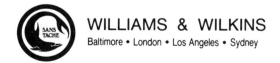

WILLIAMS & WILKINS
Baltimore • London • Los Angeles • Sydney

*Editor:* Nancy Coulter, RN, MSN
*Production:* Raymond E. Reter

Copyright © 1987—Williams & Wilkins
428 East Preston Street, Baltimore, Maryland 21202 U.S.A.

Accurate indications, adverse reactions, and dosage schedules for drugs are provided in this book, but it is possible that they may change. The reader is urged to review the package information data of the manufacturers of the medications mentioned.

*Printed in the United States of America*

**Library of Congress Cataloging in Publication Data**
Dickey, Susan B.
  A guide to the nursing of children.

  Includes bibliographies and index.
  1. Pediatric nursing. I. Title. [DNLM: 1. Pediatric Nursing. WY 159 D551g]
RJ245.D53 1986      610.73'62      86-9073
ISBN 0-683-09560-9

86  87  88  89  90      10  9  8  7  6  5  4  3  2  1

*This book is dedicated to my parents, Mary Beth and Joseph M. Dickey, whose gifts of a solid lifelong and undergraduate education made it a possibility.*

S.B.D.

**Standards of Maternal and Child Health Nursing Practice**

    I. The nurse helps children and parents attain and maintain optimum health.

    II. The nurse assists families to achieve and maintain a balance between the personal growth needs of individual family members and optimum family functioning.

    III. The nurse intervenes with vulnerable clients and families at risk to prevent potential developmental and health problems.

    IV. The nurse promotes an environment free of hazards to reproduction, growth and development, wellness, and recovery from illness.

    V. The nurse detects changes in health status and deviations from optimum development.

    VI. The nurse carries out appropriate interventions and treatment to facilitate survival and recovery from illness.

    VII. The nurse assists clients and families to understand and cope with developmental and traumatic situations during illness, childbearing, childrearing, and childhood.

    VIII. The nurse actively pursues strategies to enhance access to and utilization of adequate health care services.

    IX. The nurse improves maternal and child health nursing practice through evaluation of practice, education, and research.

---

"To revert to children. They are much more susceptible than grown people to all noxious influences. They are affected by the same things, but much more quickly and seriously, viz., by want of fresh air, of proper warmth, want of cleanliness in the house, clothes, bedding, or body, by startling noises, by improper food, or want of punctuality, by dulness and by want of light, by too much or too little covering in bed, or when up, by the spirit of management of those in charge of them."

Florence Nightingale
*Notes on Nursing*, 1860

# FOREWORD

It is unusual to find an eminently practical and pragmatic book written for the "firing line" professional that manages to include information on the leading edge. This book suggests even more. The nursing of children in an acute-care setting focuses on the interplay of psychologic, social, and biophysiologic factors that in combination affect the family's and the individual's stress tolerance, adjustment to illness, and subsequent wellness. In this timely book, these factors are considered in the context of functional health patterns and nursing diagnoses. The author's approach to the nursing of children is broad and clear. While not covering the entire waterfront of childhood illness and care, the book is clear about why it does not and indicates where to obtain information about those other areas. Most important, it takes a specifically nursing approach and permits the reader to examine nursing concerns by looking them up directly rather than through medical screens. The book should serve as a useful reference for nurses practicing in all inpatient pediatric care settings.

Claire M. Fagin
Professor and Dean,
University of Pennsylvania
School of Nursing

# Preface

*A Guide to the Nursing of Children* is designed as a ready-reference manual to assist pediatric nurses to apply the principles of nursing diagnoses in inpatient acute-care settings. Decisions about what to include and the depth of information presented were made with the audience in mind. Fundamental knowledge of nursing skills is presupposed. Medically oriented content is restricted to those diagnoses/conditions most likely to be *regularly* encountered in pediatric units. Conditions requiring intensive care or very specialized care were judged outside the scope of the book.

This book is unique in its philosophy that nursing care has basic processes that are evident regardless of a child's medical diagnosis. A given medical diagnosis, whether detailed in the following chapters or not, will necessitate certain modifications in nursing care, but the nursing approach to a child with a nursing diagnosis of *Anxiety*, for instance, will be very similar and follow basic principles whether the child has asthma or leukemia.

My hope is that *A Guide to the Nursing of Children* will help pediatric nurses integrate nursing and medical diagnoses.

Susan B. Dickey

# ACKNOWLEDGMENTS

I would like to gratefully acknowledge the help and support of many individuals in the preparation of this book. I thank each of my contributors, particularly Chris Bechtel, Donna DeSantis, Bill Fawcett, Lenny Papineau, and Judi Vessey. These individuals were responsible for sections equivalent to the size of individual chapters.

A personal thank-you goes to the following: my sister, Patrice, for her unending praise; Sylvia Fields, for introducing me to my first contact at Williams & Wilkins; Louise Nash for "Fridays"; and Linda Powell for editorial assistance.

Special recognition goes to Carol Dedov, RN, CEN (manuscript typist) whose fund of knowledge about nursing and writing provided an invaluable contribution that a typist alone could never offer.

My editor at Williams & Wilkins, Nancy Coulter, RN, MSN, has contributed a vast amount of time and creativity to the manuscript. Her personal and professional knowledge of children has added another dimension to the book.

Above all, I would like to express gratitude to Susan L. Taddei, former nursing acquisitions editor at Williams & Wilkins. Her skillful and diplomatic encouragement initiated this project. Thank you all.

S.B.D.

# CONTRIBUTORS

Christine M. Bechtel, MSN, RN. Instructor, Department of Nursing, Temple University, Philadelphia, Pennsylvania.

Prince J. Campbell, Baccalaureate nursing student, Temple University, Philadelphia, Pennsylvania.

Donna DeSantis, BSN, CEN. Staff nurse, Emergency department, St. Mary's Hospital, Langhorne, Pennsylvania.

William J. Fawcett, BSN, RN. Staff nurse, Department of Medicine, The Graduate Hospital, Philadelphia, Pennsylvania; Graduate student, University of Pennsylvania.

Harriet Wagner Ferguson, MSN, RNC. Assistant Professor, Department of Nursing, Temple University, Philadelphia, Pennsylvania; Doctoral candidate, Teachers' College, Columbia University, New York.

Mary T. Folkerth, MSN, RN. Assistant Professor, Department of Nursing, Temple University, Philadelphia, Pennsylvania.

Jo Haggerty, BSN, RN. Primary nurse, Children's Hospital of Philadelphia; Graduate student, University of Pennsylvania.

Barbara L. Hughes, MSN, RN. Assistant Professor, Department of Nursing, Temple University, Philadelphia, Pennsylvania.

Mary Lou Manning, MSN, RN, Instructor, Nursing of Children, Department of Nursing, Pennsylvania State University, Philadelphia, Pennsylvania.

Douglas B. Marshall, Esq., Attorney at Law, Philadelphia, Pennsylvania.

Lenny Papineau, BA, RRT. Respiratory Therapy Department, University Hospital, University of Maryland, Baltimore, Maryland.

Madeline Masucci Perkel, MSN, RNC. Former Head Nurse, Pediatric Intensive Care—Acute, The Children's Hospital of Philadelphia.

Judi Vessey, MSN, CRNP. Instructor and doctoral candidate, School of Nursing, University of Pennsylvania.

# Contents

# INTRODUCTION

*A Guide to the Nursing of Children* is one of the first clinical practice books to be organized strictly around a nursing model rather than around a medical model. Thus, its approach is unique.

Nurses do not plan and implement their care based on medical diagnoses per se; they provide care for the patient's problems and concerns that are a result of the medical diagnoses. Many of these problems and concerns—now classified as nursing diagnoses—occur again and again with different medical diagnoses (e.g., fluid balance, nutritional alterations, grieving). Consequently, they generate some basic or generic processes. These generic nursing processes are modified, of course, by the impact of a specific medical diagnosis on the individual. *A Guide to the Nursing of Children* presents its content in precisely this way. A basic or generic nursing care plan is presented for a given nursing diagnosis followed by supplemental care for a selected medical diagnosis.

This book utilizes Gordon's functional health patterns (FHP) and nursing diagnosis. The nursing diagnosis statements are generally from the list approved by the North American Nursing Diagnosis Association (NANDA). Each functional health pattern is a separate chapter, and nursing diagnoses that may fall within that specific pattern are included in the chapter. Not every functional health pattern or every nursing diagnosis is included; only those that relate to the most common concerns in the nursing of children. Occasionally, we have employed non-NANDA approved qualifiers for the nursing diagnosis (e.g., Temperature Instability). When this has been necessary, the qualifier is contained in parentheses.

There is an implicit conceptual model of nursing and manner of application of the nursing process associated with the NANDA list. There is room for concept-overlap in this taxonomy. For example, the nursing diagnosis "anxiety" may be closely related to another one such as ineffective airway clearance or ineffective family coping. Thus, one health problem may have several related nursing diagnoses. The reader is urged to look under several applicable diagnoses for related information.

In this book, the medical diagnoses appear as selected health problems frequently associated with a particular nursing diagnosis and are under the nursing diagnoses that have the most significant impact, and vice versa. Thus, if you want information about caring for a child undergoing cardiac surgery, you will not find it under the cardiovascular system; you will find it after the nursing diagnosis "Alteration in Cardiac Output: Decreased."

A look at chapter 7, *Activity-Exercise Functional Health Pattern* will be illustrative. The chapter opens with general information on activity and exercise, how these concepts apply to children, and some of the medical problems that affect activity and exercise. Next, the author addresses the nursing diagnosis of "Alteration in Cardiac Output: Decreased" via a generic (basic) care plan. When using the generic nursing care plan, the nurse must use judgement to select the specific assessments, interventions, and evaluations that pertain to the specific child for whom the care is planned. The growth and development, medical diagnosis, abilities, knowledge, and motivation of child and family may all affect the specific plan of care. Selected health problems that impact significantly on this nursing diagnosis (e.g., congenital cardiac anomalies) are then presented along with additional nursing care necessitated by this particular medical diagnosis. The reader is also referred to alternate or additional nursing diagnoses necessary to complete the plan of care.

Organizing nursing facts and content in this unique way is an ongoing challenge for all concerned. *A Guide to the Nursing of Children* is the first volume in the Clinical Nursing Diagnosis Series.

# SECTION I

# GENERAL CONSIDERATIONS

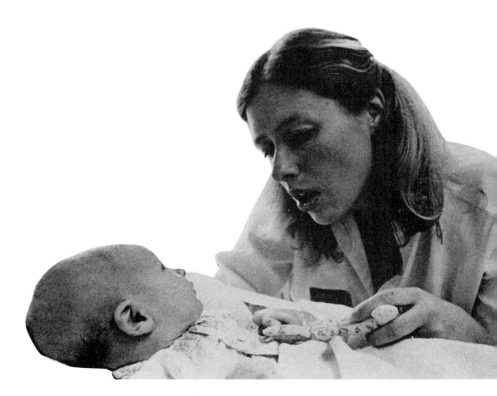

# CHAPTER 1

# THE PEDIATRIC DATA BASE

H ealth management of children begins with a health assessment. This chapter provides some basic information on assessment of infants and children in tabular form. Assessments specific to individual nursing diagnoses and selected health problems are dealt with in subsequent chapters.

Table 1.1 is a pediatric data base that encompasses information germane to the infant, young child, and the adolescent. Most infant physical parameters have been included in the head-to-toe physical examination (table 1.2). At some institutions, data bases are printed separately for specific age groups. The data base included here is a composite applicable to all pediatric age groups. Infantile reflexes are listed in table 1.3. Table 1.4 contains the range of normal vital signs by age group. Table 1.5 includes general trends in physical growth during childhood.

**Table 1.1** Pediatric Data Base

1. Informant's Name
2. Biographical Information (child)
   - Name and nickname
   - Age (in months if under 3 years); ordinal position
   - Race
   - Cultural/ethnic background; family financial resources
   - Religious affiliation
   - Number of family members
     • siblings (include sex and ages)
     • biologic vs step- or foster parents

**Table 1.1**     Pediatric Data Base (continued)

- Members of household
- Pets
3. Reason for Admission (record child's or informant's own words)
4. Health Status
   - General health for last year
   - Accidents in last year
   - Summary of present concerns
   - Illness
5. Medications Taken (before admission)
   - Prescription: dose, frequency, times, compliance
   - Over-the-counter drugs: dose, frequency, etc.
   - Vitamins
6. Developmental Status
   - One month to preschool
     - motor development (list milestones and when attained)
     - age of prehension (act of seizing or grasping)
     - cognitive milestones
     - vocalization capabilities
   - School age
     - gross motor development (milestones and when attained)
     - fine motor skills (ties shoes, uses scissors, draws with detail)
     - cognitive development (school success, special classes, learning disabilities, school difficulty, absenteeism)
     - vocalization (reading, telling time)
     - behavior (special note of thumb sucking, enuresis, lying, rocking, pica, fire setting)
   - Adolescent
     - motor development (sports interests)
     - cognitive skills (special classes, absenteeism, learning problems)
     - pubertal stage (Tanner stage)
7. Current Health Status
   - Allergies
     - drugs _____ reaction _____
     - food _____ reaction _____
     - other _____ reaction _____
   - Immunizations (list dates)
     - DPT/OPV
     - MMR
     - Tine or Mantoux tests for TB
   - Last examination (dates)
     - dental
     - ophthalmic
     - hearing
     - developmental
   - What health providers are working with the family system (e.g., community nurse)?
8. Past Status
   - Perinatal history
     - maternal health during pregnancy
     - maternal medications during pregnancy (prescription and nonprescription)
     - complications (bleeding, falls, toxemia, etc.)
     - x-rays
     - emotional state
     - pregnancy planned? paternal attitude?
     - labor and delivery (date/place, complications, anesthesia/analgesia)
     - gestational age
     - type of delivery

**Table 1.1**    Pediatric Data Base (continued)

- birth weight and length
- cry
- problems
- regular nursery/special equipment
- discharged with mother
- Neonatal history
  - feeding
  - choking, blue spells, increased crying
  - jaundice
- Growth and development
  - normality (by published standards, comparison with siblings, parental impressions)
  - mental status (mood, attention span, etc.)
- Childhood diseases (varicella, rubella, measles, mumps, pertussis, hay fever)
  - age
  - complications
- Serious illnesses/hospitalizations
- Accidents and injuries (note age)
  - head fractures
  - burns
  - trauma
  - poisonings
- Family history
  - draw genogram, including parents and grandparents. Indicate living and deceased family members, chronic illnesses, causes of death, genetic defects.
9. Review of Physiologic Systems
  - General (frequent illness, birth defects, fevers/sweats, etc.)
  - Fatigue patterns
  - Energy patterns (hyperactivity)
  - Nutrition
    - 24-hour dietary intake
    - tolerance of milk products/formula
    - feeding patterns (self, assisted, special equipment)
    - parents' perception of child's nutritional status (fad diets, etc.)
    - "junk food" consumption
  - Skin
    - chronic rashes
    - easy bruising, petechiae, bleeding
    - acne
    - pigmentation (normal, changes)
    - infections/parasites (scabies, lice, impetigo)
    - nails (texture, clubbing)
  - Eyes
    - crossing, strabismus
    - reading/visual disturbances
    - glasses/contact lenses
  - Ears
    - multiple infections
    - tube placement
    - hearing loss/aids
  - Nose
    - bleeding
    - allergies
    - postnasal drip
  - Mouth/throat
    - tonsils/tonsillitis (note frequency)

**Table 1.1**    Pediatric Data Base (continued)

- caries, bottle mouth
- malocclusion/retainers/braces
− Neck
  - swollen/tender glands
  - stiffness of neck, myalgias
− Cardiovascular
  - heart murmur, palpitations, rheumatic disease, arrhythmias and other problems
  - circulation (cyanosis, hypertension, cold extremities)
− Respiratory
  - cough, sputum
  - dyspnea, wheezing, croup, shortness of breath
− Hematopoietic
  - swelling of nodes
  - bleeding
  - easy ecchymosis
  - blood dyscrasias
  - plumbism (history)
  - sickle cell disease (trait)
  - hemophilia (active, carrier)
  - blood type (if known)
− Gastrointestinal
  - nausea, vomiting, diarrhea
  - stooling patterns
  - toilet training regimen
  - stool character/changes (e.g., worms, perianal pruritus)
  - evacuation aids
− Urinary
  - UTIs
  - suprapubic tenderness, flank pain
  - nocturia, polyuria
− Genitalia
  - discharges/odors
  - rash/irritation
  - concerns/recent changes
  - sexuality education (evaluate parental attitudes and ability to make appropriate explanations)
− Musculoskeletal
  - cramping
  - fractures, other bone/joint injuries
  - back injury, family history of scoliosis
− Central nervous system
  - perinatal anoxia
  - unusual episodic behaviors
  - diseases
  - seizure disorders
  - speech problems
  - cognitive changes
  - motor—gait disturbances
  - sensory—tingling disturbances
− Endocrine
  - known disease (diabetes mellitus, hypothyroidism)
  - skin/hair texture (changes)
  - goiter
  - precocious puberty
  - panhypopituitarism

**Table 1.1**    Pediatric Data Base (continued)

10. Psychosocial
    − Feelings about self/siblings
    − Friends
    − Extracurricular activities, hobbies, interests
    − Discipline (parental attitudes, strategies, in school)
    − Parental support systems, money, time away from children
        • primary caretakers
        • day care
    − Parental attitudes about health maintenance
    − Parental attitudes about environmental safety
    − Home hazards
        • age-appropriate toys, activities
        • poisons (including availability of alcohol and drugs to adolescents)
        • yard play, neighborhood (traffic, overcrowding, sidewalks, pollution, noise, pesticides, toxic waste dumps, water purity)
    − Room/bed (does infant sleep in bed with parents?)
    − Available transportation
    − Latchkey children

**Table 1.2**    Physical Assessment of Children

| | Assessment Objectives/Procedures | Normal Findings | Anomalies/Implications |
|---|---|---|---|
| **1. Integument**<br>**A. Inspection**<br>1) Skin | Color | Light, tan, fair, rosy, olive, pale; cyanosis normal for 4 hours postdelivery | Cyanosis: appears when the central Hgb is $\leq 5$ gm/100 ml or there is deoxygenated blood in the periphery |
| | | Physiologic jaundice: appears at 36–48 hours, peaks at 3–6 days; remission after 7–10 days | Jaundice<br>− infants: 5 mg bilirubin/100 ml blood<br>− older children: 2 mg bilirubin/100 ml blood<br>Carotenemia (infants — palms, soles beefy red): hypoglycemia |
| | Vascularities/Telangiectasis | Angiomatous spots on skin ("Stork's beak" marks); nevi Mongolian spots<br>− occur in dark-complexioned children<br>− disappear by 4–5 years<br>− located over sacrum | Hairy nevi at base of spine: r/o spina bifida<br>Hemangiomas; strawberry marks — grow until 3 months; regress by 7 years<br>Cavernous hemangiomas (grow until 1 year; regress by school age) |

**Table 1.2**    Physical Assessment of Children (continued)

| | Assessment Objectives/Procedures | Normal Findings | Anomalies/Implications |
|---|---|---|---|
| | Surface moisture | Dry → moist | Dehydration<br>– mild: < 5% body weight<br>– moderate: 5%–10% body weight, tented skin<br>– severe: 10%–15% body weight, sunken orbits and fontanels, dry membranes |
| | Edema | | Anasarca (generalized edema): pitting edema (1–4 scale — skin can be depressed 1–4 cm). |
| | Pigmentation | Even coloring Freckles | Hyperpigmentation (cafe-au-lait spots): r/o neurofibromatosis<br>Hypopigmentation (vitiligo, albinism, amelanosis secondary to trauma) |
| | Lesions | | Types<br>– primary (initial lesions, minimal changes)<br>– secondary (evolved from primary lesions) |
| 2) Nails | Color | Semitransparent; pink color reflected from vascular bed | Nailbed<br>– pale: r/o iron-deficiency anemia<br>– blue: cyanosis<br>– yellow (infants): postmaturity<br>– white spots: trauma to nailbed |
| | Size | | Micronychia: trisomy 13, 18, fetal alcohol syndrome<br>Thickening: r/o fungal infection |
| | Shape, position, angle | ~ 160 (< 180°) | Clubbing (nail angle ≥ 180°)<br>Paronychia: cuticular infection<br>Torn cuticles: r/o nail-biting, poor nutrition |

**Table 1.2**   Physical Assessment of Children (continued)

| | *Assessment Objectives/Procedures* | *Normal Findings* | *Anomalies/Implications* |
|---|---|---|---|
| **B. Palpation** | | | |
| 1) Skin | Compare contralateral parts (use back of hands on various body parts) | | |
| | Skin texture (palpate with fingertips) | Smooth, even skin | Excessive smoothness: edema  Excess roughness: allergies, vitamin A deficiency, exposure to chemical agents |
| | Turgor (pinch skin) | Skin immediately resumes original position | Poor turgor: dehydration |
| 2) Hair | Color | Blond → Black | Red streaks: kwashiorkor  No color: r/o albinism  White streak from forehead to crown: Waardenburg's syndrome |
| | Location | Prematures: lanugo over body  Infants and children: primarily on scalp  Adolescents: scalp, axillae, pubic area | Low hairline: r/o Hurler's syndrome, hypothyroidism  Alopecia (if child is pulling it out): r/o ringworm |
| | Amount | Thin → thick  Dry → oily  Coarse → fine  Soft → brittle  Infant hair replaced by 3 months | Brittle and patchy: r/o hypothyroidism, malnutrition |
| | Scalp | | Seborrheic dermatitis (cradle cap)  Lice |
| **2. Head** | | | |
| **A. Measurement** | | | |
| Occipital-frontal circumference | Usually measured from ages 0–3 years or when known neurologic problems exist  – measure above ears, over widest part of occiput and forehead  – avoid measuring over braids, barrettes  – use a nonstretchable tape measure | See head circumference growth chart | Macrocephaly (> 95th percentile for age)  Microcephaly (< 5th percentile for age) |

**Table 1.2**    Physical Assessment of Children (continued)

| | Assessment Objectives/Procedures | Normal Findings | Anomalies/Implications |
|---|---|---|---|
| **B. Inspection** | | | |
| 1) Cranium | Size, symmetry, shape<br>Confirm observations by palpation | Round and symmetrical; areas of minor depression or protrusion | Flatness (seen when infants are left supine)<br>Premature closure of the sutures: brachycephaly, acrocephaly<br>Frontal bossing: syphilis, congenital syndromes<br>Macrocephaly<br>Microcephaly<br>Swelling or molding: caput succedaneum, cephalohematomas |
| | Note head to body ratio<br><br>Head lag | Birth: 1:4<br>Young child: 1:5–1:6<br>Older child: 1:7<br>Normal until 3 months | Disproportionate head to body ratios: dwarfism, gigantism<br>Persistent lag: neurologic deficit/immaturity |
| 2) Face | Symmetry, position, and size of features | Symmetrical appearance | Asymmetry: abnormal intra-uterine lie, cranio-facial malformations<br>Facial nerve disruption: ptosis, drooping of mouth corner<br>Abnormal head angle: torticollis, vision-hearing problems<br>Lowset ears: chromosomal aberrations; congenital malformations |
| **C. Palpation** | | | |
| Skull | Suture lines, fontanels<br>Palpate systematically | Marked ridges of sutures disappear by 6 months<br>Fontanel closure<br> – posterior: 2–3 months<br> – anterior: 12–18 months<br>Mild pulsations of fontanels normal in some infants | Craniotabes (skull can be depressed, much like a ping-pong ball): long-term increased ICP, infection, rickets, osteogenesis imperfecta<br>Fontanel changes<br> – bulging: vomiting, increased ICP<br> – sunken: dehydration<br> – marked pulsation: increased ICP |

**Table 1.2**   Physical Assessment of Children (continued)

| | Assessment Objectives/Procedures | Normal Findings | Anomalies/Implications |
|---|---|---|---|
| **D. Percussion** | | | |
| Head | Check for Macewen's sign (a resonant "cracked pot" sound); must be done after fontanel closure | | Macewen's sign seen in: open fontanels, skull fractures, separated sutures |
| **E. Instrumentation** | | | |
| Cranium | Fontanels, temporal and orbital areas: auscultate for bruits | | Bruits suggest cerebrovascular abnormalities |
| | Skull (newborns): transilluminate | Frontal area: transilluminates ≤ 2 cm Posterior area: transilluminates ≤ 1 cm | Marked light rings or asymmetry: hydrocephalus, intracranial lesions |
| **3. Vision** | | | |
| **A. Inspection** | | | |
| External eyelids and lashes | | Lids should cover 1–3 mm of limbus | Entropia (lashes turned inward) Exotropia (lashes turned outward) Other abnormalities (hordeolums/sties, chalazions) Ptosis: r/o CN III damage, edema |
| | Sclerae, conjunctivae | Sclerae: white, blue-white, yellow-white | Sclerae – yellow: r/o jaundice – inflamed: r/o conjunctivitis, herpes infection |
| | | Conjunctivae: salmon pink | Inflamed conjunctivae: r/o conjunctivitis |
| | Epicanthal folds | Normal in children of Oriental descent | In nonOrientals: r/o Down's or other congenital syndrome |
| | Corneas | Clear, transparent | White, opaque with scarring |
| | Iris | Blue → brown | Red: r/o albinism Brushfield spots: r/o Down's syndrome Irregular borders: r/o iriditis |

**Table 1.2**    Physical Assessment of Children (continued)

| Assessment Objectives/Procedures | Normal Findings | Anomalies/Implications |
|---|---|---|
| Pupils: Observe direct and consensual response to light<br>Compare size, shape | | Abnormal size/response: r/o CN III damage |
| Acuity (use age-appropriate method)<br>– 3–6 years (no learning disabilities): illiterate E Chart<br>– 3–6 years: Lawson picture chart<br>– 6 years: Snellen chart<br>Place chart at 15′ rather than 20′<br>Ensure chart height is appropriate to the child's size | Newborn: 20/200–20/600<br>1 year: 20/100–20/200<br>3 years: 20/50<br>4–8 years: 20/40<br>8 years: 20/30 or less | Refractive errors/disorders<br>– myopia (nearsightedness)<br>– hyperopia (farsightedness)<br>– anisometropia (inequality of the refractive power of the eyes)<br>– astigmatism (corneal curvature < 360°) |
| Color recognition (not accurate until mental age of 3½–4 years) | Recognizes all colors | Color blindness: red-green occurs in approximately 3.5% of males and .5% of females |
| Binocularity: Hirschberg light test (corneal light reflex test) | Light directed to bridge of nose falls equally or slightly medially on both pupils | Light falls medially on 1 pupil<br>Light falls laterally on 1 pupil<br>Light falls laterally on both pupils |
| Cover test | No movement of eye when cover is removed | Lateral or medial deviation of eye when cover is removed, specifically<br>– esotropia (eye deviates medially and fixes in position)<br>– esophoria (eye deviates medially part of the time)<br>– exotropia (eye deviates laterally and fixes in position)<br>– exophoria (eye deviates laterally part of the time) |

**Table 1.2**   Physical Assessment of Children (continued)

| | Assessment Objectives/Procedures | Normal Findings | Anomalies/Implications |
|---|---|---|---|
| | Extraocular movements (6 cardinal fields of gaze) | Full movement<br>— upward, medially<br>— downward, medially<br>— medially<br>— upward laterally<br>— downward, laterally<br>— laterally | No medial downward movement: r/o CN IV damage<br>No lateral movement: r/o CN VI damage<br>All other deviations: r/o CN III damage |
| | Visual fields (difficult in children under age 8) | Nasal: 60°<br>Upward: 50°<br>Downward: 70°<br>(up and down total: 120°)<br>Lateral: 90° | Decreased fields: r/o RLF, glaucoma |
| **B. Instrumentation** | | | |
| | Ophthalmic exam<br>— in infants, elicit sucking reflex (eyes will open)<br>— always perform in a darkened room | Red reflex | Dark reflex: r/o cyanosis<br>Pale reflex: r/o anemia<br>Leukocoria: r/o cataracts, retinoblastoma |
| | | Disc to cup ratio of 1:2 | Large, uneven discs: r/o papilledema, hemorrhage, exudate |
| | | No nicking of vessels | Vascular nicking: r/o hypertension |
| **4. Ear**<br>**A. Inspection** | | | |
| | External ear: slant | Flexible pinna<br>Well developed helix | Poorly developed pinna: r/o prematurity, congenital syndromes |
| | Position relative to eye | Juncture of helix even with outer canthus of eye | Low-set ears: r/o trisomy 13, 18, various other syndromes |
| **B. Palpation** | | | |
| | Tragus | No tenderness | Tenderness: r/o otitis externa |
| | Mastoid process | No tenderness | Tenderness: r/o mastoiditis |
| | External canal | Light pink, no lesions | Edematous, white debris or inflammation: r/o otitis externa |

**Table 1.2**    Physical Assessment of Children (continued)

| | Assessment Objectives/Procedures | Normal Findings | Anomalies/Implications |
|---|---|---|---|
| **C. Instrumentation** | | | |
| | Tympanic membrane<br>– make sure otoscope is correctly positioned to prevent injury<br>– infants: pull auricle down and back<br>– young children: pull auricle straight back<br>– older children: pull auricle up and back | Pearly gray, translucent<br>Light reflex<br>– 5 o'clock in right ear<br>– 7 o'clock in left ear<br>– good mobility | Decreased light reflex, straw-colored membrane (with or without bubbles): r/o serous otitis media<br>Bright red, bulging membrane: r/o acute purulent otitis media<br>Blue, bulging membrane: r/o internal hemorrhaging |
| | Check mobility with pneumoscope; ensure external canal is well sealed | | Retracted, poor membrane mobility: r/o retracted membrane<br>White markings, opaque membrane: r/o scar tissue |
| | Hearing best checked through audiometry, tympanometry | Audiometry: 0–10 decibels (dB) at F 500–2,000 Hertz (Hz) | Audiometric indicators of hearing loss<br>– mild: 20–40 dB at F 500–2,000 Hz<br>– moderate: 40–60 dB at F 500–2,000 Hz<br>– severe: 60–80 dB at F 500–2,000 Hz |
| | May use Weber & Rinne tests with older children | Weber:<br>no lateralization<br>Rinne: air conduction 2x bone conduction bilaterally | Weber: lateralization to one ear<br>Rinne: air conduction ≤ bone conduction |
| | Gross hearing tests<br>– newborns: elicit startle reflex, use a Crib-O-Gram<br>– older children: watch test, "whisper down the lane" games | | |

**Table 1.2**   Physical Assessment of Children (continued)

| | Assessment Objectives/Procedures | Normal Findings | Anomalies/Implications |
|---|---|---|---|
| **5. Nose** | | | |
| **A. Inspection** | | | |
| | Size, shape, and position | Midline placement; small in early childhood, grows throughout lifetime Septum midline (some deviation common with aging) Saddle bridge normal in blacks, Orientals | Horizontal line above tip: r/o "allergic salute" Deviated septum: r/o fracture(s) Saddle bridge: r/o various congenital syndromes |
| | Skin | Even flesh tones Milia normal in infants | Butterfly rash: r/o systemic lupus erythematosus |
| | Nares | No flaring | Flaring: respiratory distress |
| | Nasal mucosa (color, moisture, and integrity) | Deep red, moist, no lesions | Pale, boggy mucosa: r/o allergies Inflamed, edematous mucosa: r/o URI Nasal polyps: r/o cystic fibrosis |
| **B. Palpation** | | | |
| | Naral patency: block off each side of nose separately, ask the child to exhale | Bilateral patency | Decreased patency: r/o URIs, allergy, deviated septum, foreign bodies |
| | Maxillary and frontal sinuses Evaluation not helpful until school age, when the sinuses have completed pneumonization | No tenderness | Tenderness: r/o sinusitis |
| **6. Mouth/(Oropharynx)** | | | |
| **Inspection** | External structures (lips, cheeks, nasolabial fold) Symmetry | Symmetrical features and movements | Asymmetry: r/o cranial nerve damage (CN V, VII) |
| | Lip color, condition | Pink, smooth, moist | Blue tint: cyanosis Pallor: anemia Fissures: r/o chelitis Lesions: r/o herpes |

**Table 1.2**    Physical Assessment of Children (continued)

| | Assessment Objectives/Procedures | Normal Findings | Anomalies/Implications |
|---|---|---|---|
| Mucous membranes | Moisture | Moist | Dryness: r/o dehydration, mouth breathing, specific drugs (e.g., antihistamines) |
| | Color | Pink → brown (depends upon melanin content) | Yellow tinge: r/o jaundice |
| | Lesions | | Ulcerations Thrush Mucoceles Aphous ulcers |
| | Teeth Number | 20 deciduous teeth 32 permanent teeth (begin erupting by 5–7 years) | |
| | | Order of eruption: first molars, central incisors, lateral incisors, canines, 1st bicuspids, 2nd bicuspids, 2nd molars, 3rd molars | Abnormal order of eruption |
| | Color | Pearly white/ pearly yellow | Gray, mottled: r/o tetracycline exposure Chalky: r/o caries formation/bottle mouth Black: r/o caries Brown spots: r/o plaque |
| | Position (bite) | Uppers just in front of lowers No space between upper/lower molars and bicuspids | Typical problems: malocclusion, overbite, crowding, excess spacing |
| | Gums Color, bleeding, adherence | Salmon pink → brown (depending upon melanin deposits) | Red, swollen, bleeding: r/o gingivitis, pyorrhea |
| | Tongue, salivary glands Color | Light pink | Strawberry or raspberry tongue: r/o febrile condition |

**Table 1.2**   Physical Assessment of Children (continued)

| | Assessment Objectives/Procedures | Normal Findings | Anomalies/Implications |
|---|---|---|---|
| | Texture | Velvet texture Common variants: geographic tongue (denuded papillae), hairy tongue (elongated papillae) | Smooth, slick tongue: r/o nutritional deficiency (e.g., vitamin $B_{12}$, iron, or niacin) |
| | ROM | 360° | Limited ROM: r/o cranial nerve involvement (CN XII), r/o ankyloglossia (tied) |
| | Palate | Intact Rises on "ah" | Cleft palate, submucous cleft Cranial nerve damage (CN IX) |
| | Uvula Phonation | Midline | Deviation: r/o cranial nerve damage (CN IX, X) |
| | Tonsils Size | Enlarged during middle childhood | Enlarged in infancy, adolescence (touching uvula or each other) |
| | Color | Pink | Reddened, with or without exudate: r/o tonsillitis |
| | Crypts | None | |
| **7. Neck** **A. Inspection** | | | |
| | Length | | Too short: r/o congenital hypothyroidism, gargoylism, Morquio's syndrome Webbed: r/o Turner's syndrome |
| | ROM | Side-to-side ~ 180° Down ~ 45° Back ~ 55° | Tilting: r/o brain tumors, vision problems, absent corpus callosum Stiffness: r/o infectious processes, adenitis, torticollis Hyperextension/ opisthotonus: r/o cerebral palsy, tetanus, respiratory tract infections |

**Table 1.2**    Physical Assessment of Children (continued)

|  | *Assessment Objectives/Procedures* | *Normal Findings* | *Anomalies/ Implications* |
|---|---|---|---|
|  | Symmetry | Symmetrical, no masses | Mass (lower 1/3 of neck): r/o congenital torticollis<br>Mass (oval, cystic, upper 1/3 of neck): r/o branchial cleft cysts |
|  | Pulsations | Normal in carotids and jugulars (child in supine position) | Distended/engorged veins: r/o aortic insufficiency, liver damage with cardiac failure, asthma, COPD |
| **B. Palpation** |  |  |  |
|  | Trachea, suprasternal notch | Palpable cartilaginous rings, midline to slightly right | Tracheal deviation: r/o pleural effusion, pneumothorax, tumor<br>Palpable thud over trachea: foreign body |
|  | Thyroid<br>– identify supporting structures (hyoidbone, thyroid cartilage, cricoid cartilage, trachea) to help identify thyroid isthmus | Frequently nonpalpable in children | Masses: r/o goiter, thyroid nodules |
|  | Palpate lobes In young children, use supine position Lymph nodes (see lymphatics) | Equal and small |  |
| **C. Auscultation** |  |  |  |
|  | Neck vessels (for bruits and murmurs) | None | r/o tracheal vascular rings<br>To-and-fro bruits: possible thyroid involvement<br>Bilateral bruits, low in the neck: r/o aortic stenosis<br>Unilateral bruits, high in the neck: r/o vascular insufficiency |

**Table 1.2**    Physical Assessment of Children (continued)

| | *Assessment Objectives/Procedures* | *Normal Findings* | *Anomalies/ Implications* |
|---|---|---|---|
| **8. Lymph Nodes**<br>  **Palpation** | | | |
| | Size, consistency, mobility, tenderness, temperature<br>Use tips of fingers, small circular motions<br>Adjust child's position to reduce tension of overlying skin, fascia<br>Areas to palpate<br>*Head and neck*<br>– preauricular<br>– postauricular<br>– occipital<br>– mandibular<br>– submental<br>– anterior cervical chain<br>– posterior cervical chain<br>– supraclavicular<br>*Breast/axillae*<br>– central<br>– lateral<br>– infraclavicular<br>– subscapular<br>– pectoral<br>*Elbow:* epitrochlear<br>*Groin:* inguinal | Nodes not palpable<br>Shotty nodes (cool, nontender, mobile, firm, < 1 cm are normal in cervical area of young children, inguinal area of adolescents | Enlargement<br>(> 1 cm, spongy, fixed, tender, warm or unilateral)<br>– cervical adenitis: tonsillitis<br>– submaxillary adenopathy: stomatitis<br>– occipital, postauricular adenopathy: pediculosis<br>– generalized adenopathy: infectious mononucleosis<br>– inguinal or axillary adenopathy: postvaccination<br>– unilateral adenopathy: Hodgkin's disease |
| **9. Chest**<br>  **A. Inspection** | | | |
| | Shape<br>Measure<br>Skeletal abnormalities (ribcage) | Anterior/Posterior lateral diameter<br>– newborns: 1:1<br>– 1 year: 1:1.25<br>– 6 years: 1:1.35<br>– 15–18 years: 1:2 | Pectus excavatum (frequently normal): r/o rickets<br>Pectus Carinatum: r/o COPD, rickets, postsurgical repair<br>Barrel Chest: r/o COPD (frequently associated with kyphosis) |
| | Spinal column abnormalities<br>Skin lesions | (see musculo-skeletal system) | Spider nevi: liver disease |

**Table 1.2**  Physical Assessment of Children (continued)

| Assessment Objectives/Procedures | Normal Findings | Anomalies/Implications |
|---|---|---|
| Mammary area<br>– spacing of nipples | Distance between outer areolar area is ~ 1/4 chest circumference | Wide-spaced nipples (distance between outer areolar area > 1/4 of chest circumference): r/o Turner's syndrome |
| – amount of glandular tissue | Absent/minimal in prepubertal children | Gynecomastia (common in pubertal boys) |
| – discharge<br>"Witches' milk" (neonates)<br>– extra nipples | | Supernumerary nipples: usually 5–6 cm below regular nipples |
| Respiration rate and rhythm | (see table 1.4 for normal rates) | |
| Breathing style | Abdominal breathing (infants and older males)<br>Costal breathing (children < 7) | Costal breathing in infants: r/o intra-abdominal or intrathoracic pathology<br>Retractions: r/o pneumonia, asthma<br>Bradypnea: r/o brain lesions, increased ICP, alkalosis<br>Tachypnea: r/o acute pulmonary disease, fever, acidosis<br>Hyperpnea: indicates anoxia |
| Cough | No cough | Paroxysmal with inspiratory whoop: r/o pertussis<br>Loose and productive: r/o URI, bronchitis<br>Brassy and nonproductive: r/o foreign body, croup<br>Tight and nonproductive: r/o pneumonia |

**Table 1.2**   Physical Assessment of Children (continued)

| | Assessment Objectives/Procedures | Normal Findings | Anomalies/Implications |
|---|---|---|---|
| | Fremitus (palpate) | Increased over large airways | Abnormal increases: r/o pneumonia, bronchitis, atelectasis |
| | | Decreased in lower chest | Abnormal decreases: r/o pneumothorax, asthma |
| | Chest expansion | Equal bilateral expansion | Unequal chest expansion: r/o pneumothorax, airway blockage |
| **B. Percussion** | | | |
| | Both sides of the chest (compare) Level of diaphragmatic excursion | Resonant throughout (except over heart) | Dull percussion: r/o pneumonia, atelectasis Hyperresonant percussion: r/o COPD, asthma |
| **C. Auscultation** | | | |
| | Breath sounds (throughout the chest) − generally coarser in children than adults due to thinner chest wall − to facilitate having young children take a deep breath, ask them to "blow out" the light on a penlight | Tracheal sounds (over trachea and tracheal bifurcation) Bronchial sounds (over middle lung fields) Vesicular sounds (over lung bases) | Adventitious sounds − wheezes: r/o asthma, foreign bodies − friction rubs: r/o pleurisy − rhonchi: r/o bronchitis − rales: r/o pneumonia |
| **10. Heart** | | | |
| **A. Inspection/Palpation** | | | |
| | Inspect chest wall for the apical impulse (PMI) | Infants: 4th ICS left of the LMCL 4–6 years: 4th ICS at the LMCL ~7 years: 5th ICS right of the LMCL Adolescents: 5th ICS at the LMCL | Apical impulse lateral to usual position: r/o enlarged heart |
| | Thrills − sternoclavicular area − aortic area − pulmonic area − ectopic area − apical area − epigastric area | None | Thrills − aortic region: r/o aortic stenosis, PDA − pulmonic region: r/o pulmonic stenosis |

**Table 1.2**   Physical Assessment of Children (continued)

| | Assessment Objectives/Procedures | Normal Findings | Anomalies/Implications |
|---|---|---|---|
| | | | Thrills (continued)<br>– tricuspid region: r/o VSD, any condition with increased right ventricular pressure<br>– apical region: r/o mitral stenosis with or without regurgitation<br>– epigastric region: r/o fever, anemia, hyperthyroidism, tricuspid stenosis |
| **B. Percussion** | | | |
| | Heart borders (test not always performed)<br>May use direct, mediated, or scratch percussion | Base: 3rd ICS<br>Apex: 5th ICS | Outside normal limits: r/o enlarged heart |
| **C. Auscultation** | | | |
| | Auscultate heart at aortic, pulmonic, Erb's, tricuspid, and mitral areas | | |
| | Note intensity of $S_1$ (closure of mitral and tricuspid valves) and $S_2$ (closure of pulmonic and aortic valves)<br>Systole: $S_1$ $S_2$<br>Diastole: $S_2$ $S_1$ | $S_1 > S_2$ at apex<br>$S_2 > S_1$ at base | increased $S_1$: r/o anemia, fever, exercise<br>increased $S_1$ with bradycardia: r/o mitral stenosis, atrial flutter<br>increased $S_2$: r/o coarctation of the aorta, atrial hypertension |
| | Rate | See table 1.4 for normal rates/age | Tachycardia: r/o fever, exercise, cardiac decompensation |

**Table 1.2**    Physical Assessment of Children (continued)

| Assessment Objectives/Procedures | Normal Findings | Anomalies/Implications |
|---|---|---|
| Rhythm | Regular Sinus dysrhythmia Tic-tac rhythm (when $S_1$ and $S_2$ sound the same) normal in young children Ventricular gallop ($S_1 S_2 S_3$) normal in some children | Bigeminy: r/o organic heart disease Premature beats (atrial or ventricular): r/o organic heart disease Gallop rhythms — atrial gallop ($S_1 S_2 S_4$) — ventricular gallop ($S_1 S_2 S_3$) — summation gallop ($S_1 S_2 S_3 S_4$) Atrial fibrillation Ventricular fibrillation |
| Extra sounds — $S_3$ (passive ventricular filling) directly follows $S_2$ | Occurs in 1/3 of healthy children | May signify overload |
| — $S_4$ (atrial contraction) directly precedes $S_1$ | Rarely normal in children | R/o hypertensive CV disease, aortic stenosis, pulmonic stenosis, cor pulmonale |
| Splits | Physiologic split of $S_2$ during inspiration in 1/4 to 1/3 of children | Wide $S_2$ splits: r/o left-to-right atrial shunt, pulmonic stenosis, RBBB, ASD Paradoxical $S_2$ splits: r/o PDA $S_1$ splits: r/o RBBB, aortic stenosis, pulmonic stenosis, pulmonary hypertension, coarctation of the aorta |
| Clicks | | R/o pulmonic and aortic stenosis |
| Snaps | | R/o stenotic mitral valve, left-to-right shunt |
| Pericardial friction rubs (do not vary with respiration) | | R/o pericarditis |
| Pleural pericardial friction rubs (vary with respiration) | | R/o adhesions |

**Table 1.2**   Physical Assessment of Children (continued)

| | Assessment Objec-tives/Procedures | Normal Findings | Anomalies/Implications |
|---|---|---|---|
| | Venous hums (auscultate over internal jugulars) | Frequently normal | R/o anemia, thyro-toxicosis |
| | Mediastinal crunch | | Consistent with post-surgical complica-tions |
| | Murmurs (grade intensity)<br>I: very faint, not heard all over chest<br>II: quiet<br>III: moderately loud<br>IV: loud<br>V: very loud, associ-ated thrill<br>VI: very loud, can hear with stetho-scope off chest, associated thrill<br>Quality (blowing, rumbling, harsh, musical)<br>Pitch (high, medium, low)<br>Position in cycle (systolic, diastolic, panstolic) | Grade I-II/VI systolic ejection murmur (functional murmur) (normal variant) | Systolic ejection murmurs: r/o anemia, ASD, mitral valve prolapse, aortic stenosis, pulmonic stenosis<br>Pansystolic regurgi-tant murmurs: r/o mitral regurgitation, VSD, tricuspid regurgitation<br>Early diastolic murmurs: r/o aortic or pulmonic insuf-ficiency<br>Late diastolic murmurs: r/o mitral and tricuspid stenosis<br>Panstolic murmurs: r/o PDA, systemic A-V fistula, aortic coarctation |
| **11. Abdomen**<br>   **A. Inspection** | | | |
| | Shape (supine position) | Thin musculature (compared to adults)<br>Common shapes<br>— rounded (particu-larly in young children)<br>— flat<br>— scaphoid | Bulging at flanks: r/o ascites<br>Scaphoid<br>— infants: r/o diaphragmatic hernia<br>— older children: r/o malnutrition, dehydration<br>Distention: r/o megacolon, intes-tinal duplication, organomegaly<br>Midline protrusion: r/o diastasis rectii |
| | Skin (color, vascular-ities, scars, striae) | Superficial veins (in infants) | Superficial veins (older children): r/o portal vein hypertension<br>Spider nevi: r/o liver disease |

**Table 1.2**   Physical Assessment of Children (continued)

| | Assessment Objectives/Procedures | Normal Findings | Anomalies/Implications |
|---|---|---|---|
| | Pulsations | Light midline pulsations | Diffuse epigastric pulsations: r/o ventricular hypertrophy<br>Wide midline pulsations: r/o abdominal aortic aneurysm |
| | Hair distribution | Minimal | Hirsuteness: r/o adrenocortical dysfunction<br>Abnormal hair distribution (adolescents): r/o endocrine or liver disorders |
| | Peristalsis | Normal in thin-walled infants | Hyperstalsis: r/o pyloric stenosis (infants), diarrhea, abdominal distention |
| | Umbilicus: measure size of umbilical ring | Round, indented or slightly protuberant, about 1 cm in diameter; 3 vessels evident (newborns) | Eversion: r/o increased intra-abdominal pressure, herniation (closes spontaneously in most cases by age 5)<br>Fistulas: r/o abscess, patent urachus<br>Granulomatous tissue<br>Fewer than 3 vessels |
| **B. Auscultation** | | | |
| | All quadrants for bowel sounds (should *precede* palpation, which can disturb bowel sounds) | Peristaltic sounds: high-pitched, irregularly timed, 4–6/minute; more evident before meals | Hyperperistalsis: r/o diarrhea, intestinal obstruction<br>No sounds: r/o paralytic ileus |
| | Vascular sounds | No vascular sounds (most children) | Bruits: r/o dilated, tortuous, or constricted vessels<br>Venous hums: r/o portal hypertension, liver hemangiomas<br>Murmurs: r/o aortic coarctation |

**Table 1.2**    Physical Assessment of Children (continued)

| | Assessment Objectives/Procedures | Normal Findings | Anomalies/Implications |
|---|---|---|---|
| **C. Percussion** | | | |
| | All quadrants (use mediated method) | Predominantly tympany Dullness over liver (5th–7th ICS, RMCL to or just below the costal margin); over spleen (above the 9th ICS; LMAL); over fecal masses (LLQ) | Dullness in other areas: r/o abdominal mass, enlarged liver, spleen |
| **D. Palpation** | | | |
| | All quadrants — begin with *light* palpation (circular fingertip motion), depressing the abdominal wall ½–1 cm — follow with *deep* palpation (bimanual 3–5 cm depression of the abdomen) — alternative method: place one hand on the abdomen and one hand on the back, "squeezing" the abdominal wall | Negative findings | Involuntary rigidity — with palpable nodes: r/o infection (e.g., peritonitis) — without palpable nodes: r/o abdominal distention, pain, ticklishness Palpable lymph nodes |
| | | Lower border of the liver — firm, with an even, well-demarcated edge — palpable upon deep inspiration in young children; often in older children as well | Liver hypertrophy (palpable well below costal margin) |
| | | Spleen often not palpable | Splenic hypertrophy (older children) — slight: 1–4 cm below costal margin — moderate: 4–8 cm below costal margin — severe: > 8 cm below costal margin |
| | | Kidneys rarely palpable; right kidney felt more often than left Palpable mass: pregnant uterus | Palpable kidney: r/o hydronephrosis; neoplasms, polycystic disease Palpable masses: r/o Wilms' tumor, neuroblastomas, pyloric tumor or stenosis |
| | Rebound tenderness (use two hands; press in slowly, then withdraw quickly) | Negative findings | Positive in RLQ with appendicitis |

**Table 1.2**  Physical Assessment of Children (continued)

| | Assessment Objectives/Procedures | Normal Findings | Anomalies/Implications |
|---|---|---|---|
| **12. Male Genitalia** | | | |
| **A. Inspection/Palpation** | | | |
| | Penis (retract foreskin) | Foreskin not retractable for first 3 months; completely retractable by 4 years. | Not retractable after 3 months: r/o phimosis, adhesions Paraphimosis (everted foreskin over glans) Infection: balanoposthitis Prepubertal calculus: poor hygiene |
| | Position of meatus | Opening on tip of penis | Hypospadias (opening is underneath side of glans or shaft) <br>– balanic (meatus opens on glans) <br>– penile (meatus opens on shaft) <br>– penoscrotal (meatus opens below shaft) <br>Epispadias (opening is on top side of glans or shaft) <br>– balanic (meatus opens on glans) <br>– penile (meatus opens on shaft) <br>– penopubic (meatus opens near symphysis) <br>Pinpoint meatus: r/o urinary obstruction |
| | Glans | | Warts: r/o condyloma acuminatum, c. latam |
| | Shaft (note size) | > 2–3 cm at birth | < 2–3 cm at birth: r/o microphallus, enlarged clitoris Penile hyperplasia (after 1 year): r/o adrenal tumor, hypothalamic tumor Priapism: r/o sickle cell disease, leukemia, neoplasms, thrombosis |

**Table 1.2**    Physical Assessment of Children (continued)

| | Assessment Objectives/Procedures | Normal Findings | Anomalies/Implications |
|---|---|---|---|
| | Scrotum<br>– color | Flesh-colored, slightly pigmented | Red and shiny: r/o orchitis<br>Dark: r/o adrenal hyperplasia |
| | – rugae<br>– contour | Well-formed<br>Varies; left testicle should be slightly lower than right | Enlarged scrotum: r/o hydrocele, hematocele, chylocele, variocele, hernias |
| | Testes (palpation)<br>– block inguinal canals<br>– avoid eliciting cremasteric reflex<br>– if difficulty is encountered, have child assume flexed position | Smooth, ovoid<br>1.5–2.0 cm (at birth)<br>3.5–5 cm (after puberty) | Undescended testicles at birth<br>– ½ descended by 1 month<br>– ¼ more descended by 1 year<br>Undersized: r/o Klinefelter's syndrome (at puberty), hypopituitarism, adrenal hyperplasia<br>Oversized: r/o sexual precocity, testicular tumor |
| | Epididymis (palpate): usually posterior to testes | Smooth ridge of tissue | Mass: r/o spermatocele, retention cyst<br>Tenderness: r/o epididymitis |
| | Inguinal hernia<br>– inspect for enlarged scrotal sac<br>– invaginate scrotum; follow inguinal ligament<br>– note developmental stage (in puberty) | | Bulge in inguinal canal |
| **B. Transillumination** | | | |
| | Scrotum (when swelling is present) | | Positive: hydrocele, chylocele |
| **C. Auscultation** | | | |
| | Scrotum (when mass is present) | | Positive (bowel sounds): large inguinal hernia |
| **13. Female Genitalia**<br>**Inspection/Palpation** | | | |
| | External genitalia<br>– note any abnormalities in labia majora | | Skin lesions: ulcers, chancres, herpes, condylomas<br>Swelling: r/o lymphedema, labial-inguinal hernia |

**Table 1.2**  Physical Assessment of Children (continued)

| Assessment Objectives/Procedures | Normal Findings | Anomalies/ Implications |
|---|---|---|
| Labia minora | Quite large in the newborn | Adhesions: poor hygiene |
| Clitoris | Hypertrophy common in infancy; involutes by 1 month | |
| Meatus | | Prolapse |
| Vagina | No discharge Hymen intact | Signs of abuse, e.g., lacerated labia, contusions, lacerated perineum, edema, vaginal tears, bleeding |
| Developmental stage (in puberty) | (Note: internal exam usually deferred until late puberty) | |

**14. Adolescent Developmental Stages**

| Stage | Male | Female |
|---|---|---|
| 1: Development of gonads, reproductive organs, and secondary sex characteristics | No pubic hair No increase in size of penis Testes begin to mature Acceleration in height and weight gain Changes in body composition (more fat) | No pubic hair No breast enlargement, but papillar elevation Ovaries begin to enlarge External preadolescent genitalia Vaginal pH 6–7 |
| 2: Acceleration/deceleration of skeletal growth | Early growth of testes and scrotum before pubic hair appears Height spurt accelerates Physique begins to change (increased fat, muscle) Areolae increase in size and darken slightly | Breast bud formation followed by early pubic hair growth Acceleration in the deposition of total body fat Hips widen |
| 3: Altered body composition (skeletal and muscular growth); changes in the quantity and distribution of fat | Testicular, scrotal enlargement Lengthening of penis Spreading, darkening pubic hair Facial hair at upper corner of lip Further acceleration of height spurt Shoulders broaden General increase in physical definition Increased muscle mass (relative to fat) Circumanal hair | Further breast enlargement Further spread of pubic hair Enlarged vagina Increased thickness of vaginal epithelium with glycogen deposition (response to estrogen stimulation from maturing ovaries) Appearance of Doderlein's (lactic-acid producing) bacilli; vaginal mucosa becomes acid (pH 4–5) Height spurt peaks (early stage 3) Menarche may begin (late stage 3) |

**Table 1.2**  Physical Assessment of Children (continued)

| Stage | Male | Female |
|---|---|---|
| | Cartilage of the larynx enlarges; voice may begin to deepen<br>Transient gynecomastia with slight projection of the areolae | |
| 4: Increased strength and endurance | First axillary hair<br>Continued enlargement (breadth) of scrotum, testes, and penis<br>Pubic hair begins to take on adult characteristics<br>Facial hair (limited to upper lip and chin)<br>Considerable growth of prostate gland; first ejaculation<br>Sebaceous glands approach adult size and function<br>Voice deepens further | Menarche occurs (if not in stage 3)<br>Axillary hair appears around menarche<br>Areolar mound may appear (75% of the time), persisting into stage 5<br>Breasts, pubic hair, ovaries continue enlargement<br>Ovulation may occur |
| 5 | Genitals (size) and pubic hair (distribution) are adult in appearance<br>Hair appears on the side of the face<br>Gynecomastia<br>Deceleration of height spurt<br>Mature physique | Adult-appearing breasts and pubic hair<br>Growth decelerates (after menarche may grow 2–4 inches)<br>Ovulation regulated some 2 years after menarche |
| 6 | Further spread of pubic hair up linea alba (80% of all males) | Further spread of pubic hair (10% of females) |

| | Assessment Objectives/ Procedures | Normal Findings | Anomalies/ Implications |
|---|---|---|---|
| **15. Musculoskeletal System**<br>**A. Inspection/Palpation** | Size and shape<br>— measure height and weight<br>— plot on appropriate growth chart<br>Symmetry<br>— compare level, size, shape, and number of corresponding parts (specifically shoulders, iliac crest, knees, ankles, arms) | Height, weight, and weight/height measurements between the 5th and 95th percentiles<br>Bilateral symmetry throughout | Height or weight < 5th percentile or > 95th percentile<br>Weight/height < 5th percentile or > 95th percentile |

**Table 1.2**     Physical Assessment of Children (continued)

| Assessment Objectives/ Procedures | Normal Findings | Anomalies/ Implications |
|---|---|---|
| – anterior and posterior views (compare) | | |
| Spine – shoulder and iliac crest height (compare), ribcage symmetry – bend child over, mark spinous processes, note curves | Double S curve – lordotic cervical curve – kyphotic thoracic curve – lordotic lumbar curve – kyphotic sacral curve | Kyphosis Gibbus Lordosis (normal in toddlers) Scoliosis |
| Neck and spine (ROM) | Cervical rotation ~ 170° | Cervical rotation < 170°: r/o torti- collis, muscle spasm |
| | Spinal flexion and extension ~ 45° each Lateral flexion ~ 45° Lumbar-sacral flexion ~ 75°–90° Lumbar-sacral lateral flexion ~ 30°–35° | Limited ROM: r/o back injury, spinal deformity or fusion |
| Sacral-coccygeal dimple | None | If present: r/o spina bifida occulta |
| Upper extremities – compare arms, shoulders (bilat- erally) | Bilateral symmetry | |
| – observe ROM of rotator cuff | External rotation ~ 90° Internal rotation ~ 90° Flexion ~ 180° Extension ~ 50° Adduction ~ 50° Abduction ~ 180° | Limited ROM: r/o frozen shoulder, previous injury, joint inflammation, Sprengel's syndrome |
| Crepitus (joint) | None | Crepitus: r/o degenerating cartilage |
| Elbow (inspect), epicondyles (palpate) | Flexion ~ 160° Rotation ~ 180° Limited ROM: r/o injury or inflamma- tion | Excessive carrying angle: r/o gonadal dysgenesis |

**Table 1.2**   Physical Assessment of Children (continued)

| Assessment Objectives/ Procedures | Normal Findings | Anomalies/ Implications |
|---|---|---|
| Hand Test ROM of wrist, fingers | Radial deviation ~ 20° Ulnar deviation ~ 55° Wrist extension ~ 70° Wrist flexion ~ 90° Metacarpo-phalangeal flexion ~ 90° Metacarpo-phalangeal hyper-extension ~ 30° Proximal interphalangeal flexion ~ 120° Distal interphalangeal flexion ~ 80° | Limited ROM: r/o inflammation, injury Clawlike hands: r/o Hurler's syndrome |
| Joints (palpate) | No tenderness | Swelling and tenderness: r/o rheumatoid arthritis |
| Fingers: number, dermatoglyphics | | Syndactyly, polydactyly Unusually short fingers: r/o genetic abnormalities Simian crease: r/o Down's syndrome |
| Lower extremities – gait | Acceleration → midswing → decel-eration | Limp: r/o dislocated hip, knee or foot injury |
| – stance | Heel strike → foot flat → midstance → push off | |
| Buttocks folds (shape and contour) | Bilateral symmetry | |
| ROM of hip | Flexion with knee extension ~ 80–90° Flexion with knee flexion ~ 120° Abduction ~ 45° Adduction ~ 30° Newborns' hips rotate ~ 160–175° (bilaterally) | Limited ROM: r/o injury, inflammation Pain on rotation: r/o Legg-Calvé-Perthes disease, dislocated hips (infants) |

**Table 1.2**    Physical Assessment of Children (continued)

| | *Assessment Objectives/ Procedures* | *Normal Findings* | *Anomalies/ Implications* |
|---|---|---|---|
| | Ortolani's test<br>— abduct hips and listen/palpate for clicks over the joints | No clicks | Clicks: r/o dislocated hip |
| | Allis Test<br>— flex knees and hips, look at knee height | Knees of equal height | Knees > 2 cm apart with medial maleoli touching: genu varum |
| | Knees | Knees and medial maleoli should touch in older child<br>— mild genu varum normal under 2 years<br>— mild genu valgum normal 2 years to school age | Knees > 2 cm apart with medial maleoli touching: genu varum<br>Medial maleoli > 2 cm apart with knees touching: genu valgum |
| | — ROM | Flexion ~ 130°<br>Hyperextension ~ 15°<br>Internal rotation ~ 40°<br>External rotation ~ 45° | Limited ROM: r/o injury, inflammation<br>Excessive ROM: r/o injury |
| | — crepitance, fluid effusion | | Pain over tibial head: r/o Osgood-Schlatter's disease |
| | ROM of ankles and feet (note positioning) | Ankle inversion ~ 30°<br>Ankle eversion ~ 20°<br>Dorsiflexion ~ 20°<br>Plantar flexion ~ 45° | Limited ROM: r/o inflammation, infection, shortened Achilles tendon<br>Pes valgus<br>Pes varus<br>Pes planus<br>Pes cavus<br>Metatarsus adductus<br>Talipes |

**16. Neurologic**
   **A. Mental Status**
(In a young child, most neurologic assessment can be done through the Denver Developmental Screening Test.)

| | | |
|---|---|---|
| | Level of consciousness, orientation | Child oriented first to person, then place, then time |
| | Memory (short/long term, recall/recognition) | Digit recall<br>— 4 years: 3 digits<br>— 5 years: 4 digits<br>— 6 years: 5 digits |

**Table 1.2**    Physical Assessment of Children (continued)

| | Assessment Objectives/ Procedures | Normal Findings | Anomalies/ Implications |
|---|---|---|---|
| | Ask age-appropriate questions, e.g., "What did you do in school?" | | |
| | Language and speech (both receptive and expressive language) | 4 months: babbling 7–9 months: nonspecific words 12–15 months: specific words 18 months: 3 words 2 years: 2-word sentences 3 years: 3-word sentences | Poor language: r/o hearing loss, cerebral palsy |
| | Abstract reasoning (cannot test until adolescence) | | Poor mental skills: r/o mental retardation, developmental delay |
| **B. Cranial Nerves** | Olfactory (I) | Intact from birth | |
| | Optic (II) | | |
| | – acuity (children over 3): use Lazy E or symbol charts | Neonates: 20/600 Infants: 20/200 1 year: 20/100 4–5 years: 20/40–20/50 6–8 years: 20/20 | Common problems: myopia, hyperopia, amblyopia (from uncorrected esotropia, exotropia, unequal bilateral acuity) |
| | – fixation | Present from 6 weeks of age | |
| | – visual fields | 60° nasally 130° vertically 100° temporally | Disturbed visual fields: r/o glaucoma, RLF |
| | – optic fundi | Red reflex | Leukocoria: r/o RLF, retinoblastoma, cataracts |
| | Oculomotor (III) | | |
| | Trochlear (IV) | | |
| | Trigeminal (V) | | |
| | – sensory function: touch face with cotton | Bilateral sensory function | |
| | – masseter muscle strength: have child bite on tongue blade | Blade removal should be difficult | |
| | Abducens (VI): ocular ROM | Full ROM in each of the 6 cardinal fields of vision | |

**Table 1.2**  Physical Assessment of Children (continued)

| | Assessment Objectives/ Procedures | Normal Findings | Anomalies/ Implications |
|---|---|---|---|
| | − pupillary response | Pupils equal and round, reactive to light and accommo-dation | Fixed or sluggish response: r/o brain lesion or trauma |
| | | Lid covers 1−3 mm of limbus | Ptosis: r/o CN III damage |
| | Facial (VII) − symmetry: have child puff cheeks, purse lips, show teeth, wrinkle forehead, raise eyebrows | Bilateral symmetry | Asymmetry: r/o facial palsy |
| | − taste: test on anterior 2/3 of tongue | Intact | |
| | Acoustic (VIII): hearing assess-ment in young children best done by audiometry | Intact | Conductive loss: r/o middle ear effusion, impacted cerumen |
| | Glossopharyngeal (IX) Vagus: − taste: assess on 1/3 posterior of tongue | | |
| | − palate, movement | With "ah," palate moves upward; uvula midline | |
| | − gag reflex | Intact | |
| | Accessory (X): ROM of neck, shoulder (shrug) | Full ROM | Limited ROM: r/o torticollis |
| | Hypoglossal (XII) − tongue: ROM, strength | Full ROM | |
| **C. Motor Function** | | | |
| | Motor function | Knee bends: 12 months Jumping: 2½−3 years Balancing on 1 foot: 2½ years Hopping: 4½ years Tandem walking: 5 years Skipping: 5−6 years Rapid supination/ pronation of hands: 5−6 years Finger touching: 5−6 years | Inability to perform activities at appro-priate ages is consistent with the neurologic "soft signs" seen in learning disabilities |

**Table 1.2**    Physical Assessment of Children (continued)

|  | Assessment Objectives/ Procedures | Normal Findings | Anomalies/ Implications |
|---|---|---|---|
|  | Muscle strength | Full ROM of all joints against gravity and additional resistance; bilateral strength | Increased tone: r/o upper motor neuron disease Decreased tone: r/o lower motor neuron disease |
| **D. Sensation** |  |  |  |
|  | Sensation (across body parts) Stereognosis, graphesthesia, kinesthesia (cannot evaluate until school age) | Intact |  |
| **E. Reflexes** |  |  |  |
|  | Deep tendon reflexes<br>– triceps<br>– biceps<br>– brachioradialis<br>– patellar<br>– Achilles<br>Superficial reflexes<br>– plantar<br>– corneal<br>– gag<br><br>Primitive reflexes (table 1.3) | 2 + reflexes all around<br><br><br><br><br><br>Bilateral plantar flexion<br>Eye blink<br>Gag | 4 + reflexes: r/o cerebral palsy |

*Abbreviations Used*

| | | | |
|---|---|---|---|
| ASD | atrial septal defect | LUQ | left upper quadrant |
| A-V | atrioventricular | PDA | patent ductus arteriosus |
| CV | cardiovascular | PMI | point of maximum impulse |
| dB | decibels | RBBB | right bundle branch block |
| Hz | Hertz | RLF | retrolental fibroplasia |
| ICP | intracranial pressure | RLQ | right lower quadrant |
| ICS | intercostal space | RMCL | right midclavicular line |
| LLQ | left lower quadrant | r/o | rule out |
| LMAL | left midaxillary line | ROM | range of motion |
| LMCL | left midclavicular line | VSD | ventricular septal defect |

**Table 1.3**    Infantile Reflexes

| Type | Appears | Disappears | Noteworthy Assessments |
|------|---------|-----------|------------------------|
| Localized, protective: | | | |
| pupillary | At birth | — | Unique responses; fixed, dilated pupils |
| corneal | At birth | — | Absence (possible damage to CN V, III) |
| sneeze | At birth | — | Absence, continuous sneezing |
| gag | At birth | — | Hyperactive, absence (possible damage to CN IX) |
| yawn | At birth | — | Absence |
| cough | At birth | — | Absence |
| Localized, primitive: | | | |
| oculovestibular (Doll's eye) | At birth | With fixation, 6 weeks | Asymmetry (paralysis of CN VI) |
| sucking | At birth (28 weeks) | 6 months | Weak, absent suck (suggests general CNS depression) |
| rooting | At birth | 3–4 months | Absence |
| palmar grasp | At birth | 3–4 months | Absence/asymmetry (indicates brachial plexus damage or Klumpke's paralysis) |
| plantar grasp | At birth | 8 months | Absence or asymmetry |
| Babinski | At birth | With walking | Persistence (possible pyramidal lesion) |
| Generalized, primitive: | | | |
| Moro | At birth (28 weeks without flexion) | 3–4 months | Persistence after 6 months (brain damage) Asymmetry (injury to brachial plexus, humerus, or clavicle) Cortical thumbs (cortical damage) |
| startle | At birth | 3–4 months | Absence (suggests hearing loss) |
| asymmetric tonic neck reflex (fencing) | At birth | 3–4 months | Absence or persistence (CNS damage) Obligatory responses |
| Galant's reflex | At birth | 4 weeks | Absence (indicates reflex spinal cord lesion) |
| neck-righting | At birth (34–37 weeks) | 10 months | Absence |
| Perez | | 4–5 months | Persistence (possible brain damage) |
| stepping (dance) | At birth (36 wk) | 3–4 month | Asymmetry |
| crawling | At birth | 6 weeks | Asymmetry |

**Table 1.4**    Range of Normal Vital Signs

| Age | Pulse | Respirations | Systolic BP |
|---|---|---|---|
| Newborn | 125 | 64–70 | |
| 1 year | 120 | 35–40 | |
| 2 years | 110 | 31–35 | 96 |
| 4 years | 100 | 26–31 | 96 |
| 6 years | 100 | 23–26 | 96–98 |
| 8 years | 90 | 21–23 | 104 |
| 10 years | 90 | 21 | 110 |
| 12 years | 85–90 | 21 | 115 |
| 14 years | 80–85 | 21–22 | 118–120 |
| 16 years | 75–80 | 20 | 120–124 |

**Table 1.5**    General Trends in Physical Growth During Childhood

| Age | Weight* | Height* |
|---|---|---|
| Infant | Weekly gain: 140–200 gm (5–7 oz) | Monthly gain: 2.5 cm (1 in) |
| • Birth–6 months | Birth weight doubles by end of first 6 months** | |
| • 6–12 months | Weekly gain: 85–140 gm (3–5 oz) Birth weight triples by end of first year | Monthly gain 1.25 cm (0.5 in) Birth length increases by approximately 50% by end of first year |
| Toddler | Birth weight quadruples by age 2½ Yearly gain: 2–3 kg (4.4–6.6 lb) | Height at 2 years is approximately 50% of eventual adult height Gain during second year: about 12 cm (4.8 in) Gain during third year: about 6–8 cm (2.4–3.2 in) |
| Preschooler | Yearly gain: 2–3 kg (4.4–6.6 lb) | Birth length doubles by age 4 Yearly gain: 6–8 cm (2.4–3.2 in) |
| School-age child | Yearly gain: 2–3 kg (4.4–6.6 lb) | Yearly gain after age 7: 5.0 cm (2 in) Birth length triples by about age 13 |
| Pubertal growth spurt • Females (10–14 years) | Weight gain: 7–25 kg (15–55 lb) Mean: 17.5 kg (38.1 lb) | Height gain: 5–25 cm (2–10 in) Mean: 20.15 cm (8.2 in) Approximately 95% of mature height achieved by onset of menarche or skeletal age of 13 years |
| • Males (11–16 years) | Weight gain: 7–30 kg (15–65 lb) Mean: 23.7 kg (52.1 lb) | Height gain: 10–30 cm (4–12 in) Mean: 27.5 cm (11 in) Approximately 95% of mature height achieved by skeletal age of 15 years |

*Yearly gains for each group represent averaged estimates from a variety of sources.
**A recent study has shown the mean time for doubling of birth weight to be 3.8 months (Neumann & Alpaugh, 1976).
Note: From *Clinical handbook of pediatric nursing,* p. 63, by D. Wong and L. Whaley, 1981, St. Louis: Mosby. Copyright 1981 by Mosby. Reprinted with permission.

To estimate developmental status, refer to the tables of developmental tasks, stages, and milestones in Chapters 8 and 9. In addition, the Denver Developmental Screening Test may be used.

Each child must be evaluated within the context of the family situation. Therefore, information concerning the family constellation is of paramount importance in the delivery of family-centered care. The stages of family development are discussed in Chapter 10.

The assessment data collected for children is similar to that obtained from adults; however, some questions must be asked about young children that would not ordinarily be asked of older clients.

Whenever possible, include the child as an informant. This practice gives insight into the child's intelligence, verbal skills, and emotional status, and it enhances understanding of the health of the entire family constellation. It is also helpful to have the child's mother provide information about the prenatal and puerperal course. The father, if present, can also contribute to the assessment and should certainly be made aware of the importance of his contributions to child care. Always identify the informant in the written history.

Thoroughness is critical when eliciting a pediatric health history. For instance, when inquiring about allergies (table 1.6), it is important to cover drug, food, insect, and detergent allergies and their specific reactions (Rosen & Viau, 1977). Do not ask if immunizations are "up to date"—the answer will usually be yes. It is better to request the specific ages at which immunizations were administered.

When doing a data base for preteens and adolescents, be sure to set time aside for private discussion with the patient. The teen may wish to obtain or reveal information of a sexual nature or to discuss other private concerns. Such an exchange may not occur at all unless privacy is respected.

# The Vital Signs

Blood pressure and temperature monitoring in children deserve special consideration. Vital signs must be interpreted by the standards appropriate to the child's age. Pulse and respiratory rates decrease as a child gets older, whereas blood pressure gradually increases with age.

**Blood Pressure.**    Blood pressure may be taken in any of the four extremities with a cuff by auscultation, palpation, or Doppler, or in multiple arterial locations via an indwelling arterial catheter. Common locations for arterial lines include the umbilical, radial, and dorsalis pedis arteries. Do not measure blood pressure or draw blood from an extremity upon which vascular surgery has been performed—e.g., after creation of an arteriovenous fistula, Blalock-Taussig, or Blalock-Hanlon procedure—since it can cause injury to the created structure or interfere with venous drainage.

**Temperature.**    *Oral* temperature taking is recommended only for children who are emotionally or developmentally capable of cooperation. Normal children 5–6 years of age are usually able to cooperate. The mentally retarded child, on the other hand, is an excellent candidate for axillary measurement.

**Table 1.6**    Components of an Allergy History

1. Family History
   - Food/drug/substance (dander, insect, detergent) allergies
   - Hay fever, eczema, hives, asthma, migraine, rhinitis, sinusitis
2. Infancy
   - Formula intolerance, colic, fussiness, choking, eczema, diarrhea, rashes, recurrent illnesses, croup
3. Symptoms (asthma, dermatitis, hives, etc.)
   - Weather conditions, season, year, time of day, geographic location (shore vs inland), climate, and age at symptom onset
   - Previous treatment (prescriptions, home remedies)
   - Hospitalization for symptoms
   - Activity restrictions
4. Exposure to Related Factors
   - Dust (housemites)
   - Plants (pollen sources): trees (spring), grasses (summer, fall), weeds (fall)
   - Respiratory infections (winter)
   - Animals (dander): pets, farm animals, clothing of animal origin (wool, alpaca)
   - Cosmetics, perfumes
   - Aerosols
   - Fresh paint
   - Molds, mildews, damp (shoreline) climates with high mold counts
   - Cold-induced reactive airway disease
   - Medicines: aspirin, antibiotics
5. Environment
   - Heat source (electric; old ducts and vents; kerosene, oil, or wood stoves)
   - Age of house
   - Location of affected individual in house (bedroom, location at time of allergy attacks)
   - Flora (house and yard)
   - Type of pillow (down from fowl or kapok vs foam rubber)
   - Stuffed animals
   - Dusty rags

A study measuring the effect of oxygen inhalation on oral temperature noted no significant effect (Lim-Levy, 1982). Oral temperatures should be taken for eight minutes (Nichols & Kucha, 1972).

Many people interested in protecting children, particularly toddlers, from the trauma of intrusive procedures, have recommended axillary thermometry. When fevers or subnormal temperatures are reported by this method, however, unnecessary requests are often made by physicians for rectal retakes to ensure an "accurate" reading. Eoff and Joyce (1981) state "for hospitalized toddlers and preschoolers, there is no clinically important difference in accuracy between axillary and rectal temperatures." In another study, Schiffman (1982) found "a strong positive relationship . . . between axillary and rectal temperatures" in full term newborns, and therefore recommended the axillary method (Eoff & Joyce; Schiffman, 1982; Takacs & Valenti, 1982). No study recommended an optimum length of time for axillary thermometry, but all seemed to concur that a minimum of 7–10 minutes was appropriate. Critically ill children with peripheral vasoconstriction may be poor candidates for this method. No studies were found that correlate core and axillary temperatures in the critically ill.

One study of temperature measurement with glass thermometers recommended that *rectal* readings be taken for five minutes (Takacs & Valenti).

*Electronic* thermometry, when available, was supported by one research group (Takacs & Valenti) that sampled oral, rectal, and axillary temperature taking. There are many advantages of electronic thermometry, but two decided disadvantages do exist: the tendencies of nurses to place the instrument on the children's beds and to avoid washing hands between children.

# References

Behrman, R., & Vaughan, V. (1982). *Nelson's textbook of pediatrics.* (12th Ed.) Philadelphia: Saunders.

Eoff, M., & Joyce, B. (1981). Temperature measurements in children. *American Journal of Nursing, 81,* 1010-1011.

Lim-Levy, F. (1982). The effect of oxygen inhalation on oral temperature. *Nursing Research, 31,* 150-152.

Nichols, G., & Kucha, D. (1972). Oral measurements. *American Journal of Nursing, 72,* 1091-1092.

Rosen, E., & Viau, M. (1977). Pediatric allergy nursing assessment and history guide. *Pediatric Nursing, 2,* 37-39.

Schiffman, R. (1982). Temperature monitoring in the neonate: A comparison of axillary and rectal temperatures. *Nursing Research, 31,* 274-277.

Takacs, K., & Valenti, W. (1982). Temperature measurement in a clinical setting. *Nursing Research, 31,* 368-370.

Waring, V. et al. (1977). *Disorders of the respiratory tract in children.* Philadelphia: Saunders.

# CHAPTER 2

# ADMINISTRATION OF MEDICATIONS

N urses who administer medications to children must do so with great caution. Even therapeutic levels of certain drugs may be toxic to some children. Although it is the physician's responsibility to order the drug, route, dose, and administration schedule, it is the legal and ethical responsibility of the pediatric nurse to know each drug and its implications. A nurse practicing in a pediatric setting is expected to have this professional knowledge.

The "Five Rights" can be a useful set of guidelines for administering drugs in any setting.

1. **Right Patient:** Check identification band. Verify identity with verbal children or parents of nonverbal children.
2. **Right Drug:** Check container label against orders or Kardex three times.
3. **Right Dose:** Check concentrations per capsule, tablet, cubic centimeter, and container.
4. **Right Route:** Check physician's orders for the specific administration procedure: Oral, IM, IV, subcutaneously, topically, per oculus dexter (od, right eye), oculus sinister (os, left eye), oculi unitas (both eyes).
5. **Right Time:** Ensure that the medication is administered within 30 minutes before or after it is scheduled.

Care providers other than licensed professional nurses or physicians and dentists should not be asked to administer medications, including vitamin and iron solutions, in an inpatient pediatric setting. Never assume that parents will give medications, or give them accurately. Many teaching hospitals with multiple affiliating schools of nursing do not permit nursing students to administer medications to children. This may not facilitate learning, but it protects the patients.

**Table 2.1**   Drugs to Be Checked by Two RNs

| Vasoactive Drugs | Cardiac glycosides | Digoxin |
| | Antihypertensives | Inderal (propranolol) |
| | | Hyperstat (diazoxide) |
| | | Hydralazine |
| Respiratory depressants | Narcotics | Morphine |
| | | Codeine |
| | | Demerol (meperidine) |
| | Sedatives | |
| | Barbiturates | Phenobarbital |
| | | Nembutal |
| | Benzodiazepines | Valium (diazepam) |
| Central vasopressors | Catecholamines | Epinephrine |
| | | Levophed (levarterenol, norepinephrine) |
| | | Isuprel (isoproterenol) |
| | | Intropin (dopamine) |
| | | Dobutrex (dobutamine) |
| Miscellaneous | Insulins | |
| | Heparin | |
| | Intravenous methylxanthines | Aminophylline |

Drugs that can be particularly dangerous to children must be checked by two RNs (table 2.1). A few minutes to double-check may avoid a serious drug error and may save the nurse, the child, and the family incalculable hours of regret and pain. Documented double-checking also provides additional legal protection to the nurse and the hospital, since an unexpected occurrence or adverse drug reaction often results in a thorough analysis of the drug and its concentration in the syringe used to administer it.

## Pediatric Physiology and Drug Metabolism

Physiologic considerations must be taken into account when giving medications to children. It is not unusual for children to experience paradoxical reactions to a drug. For instance, methylphenidate HCl (Ritalin), given in an attempt to regulate hyperactivity, can trigger a state of excitement rather than the desired calming effect. Another example of an unexpected drug response would be asystole following a dose of phenytoin (Dilantin) administered by intravenous push. It is never wise to administer any drug rapidly by IV push.

Children absorb, distribute, metabolize, and excrete drugs in a manner much different from adults, owing to their immature organ systems (particularly in neonates) and concentration of body water. Fluid and electrolyte balance is discussed in chapter 5, but an important point to remember is that the body weight of full-term neonates is approximately 73% water. Other variables that determine how a drug will be handled include children's "increased tissue responsiveness to many drugs and acceptance and ease of drug administration" (Malseed, 1983, p. 22).

Some children have been called "rapid metabolizers." These children may have a more rapid heart rate, which results in faster metabolism of a drug. They may weigh the same as their peers but do not derive the same amount of benefit from a standardized drug dose. Conversely, some children develop a tolerance to drug levels that may be toxic in others.

Periods of rapid growth and development in the child, such as the neonatal period, infancy, toddlerhood, and puberty, are sensitive periods in which negative side effects of drugs may be enhanced. It is particularly difficult to recognize adverse effects of drugs in preverbal children, since they are unable to report such sensations as "ringing in the ears," pain, or laryngeal edema in preanaphylactic reactions.

## Special Monitoring

Some drugs require special monitoring of vital signs both before and after administration. Continuous monitoring equipment, such as cardiorespiratory oscilloscope monitors, indwelling arterial lines to give continuous transducer readings of blood pressure, or a Dinamapp (intermittent blood pressure cuff that self-inflates at preset intervals) may be utilized.

- When administering any dangerous drugs, ensure that emergency airway and other advanced life-support equipment is available and *ready to function.*
- Children with head trauma or increasing intracranial pressure should not be given narcotics. Trauma to the brain does not cause pain, and administration of narcotics may mask symptoms of deteriorating neurologic status.
- Barbiturates should be administered cautiously to children with brain injuries. Phenobarbital may be used as an anticonvulsant, or pentobarbital (Nembutal) may be used to place the child in a "protective coma."
- Catecholamines, even in the form of an inhalant such as isuprel, should never be administered without advanced monitoring equipment.
- Nitroprusside, an antihypertensive given by infusion, needs arterial line monitoring. If this equipment is unavailable, it is even more important that the nurse monitor the child's status accurately and frequently, since the child is receiving a drug with potential serious side effects.

Table 2.2 lists medications that require close monitoring.

**Table 2.2**    Medications Requiring Vital Signs Measurement Before Administration

| Medication | Vital Signs to be Checked |
|---|---|
| Antihypertensives | Blood pressure prior to administration and routinely as appropriate |
| Aminophylline, IV | Blood pressure: Every 2 hours for continuous infusion; every 5 minutes for bolus doses, which are usually given over 20 minutes, or place child on cardiorespiratory monitor. |
| Antipyretics | Temperature |
| Digoxin, IV or PO | Pulse: Do not give dose if apical pulse is less than 100 beats/minute in children or infants |
| CNS depressants (e.g., barbiturates, narcotics, benzodiazepines) | Respirations |
| Blood products | Blood pressure, temperature, pulse, respiration |
| Pain medications (particularly narcotics) | Level of consciousness, pupillary reactions, respirations |

## Calculations and Dose Determinations

The professional nurse determines whether an ordered dose of a medication is safe before administering the drug. Many institutions have therapeutic standards committees to establish standard guidelines for drug orders. Orders deviating from hospital formulary guidelines should be cosigned by a chief resident or an attending physician. In institutions where a hospital formulary is not in existence, it is even more important for the nurse to administer drugs according to a standardized dose and administration protocol such as the *National Formulary* (NF), or the *United States Pharmacopeia* (USP). When the ordered dose does not fall within the therapeutic range (i.e., is less or greater than), the nurse must consult with the physician who has ordered the drug. Clinical pharmacists are also valuable in answering questions related to drug usage.

Accurate determinations of a child's height and weight are a nursing responsibility. Medication doses, fluid and electrolyte requirements, doses for anesthetic agents, and watt seconds for cardioversion are frequently calculated in terms of dose per kilogram of body weight or per body surface areas (BSA). It is the nurse's responsibility to verify that these measurements are correct.

**NURSING TIPS: Check calculations carefully in any medication situation. An error in placement of a decimal point during calculations can result in a tenfold or greater drug under- or overdose.**

**Body Surface Area (BSA).**    Body surface area ($m^2$) is a calculation based on height and weight. It is most easily determined by using a nomogram (see Appendix IV). BSA can be used to determine drug doses by applying the formulae found in table 2.3.

**Table 2.3**    Verifying Dose Accuracy Using Body Surface Area to Calculate Dosage

a.    $\dfrac{\text{BSA of child}}{\text{BSA of adult}} \times$ adult dose = estimated child's dose

b.    BSA ($m^2$) $\times$ dose/$m^2$ = child's dose

**Table 2.4**    Verifying Dose Accuracy Using Recommended Dose per Kilogram

**Example 1**

An order reads, "Give ampicillin 175 mg IV q6h."

Infant's weight = 3.5 kg
Recommended dose is 150–200 mg/kg/24 hours

Low end of dose range:
150 mg $\times$ 3.5 kg = 525 mg/24 hours
525 mg divided into 4 doses = 131.25 mg/dose

High end of dose range:
200 mg $\times$ 3.5 kg = 700 mg/24 hours
700 mg divided into 4 doses = 175 mg/dose

The dose ordered for this infant falls on the high end of the normal range.

**Example 2**

An order reads, "Give digoxin elixir, 46 mcg PO q12h."

Infant's weight = 3.5 kg
Recommended total digitalizing dose (TDD) for children under 2 years is 60–80 mcg/kg.
A maintenance dose like the one ordered would be one-third to one-fifth of the TDD daily in two divided doses.

This problem involves several steps.

*Step 1:* Calculate TDD
60 mcg $\times$ 3.5 kg = 210 mcg (low end of range)
80 mcg $\times$ 3.5 kg = 280 mcg (high end of range)

*Step 2:* Calculate safe range for maintenance doses
210 mcg divided by 5 = 42 mcg (low end)
280 mcg divided by 3 = 93.33 mcg (high end)

46 mcg q12h falls within the safe range (92 mcg/24 hours).

**Metric Calculations.**    Metric calculations furnish a safe and simple method of determining a therapeutic dose. They may also provide a safe range within which a medication such as digoxin may be prescribed. The formula, based on recommended pediatric dosage per kilogram of body weight, is

$$\text{Milligrams} \times \text{kilograms of child's body weight} = \text{safe dose for 24-hour period}$$

Table 2.4 gives some examples of how this formula can be applied.

**Digitalization.**    The entire process of digitalization begins with three loading doses of digoxin. The first is usually one-half the total digitalizing dose (TDD).

TDD = 60–80 mcg/kg (children under 2 years of age)
Low TDD divided by 2 = low first digitalizing dose (DD)
High TDD divided by 2 = high first DD

The second and third digitalizing doses are usually one-fourth the TDD and are generally given 8 and 16 hours after the first DD, respectively.

Low TDD divided by 4 = low second and third DD
High TDD divided by 4 = high second and third DD

There are many exceptions to this protocol from the *Hospital Formulary*, Children's Hospital of Philadelphia, for digitalization maintenance therapy and for the safe dosage range changes for children under 2 weeks of age and over 2 years, which may be perfectly acceptable.

Children may outgrow their maintenance levels of digoxin, and should be evaluated periodically. They are also susceptible to digoxin toxicity, which can be manifested by electrolyte (potassium) deficiencies, weakness, nausea, and visual and neurologic disturbances. In children, nausea and vomiting and visual disturbances are unusual; the most common symptom of digoxin toxicity is the appearance of atrial dysrhythmias.

## Medication Administration

When giving medications to children, approach is all-important. The nurse should expect success and work to ensure it by

- Providing developmentally appropriate explanations
- Allowing choices (such as "plain or with water" for oral medications or choosing injection and catheter site for parenteral meds)
- Being honest about expected hurts
- Providing distractions
- Permitting expression of anger
- Praising cooperation

- Accepting reactions (Whaley & Wong, 1983, p. 917)
- Never treating medications as candy, rewards, or punishment

**Oral Medications.**    Children under 5 years of age should not be given pills or capsules, owing to the danger of aspiration. Even preschoolers who are well able to handle solid foods may resist a tablet administered by an unfamiliar nurse. Liquid medicines are therefore particularly valuable in pediatric care.

- Choose an appropriate vehicle for delivery of oral medications.
- Spoons, syringes, cups, droppers, and nipples are well suited to infants, toddlers, preschoolers, or profoundly retarded patients of any age.
- Avoid mixing liquid medications in large volumes of formula or other liquid. The child may refuse to take all the liquid, resulting in an incomplete dosage.
- Do not force oral medications because of possible aspiration.
- Never administer oral medications—liquid or tablet—while the child is supine; the child's head should be elevated to a 45° angle.
- Infants and small children may need restraining (see figure 2.1).
- Squirting a small amount of liquid into the cheek pouch and stroking gently but firmly under the chin allows a liquid to be swallowed down an infant's lateral food channels with greater safety. This also avoids triggering the cough and gag reflexes.

**Table 2.5**    Liquid Equivalents

| Household | Apothecaries' | Metric |
|-----------|---------------|--------|
| 1 tsp | 1⅓ fl dram | 5.0 cc |
| 1 tbsp | ½ fl oz | 15 cc |
| 1 teacup | 4 fl oz | 120 cc |
| 1 glass | 8 fl oz | 240 cc |
| | 1 minim | 0.06 cc |
| | 15 minims | 1.0 cc |
| | 1 fl oz | 30 cc |
| | 1 pt | 500 cc |
| | 1 qt | 1 liter |

(Ross Laboratories, 1966)

Administer dangerous *liquid oral medications* such as digoxin elixer in carefully calibrated vehicles (e.g., tuberculin syringes).

*Tablets* that have been crushed with a mortar and pestle or between two souffle cups may be administered in a small amount of strained applesauce (or other fruits, gelatin, pudding, or ice cream), as may the contents of capsules (e.g., Pancrease or Theo-Dur sprinkles).

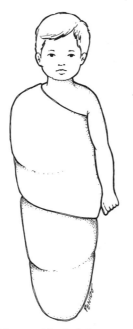 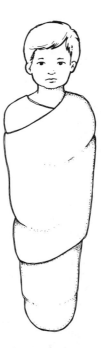

**Figure 2.1** Mummy Restraint

A mummy restraint is used for safe administration of medications to an uncooperative infant or toddler. Thigh may be left exposed if an intramuscular medication is to be administered. A "papoose" board may also be used, freeing extremities for IV catheter sites.

**Table 2.6** Liquid Measures

| Apothecaries' | Apothecaries' | Metric |
|---|---|---|
| 1 fl dram | 60 minims | 3.697 cc |
| 1 fl oz | 8 fl drams | 29.573 cc |
| 1 pt | 16 fl oz | 473.2 cc |
| 1 qt | 32 fl oz | 946.3 cc |
| 1 gal | 128 fl oz | 3,785 cc |

| Metric | English | Metric |
|---|---|---|
| 1 cc (ml) | 0.061 cu in | 1 ml |
| 1 cl | 0.61 cu in | 10 ml |
| 1 dl | 6.1 cu in | 100 ml |
| 1 liter | 61.02 cu in | 1,000 ml |

(Burroughs-Wellcome, 1982)

- Tablets in unit dose packages may be crushed easily by rolling a hard object, such as a 4 oz bottle of sterile water, over the plastic bubble of the package.

- Crushed or powdered medications can also be mixed in syrup or juice.
- Do not break a tablet for a partial dose if it is not scored. Instead, crush the tablet, mix it in liquid, and give the appropriate proportion of the solution.
- Do not crush or divide timed-release medications.

**Table 2.7**  Equivalent Weights

| Apothecaries' | Apothecaries' | Metric |
|---|---|---|
| 1 scruple | 20 grains | 1.296 g |
| 1 dram | 60 grains | 3.88 g |
| 1 oz | 480 grains (8 drams) | 31.1 g |
| 1 lb | 5,760 grains (16 oz) | 453.49 g |

| Metric | Apothecaries' | Metric |
|---|---|---|
| 1 mg | 1/65 grain | 0.001 g |
| 1 cg | 1/6 grain | 0.01 g |
| 1 dg | 1½ grains | 0.1 g |
| 1 g | 15.432 grains | 0.001 kg |
| 1 kg | 2.2 lb avdp | 1,000 g |

| Avoirdupois | Apothecaries' | Metric |
|---|---|---|
| 1 oz | 437.5 grains or 480 minims | 28.35 grams 30 cc |
| 1 lb (16 oz) | 7,000 grains | 453.59 g |

(Burroughs-Wellcome, 1982)

**Table 2.8**  Miscellaneous Equivalents

| Metric | Apothecaries' |
|---|---|
| 1.0 g | 15 grains |
| 0.3 g | 5 grains |
| 0.2 g | 3 grains |
| 60 mg | 1 grains |
| 30 mg | ½ grains |
| 10 mg | 1/6 grains |
| 1.0 mg | 1/60 grains |
| 0.4 mg | 1/150 grains |
| 0.3 mg | 1/200 grains |
| 1.0 cc | 15 minims |
| 0.6 cc | 10 minims |
| 0.06 cc | 1 minim |
| 0.03 cc | ½ minim |
| 1 drop (gutta, gtt) | 1 minim |

(Burroughs-Wellcome, 1982)

**Topical Medications.** Antifungal and antibiotic *creams and ointments* should be applied in thin layers as directed (family members may think "the more the better"). Significant and toxic levels of medications (or poisons such as insecticides) may be absorbed through children's skin. Steroid creams are a prime example. Remember not to leave containers at the bedside; a child may remove the cap and choke on it or ingest the medicine.

*Nose and eye drops* are administered to children in the same manner as to adults. Read labels carefully to determine whether an ointment, for example, is an ophthalmic preparation. Many topical antibiotic ointments are not considered safe for eyes.

*Ear drops* are administered to children less than 3 years of age by gently pulling the pinna downward and straight back. In children older than 3 years, the pinna is pulled upward and back.

**Rectal Medications.** Rectal administration of a medication should be avoided, if possible, because of the possibility of incomplete absorption. Some conditions, such as pediatric cancers, irritable bowel syndrome, a tendency for GI bleeding, or rectal fissures preclude rectal medication administration altogether.

### Procedures for Rectal Administration of Medications
- Dilute retention enemas such as Kayexalate or aminophylline enemas in the smallest possible amount of solution to diminish the urge to expel them.
- Position the child on the left side.
- Assess the length of time that the fluid inserted was retained and the approximate output.
- If a suppository must be divided, cut it lengthwise.
- Hold buttocks or tape them together firmly for 5–10 minutes to minimize the urge to expel the suppository.

**Aerosol Medications.** Nebulized droplets of medication may be distributed throughout the tracheobronchial tree via continuous or intermittent treatments. Continuous mist may be delivered by tent, collar, or mask; intermittent ventilation via an electric air compressor or a positive pressure apparatus. The more sophisticated the equipment, the smaller the particles (droplets) and the greater likelihood of reaching the bronchioles and alveoli.

Within the hospital environment, aerosol medications will most likely be propelled by oxygen. Since oxygen (greater than 21%) is a drug in itself and is particularly insidious to the infant and young child (leading to retrolental fibroplasia, $O_2$ toxicity), a physician's order must be specific regarding the propelling mode. Alternatives include air via compressor, which can be contaminated by dust and oil droplets, and the self-administered small pressure nebulizers, which use Freon as a propellant. There seems to be an increased incidence of psychologic dependence, rebound bronchospasm-asthma, and even fatal dysrhythmias from the overuse of the Freon-based bronchodilators. Once the physician has ordered an appropriate source of the aerosol treatment, the medication itself must be carefully considered. (See table 2.9 for a summary of respiratory medications administered by aerosol.)

**Table 2.9**    Drugs Used for Aerosol Nebulization and Inhalation Therapy

| Drug | Side Effects |
|---|---|
| Bronchodilators<br>  racemic epinephrine (Vaponephrine)<br>  ephedrine<br>  isoproterenol (Isuprel)<br>  isoetharine HCl (Bronkosol) | Laryngospasm, bronchospasm (racemic epinephrine)<br>Anxiety<br>Tremulousness<br>Cardiovascular instability |
| Mucolytics<br>  acetylcysteine (Mucomist)<br>  pancreatic dornase (Dornavac)<br>  propylene glycol | Secretions may be liquified very rapidly and drowning may occur.<br>Bronchospasm may occur in asthmatics. |
| Surface-acting agents<br>  saline<br>  tyloxapol (Alevaire) | |
| Antimicrobial agents<br>  neomycin<br>  polymyxin B<br>  tetracycline<br>  erythromycin | Rash, urticaria<br>Nausea, vomiting<br>Anaphylaxis |
| Corticosteriods, anti-inflammatory agents<br>  dexamethasone (Decadron)<br>  hydrocortisone (Solu-cortef)<br>  methylprednisolone<br>  sodium succinate (Solu-medrol) | Behavioral lability, Cushinoid changes |

(Whaley & Wong)

In many institutions, respiratory therapists or technicians are responsible for delivery of treatment and equipment maintenance. The nurse, however, monitors the child on a continuing basis and must be aware of the special needs of the child in inhalation therapy.

### Nursing Actions for Aerosol Administration
- Use sterile, distilled water to replenish delivery system reservoirs to prevent mineral buildup and bacterial colonization.
- Be sure that percussion and segmental bronchial drainage follow within minutes of intermittent nebulization treatments.
- Measure blood pressure and pulse prior to and every two minutes during treatment with isoproterenol, since dramatic cardiovascular changes may result within seconds of administration. Use a cardiorespiratory monitor and Dinamapp, if available.

## Intramuscular Medications.
- The vastus lateralis and outer aspect of the rectus femoris muscles are safe injection sites for all ages.

- Children with muscle-wasting problems, prematurity, or malnutrition are particularly vulnerable to nerve damage in the deltoid, the ventrogluteal area, or the gluteus medius, although some authorities consider these sites conditionally safe.
- Anterolateral thigh muscles may be used with care for infants and children.
- Use of buttocks muscles in children under 2 years is always contraindicated because of close proximity to the sciatic nerve.
- Aspirate before injecting into any muscle to ensure you are not injecting into a blood vessel.
- If the child is too strong to restrain, use a papoose board or additional helpers (preferably not parents) to prevent accidents.
- Determine needle size by assessing the patient's muscle mass. A ⅝" needle is appropriate for IMs administered to a term newborn, whereas an intradermal needle may be large enough for an early preterm infant. See figures 2.1 and 2.2 for restraining techniques and recommended sites.

**Intravenous Medications.**    Intravenous (IV) access is preferred for parenteral medications, such as antibiotics, that must be given in divided doses over an extended period. A child can be spared the repeated trauma of an intrusive procedure such as an IM injection by receiving parenteral IV medications, and the response to hospitalization may be more positive. Children who do not need additional fluid maintenance can enjoy relative freedom if a heparin lock is used rather than a "keep vein open" (KVO) low-volume continuous infusion. KVO infusions decrease a child's mobility considerably, and expose the child to becoming fluid overloaded if the drip rate changes with position.

Determine patency of a heparin lock before injecting the medicine by flushing it with approximately heparin flush solution or bacteriostatic normal saline according to hospital policy.

- Flush lock every 2–4 hours to ensure patency, if no IV medications are being given.
- Maintain pressure on plunger of syringe as it is withdrawn to permit some of the flush solution to remain in the catheter.
- Avoid flushing clots.
- Do not inject into a site that may be infiltrated.
- Do not administer caustic medications into tiny surface or scalp veins.
- Give IV medications slowly over the longest safe amount of time for the medication being administered. For example, the aminoglycoside antibiotics must be administered over a minimum of 30 minutes.

IV absorption occurs very rapidly and adverse reactions such as anaphylactic shock may develop in minutes. Some IV drugs form insoluble precipitates when administered simultaneously with stock IV fluids or other IV drugs. If unsure, refer to a formulary. Incompatibility charts are useful to help prevent such complications and should be available on the pediatric unit. Most anti-

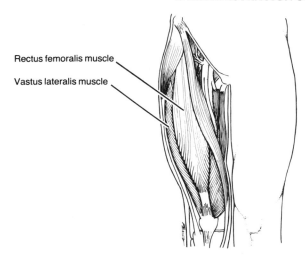

Rectus femoralis muscle

Vastus lateralis muscle

**Figure 2.2**    Recommended IM Injection Sites for Children

biotics are incompatible when given at the same time, and phenytoin (Dilantin) is incompatible with everything except physiologic saline.

When giving IV medications in a volutrol or soluset, it is important to remember that unless the tubing has been flushed completely after the medication is emptied from the chamber, part or all of the medication will remain in the tubing. Record fluids given with IV medications in the intake and output record.

**Table 2.10**    IV Insertion in Children

**Equipment**

- Armboards
    - immobilize extremity so that flexion of a joint will not dislodge the catheter
    - the line may be better protected in some instances when the extremity is not restrained
    - padded splints are useful
- Cannulas (use smallest size to meet needs)
    - winged or butterfly needle
        * 23- to 25-gauge
        * 27-gauge butterflies are available for extremely small veins
        * easier to insert and the vein heals faster
    - "Over-the-needle" catheters
        * 14- to 24-gauge
        * usually last longer
- Tape
    - use clear tape for infants less than 3 months old
    - use white porous tape for older children
    - use white water-proof tape to maintain integrity in very active children who tend to pull out lines
    - use paper (nonallergenic) tape when gloves must be worn or skin is fragile

**Table 2.10**    IV Insertion in Children (continued)

**Procedure**

Choose site
- It is best to use an extremity site for a peripheral IV if at all possible, as this permits more mobility and less danger than scalp or umbilical vein sites.
- Attempt to use the most distal veins first and work proximally.
- Use only superficial veins.
- Dorsal veins of the hands and feet make the best sites.
- The infant's scalp offers six to eight sites, most prominent being the temporal and forehead areas. If an infiltration and slough occur, the child may be permanently disfigured.
- Shaving the hair is necessary, but many parents find this completely objectionable.
- Avoid using antecubital fossa and dorsal feet veins if at all possible. These sites are difficult to immobilize and prone to sloughs and infiltrations
- Contraindicated IV sites include
  • scalps of children with possible or actual hydrocephalus who may need shunt placement/revision
  • affected arms of children who have had a Blalock-Taussig procedure (usually done on right, but occasionally on left or bilaterally)
  • extremity affected with cellulitis, osteomyelitis, thrombophlebitis, infection, necrosis, or disseminated intravascular coagulation
  • leg of child who has had a cardiac catheterization or angiogram site on affected femoral triangle area
  • affected extremity where vasospasm has occurred (deep lines of discoloration present)
  • arteries (palpate carefully to preclude and, once vessel has been entered, assess for pulsatile backflow and bright red color)

Enter vein
- have all tubing (t-connector, adapters, etc.) primed with appropriate solution and ready to "plug in"
- safely restrain child
- save hair shaved from infant's scalp and offer to parents
- prep site with povidone-iodine solution followed by alcohol swab
- apply tourniquet (rubber bands are useful for scalp veins)
- use prestick to ease insertion: 21- to 22-gauge needle for a 22- to 24-gauge catheter
- insert cannula in same direction as blood flow and check constantly for blood return (slower in infants)

NOTE: Pull gently on syringe to prevent collapse of the vein when checking for blood return.

- if blood return is not evident, gently instill IV fluid and observe for swelling at insertion site
- begin infusion when patency is determined

Secure site

- tape into place, but not too tightly in order to avoid pressure sores
- use a "chevron" approach to taping butterfly or catheter, placing tape first underneath wings or hub (sticky side up), then criss-crossing them over top
- apply povidone-iodine ointment to insertion site
- cover with clear plastic container (half a drinking cup or med cup) if appropriate to protect site and permit inspection
- write date IV was inserted on the tape

**Table 2.11**    IV Infusion Rate Calculation

*Calculation of Gravity IV Drip Rates*

Drops per minute

$$\frac{\text{total volume/hour} \times \text{gtts/ml}}{\text{total infusion time in minutes}} = \text{gtts/minute}$$

Example: An order reads 1,000 cc IV D5NS at 100 ml/hour

macrodrip:

$$\frac{100 \text{ ml} \times 15 \text{ gtts/ml}}{60 \text{ minutes/hour}} = 25 \text{ gtts/minute}$$

microdrip:

$$\frac{100 \text{ ml/hour} \times 60 \text{ gtts/ml}}{60 \text{ minutes/hour}} = 100 \text{ gtts/minutes}$$

blood administration sets:

$$\frac{100 \text{ ml} \times 10 \text{ gtts/ml}}{60 \text{ minutes/hour}} = 17 \text{ gtts/minutes}$$

Infusion time

$$\frac{\text{total volume to be delivered}}{\text{ml delivered/hour}} = \text{hours}$$

$$\frac{1,000 \text{ cc}}{100 \text{ ml/hour}} = 10 \text{ hours}$$

**Table 2.12**    IV Catheter Maintenance

| Procedure | Frequency |
|---|---|
| Maintain sterile technique | Always |
| Check IV site | Every hour |
| Check rate of infusion (by pump, bottle, or Soluset) | Every hour |
| Check central line site for leaking or bleeding | Every shift |
| Change IV tubing (do not allow air in line; tape all tubing connections) | Every 24 hours |
| Change dressing | 3 times a week or when contaminated or nonocclusive |
| Change IV site (peripheral infusion) | Every 3 days |

**Vasoactive Drugs.**    Infusion doses of major vasoactive drugs are based on the patient's weight, and are generally administered in micrograms per kilogram per minute (mcg/kg/min). Drugs in this category include

- Epinephrine
- Isoproterenol
- Dopamine
- Dobutamine (all central vasopressors)
- Lidocaine
- Bretyllium
- Nitroprusside

Theophylline infusions are considered later in this chapter.

## Nursing Responsibilities

- Know the patient's weight, the medication's usual dose range, commonly employed concentrations, side effects, special precautions.
- Two nurses should independently calculate all steps of the preparation process and then compare.
- Both nurses should be present when the doses are drawn up.
- Keep the paper used for calculating, so that if the dose is questioned, the information is available.

The notion of highly concentrated medications is germane to pediatrics where minimizing fluid volume for administration is especially important. Concentration in each milliliter of fluid is equal to the patient's weight multiplied by a concentration multiple, e.g., 1, 10, or 100. Administer major vasoactive drugs with an infusion pump that has an electric eye to monitor the rate. The recommended solution for administration is 5% dextrose in water. Syringe (or soluset) preparation of highly concentrated medications.

Sample order:
Epinephrine at 2 mcg/kg/minute, desired concentration, multiple = $10 \times$. Based on weight of 5.0 kg.

A.   Calculate the *concentration of the drug* in mcg/ml based on patient's body weight and ordered concentration multiple.

body weight $\times$ 10 = 50 mcg/ml

B.   *Calculate the total amount of drug in syringe.* For this example, a 50 ml syringe is used. Concentration (step A) times syringe capacity equals total amount of drug in syringe

50 mcg/ml $\times$ 50 ml = 2,500 mcg/50 ml

C.  *Convert to mg/50 ml* by dividing by 1,000; this is helpful when drawing up the drug.

$$\frac{2,500\ \text{mcg}}{1,000} = 2.5\ \text{mg/50 ml}$$

D.  Draw up the calculated amount of medication.

E.  In a separate syringe, draw up the diluent needed so that the total volume of diluent and medication equals desired capacity of the syringe. Add drug. You may use a smaller syringe to regulate administered fluid volume more carefully.

Label the syringe with the drug name, amount, concentration multiple, amount per syringe, names of both nurses preparing the drug, preparation date and time, and expiration date and time. Tubing and setup changes should be done routinely according to hospital policy, usually every 24 hours unless the infusion dose is changed. Infusion rate calculation (using the same example values as above)

A.  ml/min      $\dfrac{\text{mcg/kg/ml (ordered dose)}}{\text{Concentration multiple}}$    $\dfrac{2.0}{10} = 0.2\ \text{ml/minute}$
    *Divide:*

B.  mcg/min
    *Multiply:*
    Concentration of solution (mcg/ml) × volume infused/minute (ml/min)
    $$50\ \text{mcg/ml} \times 0.2 = 10\ \text{mcg/min}$$

C.  mcg/kg/min
    *Divide:*     $\dfrac{\text{mcg/minute}}{\text{weight (kg)}} = \text{mcg/kg/minute}$
                  $\dfrac{10\ \text{mcg/minute}}{5} = 2\ \text{mcg/kg/minute}$

Administer only one drug per intravenous site to prevent the occurrence of insoluble precipitates or alterations of these dangerous drugs. Do not mix vasoactive drugs with hyperalimentation fluids or IV antibiotics. Anyone ill enough to require the administration of these drugs should be monitored in an intensive care unit, but you may be required to prepare the drugs before transferring the child to critical care.

Record infusion information hourly or as often as the dose changes. It can be charted on a sample flow sheet and should include:

| Concentration | | | |
|---|---|---|---|
| Multiple | Date | Time mcg/ml | ml/syringe |

| Rate | | |
|---|---|---|
| ml/minute | mcg/minute | mcg/kg/minute |

Additional flow sheet information includes signatures of both nurses who prepared the drug infusion and comments related to the infusion, such as dose changes.

*Theophylline infusions* are considered separately from the central vasopressors and antihypertensives because they are generally administered in doses of milligrams per kilogram per hour (mg/kg/hour). The recommended dose for younger children is higher than that for adolescents, since younger children have higher metabolic rates and metabolize the drug more quickly. Some children are "rapid metabolizers" and may require even more than the recommended dosages. They may even be refractory to the drug and require something more potent such as isoproterenol or epinephrine infusions (requiring ICU observation and care).

The Children's Hospital of Philadelphia *Formulary* (Sporing, Walton, & Cady, 1984) recommends the following dose schedule:

> Preadolescent: 0.9 mg/kg/hour
> Adolescent:    0.7 mg/kg/hour

Example:
> A 15 kg child, age 3 years
> 15 kg × 0.9 mg/kg/hour = 13.5 mg/hour

To determine *milliliters* per hour, divide the child's dose per hour by the amount of milligrams available in commercially available solutions.

Example:
> If solution comes in 1.6 mg/ml:
> 13.5 mg/hour divided by 1.6 mg/ml = 8.43 or 8.0 ml/hour

The pharmacy can prepare a solution of 100 mg of theophylline in a 100 cc aliquot of D5W. Since 1 cc IV fluid would contain 1 mg of theophylline, the IV rate per hour would be the same as the ordered milligram per hour of theophylline.

When a theophylline infusion is given, record vital signs every two hours. The clinical asthma score (see chapter 7) can be used as an adjuvant assessment tool. Theophylline is frequently administered as a bolus IV drip dose, in which case vital signs should be recorded every five minutes, with a baseline set of signs determined before the drug is started. It is helpful to have a cardiorespiratory monitor, so that the alarm limits can be set for tachycardia.

Toxic side effects of theophylline include

- Tachycardia
- Blood pressure lability
- Cardiac dysrhythmias
- Nausea
- Vomiting
- Restlessness
- Irritability

If other medications are being administered, it is helpful to have two intravenous access lines. When it is necessary to infuse a piggyback medication, do not discontinue the theophylline (Sporing, Walton, & Cady).

**Table 2.13**    Prototype Drugs Used in Inpatient Pediatrics

| Generic Name | Trade Name | Dose | Route | Comments |
|---|---|---|---|---|
| Acetaminophen | Tylenol, Tempra, Liquiprin | 10–15 mg/kg/dose q4h | PO/PR | Antipyretic and analgesic |
| Aminophylline | Somophyllin | varies with age, weight | IV/PO | Bronchodilator |
| Aluminum hydroxide gel | Amphogel | 5–15 ml q3–6h | PO | Antacid |
| Aluminum hydroxide gel with magnesium | Maalox | 5–15 ml q3–6h | PO | Antacid |
| Aspirin, acetylsalicylic acid (ASA) | | 10–15 mg/kg/dose q4h | PO/PR | Antipyretic, antiinflammatory and analgesic (associated with Reye's syndrome—contraindicated for fevers of viral or unknown origin) |
| Calcium gluconate, Calcium gluceptate | | 50–100 mg/kg/dose | IV | Various indications |
| Chlorpromazine | Thorazine | 0.5–1.0 mg/kg/dose | IV/IM PO/PR | Antianxiety Antipsychotic |
| Cimetidine | Tagamet | 5–10 mg/kg/dose q6h | IV/PO | Antihistamine ($H_2$-receptor antagonist). Inhibits gastric acid secretion. |
| Codeine | | 0.5–1.0 mg/kg | IM/PO SC | Analgesic |
| Digoxin | Lanoxin | Varies with weight, age, and indication | IV/PO | Cardiac glycoside |
| Docusate sodium (Dioctyl sodium sulfosuccinate, DSS) | Colace | 5 mg/kg/day | PO | Stool softener |
| Diphenhydramine | Benadryl | 0.5–1 mg/kg/ dose q4–6h | PO/IV IM | Antihistamine ($H_1$-receptor antagonist) |
| Dobutamine | Dobutrex | 2–15 mEq/kg/ min; titrate to effect | | Cardiac stimulant |
| Dopamine | Intropin | 2–15 mEq/kg/ min; titrate to effect | | Cardiac stimulant, vasodilator except at higher doses |

**Table 2.13**   Prototype Drugs Used in Inpatient Pediatrics (continued)

| Generic Name | Trade Name | Dose | Route | Comments |
|---|---|---|---|---|
| Epinephrine | Adrenalin | Varies with indication | IV/SC inhalant | Bronchodilator, cardiac stimulant |
| Furosemide | Lasix | 1 mg/kg/dose | IV/PO IM | Diuretic |
| Hydralazine | Apresoline | 0.1–0.5 mg/kg/dose q4–6h | IV/PO IM | Antihypertensive |
| Insulin, regular | Various | Varies with blood and urine glucose concentrations | SC IV | Antidiabetic agent |
| Isoproterenol | Isuprel | Varies with indication | IV/SL inhalant | Bronchodilator, cardiac stimulant |
| Milk of magnesia (MOM) | | 0.5 ml /kg/dose | PO | Antacid, laxative |
| Mannitol | | 0.25–1 gm/kg/dose | IV | Osmotic diuretic (for cerebral edema) |
| Meperidine | Demerol | 1–1.5 mg/kg/dose q3–4h | IV/IM PO/SC | Analgesic |
| Methyldopa | Aldomet | 10–400 mg/kg/day q6–12h | IV/PO | Antihypertensive |
| Morphine | | 0.1–0.2 mg/kg/dose q2–4h | IM/IV SC/PO PR | Analgesic |
| Nitroprusside | Nipride | 0.5–10 mEq/kg/min; titrate to effect | IV | Antihypertensive |
| Pancreatic enzymes | Pancrease, Viokase, Cotazym | Determined by caloric intake | PO | Digestive enzymes (cystic fibrosis) |
| Pancuronium | Pavulon | 0.06–0.1 mg/ kg/dose | IV | Neuromuscular blocker (non-depolarizing) |
| Paraldehyde | | 0.15–0.3 ml/ kg/dose | PR | Sedative, anticonvulsant |
| Phentolamine | Regitine | 0.05–0.1 mg/ kg/dose | IV | Catecholamine antagonist; vasodilator |
| Promethazine | Phenergan | 0.25–1 mg/ kg/dose (varies with indication) | IM/IV PO/PR | Phenothiazide |
| Propranolol | Inderal | 0.5–2.0 mg/kg/day in three-four divided doses (varies with indication) | IV/PO | B-adrenergic blocker |
| Sodium polystyrene sulfonate | Kayexalate | 1 gram/kg/ dose | PO/PR | Potassium-removing resin |

**Table 2.13**    Prototype Drugs Used in Inpatient Pediatrics (continued)

| Generic Name | Trade Name | Dose | Route | Comments |
|---|---|---|---|---|
| Spironolactone | Aldactone | 1–3.3 mg/kg/day in two-four divided doses | PO | Antihypertensive, potassium-sparing diuretic |
| Succinylcholine | Anectine | 0.3–0.6 mg/kg/ dose | IV | Neuromuscular blocker (polarizing) |
| Terbutaline | Brethine | 0.05–0.1 mg/ kg/ dose q8h | PO/SC | Bronchodilator |
|  | Bricany | 0.005–0.10 mg/ kg/ dose | SC |  |
| Theophyllines | Various | Varies with age, weight | IV/PO | Bronchodilator |
| Thiopental | Pentothal | 1–2 mg/kg/dose | IV | Barbiturate (general anesthetic) |
| Tolazoline | Priscoline | 1–2 mg/kg/dose or 1–2 mg/kg/hr | IV/IM SC | Vasodilator |
| Vasopressin (antidiuretic hormone) | Pitressin | 2–10 units/dose q6–8h | IM/SC | Pituitary hormone |
| Vitamin K-1 (phytonadione) | Aquamephyton | 1–10 mg (varies with indication) | IM/IV SC | Facilitates clotting cascade (vitamin K-dependent clotting factors) |
| Vitamins | Various | Varies | IV/PO | Dietary supplement (vitamin replacement therapy) |
| **Adrenocorticosteroids** |  |  |  |  |
| Cortisone | Cortone | Depends on use | PO | Anti-inflammatory. All corticosteroids may result in Cushing's syndrome and related physical conditions. Steroids should be withdrawn in tapered decreasing doses. Decadron is used for neurologic injuries and decreasing intracranial pressure |
| Dexamethasone | Decadron | Depends on use | IV/IM PO | |
| Hydrocortisone | Cortef | Depends on use | IV/IM PO | |
| Hydrocortisone sodium succinate | Solu-Cortef | Depends on use | IV/IM | |
| Methyl-prednisolone | Medrol | Depends on use | PO | |
| Methyl-prednisolone sodium succinate | Solu-Medrol | Depends on use | IV/IM | |
| Prednisolone | Delta-Cortef | Depends on use | PO | |
| Prednisone | Deltasone | Depends on use | PO | |

**Table 2.13**    Prototype Drugs Used in Inpatient Pediatrics (continued)

| Generic Name | Trade Name | Dose | Route | Comments |
|---|---|---|---|---|
| **Anticonvulsants** | | | | |
| Carbamazepine | Tegretol | Doses are pre- | PO | |
| Clonazepam | Klonopin | scribed by age, | PO | Benzodiazepine |
| Diazepam | Valium | weight, indication. | | Benzodiazepine |
| Ethosoximide | Zarontin | | | |
| Mephobarbital | Mebaral | | | Barbiturate |
| Methsuximide | Celontin | | | |
| Phenobarbital | Luminal | Maintenance: 3–5 mg/kg/day | IV/PO | Barbiturate |
| Phenytoin | Dilantin | Loading: 10–15 mg/kg Maintenance: 5 mg/kg/day | IV/PO | Do not infuse greater than 0.5 mg/kg/min |
| Primidone | Mysoline | Doses are pre- | PO | |
| Valproic acid | Depakene | scribed by age, weight, indication. | PO | |

**Table 2.14**    Antibiotics Used in Pediatrics (IV and IM)

| Generic Name | Trade Name | Comments |
|---|---|---|
| **Aminoglycosides** | | |
| Amikacin | Amikin | Doses are prescribed by age, weight, renal clearance. Give IV *slowly* (over 20–30 min). Monitor renal function and serum levels. May cause ototoxicity and nephrotoxicity. |
| Gentamicin | Garamycin | |
| Kanamycin | Kantrex | |
| Tobramycin | Nebcin | |
| **Cephalosporins** | | |
| Cefazolin | Ancef, Kefzol | First generation. |
| Cephalothin | Meflin | First generation. |
| Cefoxitin | Mefoxin | Second generation. |
| Cefotaxime | Claforan | Third generation. |
| Ceftazidine | Fortaz | Third generation. |
| Cefuroxime | Zinacef | Second generation. |
| **Chloromycetin sodium succinate** | Chloramphenicol | Can cause bone marrow depression. Monitor serum levels. |
| **Penicillins** | | |
| Ampicillin | Omnipen, Polycillin, Totacillin | Very unstable. Give within two hours of reconstitution. |
| Carbenicillin | Geopen, Pyopen | High sodium content. |
| Methicillin | Staphcillin | |
| Nafcillin | Nafcil, Unipen | |
| Oxacillin | Bactocill, Prostaphlin | |

**Table 2.14**   Antibiotics Used in Pediatrics (IV and IM) (continued)

| Generic Name | Trade Name | Comments |
|---|---|---|
| Penicillin G | Pfizerpen | |
| Ticarcillin | | |
| **Miscellaneous** | | |
| Clindamycin | Cleocin | |
| Vancomycin | Vancocin | Monitor serum levels. |

**ANTIBIOTICS CONTRAINDICATED FOR NEONATES**
Chloramphenicol, erythromycin, lincomycin, nalidixic acid, nitrofurantoin, novobiocin, streptomycin, sulfonamides, and tetracyclines.

## NURSING TIPS

- Infuse TPN solutions with an infusion pump equipped with air, occlusion, battery, and infusion-complete alarms to preclude some of the life-threatening side effects of central line therapy.
- Do not infuse medications and blood products simultaneously; thoroughly flush the ports with normal saline to avoid precipitates.
- Draw blood samples from the inlet closest to the child when this port is covered by an intermittent infusion cap. Deliver blood products via this port.
- Keep the line patent by running a continuous infusion of solution using Y-connector setups, unless blood products are being delivered.
- Do not put a heparin lock on a central line.
- Central catheters, such as Broviacs, may be flushed and capped.
- Clamp the line with a rubber-tipped hemostat, and overpour fluid into the line to preclude air entry during daily tubing change.
- Ask a cooperative child to do the Valsalva maneuver while the tubing is being changed as an alternative to the use of hemostats.
- Tape all connections with waterproof tape.

# Central Venous Lines

Central venous lines are used when peripheral venous access is not available, or when particularly caustic drugs and solutions must be infused. They are helpful for the acute post-trauma or postsurgical patient and for oncology or total parenteral nutrition patients.

# Complications and Interventions

**Disconnections.**    Ensure that a hemostat is always close at hand in the event that the central venous line becomes disconnected. Affix the hemostat to the pump if portable and put latex tubing on the ends of the hemostat to prevent damage to the line.

**Air Emboli.**    Air emboli may be a life-threatening emergency. Remove any air in the child's tubing with a 23-gauge needle inserted into the Y-connection's rubber stopper or T-connector. Manipulate air to a site where it may be withdrawn by holding tubing taut and flicking briskly with a pen to assist the air to rise. If air has entered the child, place him/her in Trendelenburg's position (head down) on the left side immediately, in order to trap the air in right atrium, where it may be slowly absorbed. The administration of 100% oxygen will facilitate this absorption. Notify the physician immediately.

**Site Complications.**    Site complications include swelling and leakage of solution, blood, or excreta on dressing or tape. If an asymmetrical chest, chest pain, or unexplained dyspnea occur, obtain a stat chest x-ray and notify the physician immediately. Report loss of capillary refill or dusky color of the extremity of insertion in a child with a femoral line (Sporing, Walton, & Cady).

**Dressing Changes.**    Most institutions currently have a dressing change schedule that is either "every 3 days" or Monday/Wednesday/Friday, or whenever dressings are soiled or wet.

Changing a central line dressing is a sterile procedure, and includes the use of a mask. A prepackaged dressing change kit including sterile gloves, acetone-alcohol swabs, povidone-iodine swabs, povidone-iodine ointment, gauze sponges, a silk tape or elastic bandage, scissors, tape, and tincture of benzoin makes the process quick and simple.

*Procedure*   (Schmidt, 1982)

- Wash hands.
- Wear mask.
- Open dressing change kit.
- Put on sterile gloves.
- Swab around insertion site with acetone-alcohol (out to a 3-inch circumference) and along the catheter to the cap or connection site. Do the same with povidone-iodine swabs, using each swab only once (four alcohol and three iodine swabs).

- Squeeze povidone-iodine ointment onto sterile 2x2 gauze and place over catheter insertion site.
- Apply benzoin on skin around perimeter of gauze.
- Cut bandage with sterile scissors and place over gauze.
- Place tape around perimeter of bandage.

## Administration of Blood Products

The introduction of foreign protein into a child's system may have profound implications if negative sequelae arise. Table 2.15 includes a description of commonly administered blood components. Table 2.16 describes the precautions necessary for safe administration of a blood transfusion. Table 2.17 summarizes the four major categories of transfusion reactions, as well as other undesirable outcomes of blood product transfusion. Table 2.18 summarizes nursing interventions in the event of a transfusion complication.

Handwashing after the administration of blood products is essential to reduce the risk of contracting blood-borne diseases. Factor VIII and Factor IX concentrates, both manufactured from pooled human plasma, have been implicated in the transmission of hepatitis and AIDS. Children who have received multiple transfusions (e.g., for hemophilia or oncologic conditions) should be placed on standard blood precautions (see chapter 4).

**Table 2.15** Blood Products

| Product | Use | Contra-indications | Crossmatch | Usual Adminis-tration Rate | Recommended Needle Gauge | Equipment for Administration | Adverse Reactions |
|---|---|---|---|---|---|---|---|
| Whole blood | Restore blood volume and elevate hemoglobin and hematocrit; hypovolemic shock; exchange transfusions | Availability of specific component or adequacy of circulating volume | Yes | Infant/child: over 3–4 hours (ml/hour based on child's weight and other fluid balance adjust-ments); Adolescent: over no more than 4 hours | Infant/child: 22 ga; Adolescent: 18–20 ga | Straight: Y-type with microag-gregate recipient set (filter resolu-tion less than 40 microns); may be dripped; syringe pump for aliquots of less than 100 ml; infusion pump for greater than 100 ml | Hemolytic reaction, hives, chills, fever, shortness of breath, back or chest pain, circu-latory overload, allergy, anaphy-laxis, hepatitis |
| Red blood cells (RBCs) (packed; frozen-thawed) | Replace RBCs lost; treat severe anemia; prevent circulatory overload if a danger with whole blood transfusion | Nutritional anemias (unless patient is in heart failure related to severe anemia) | Yes | Infant/child: over 3–4 hours (ml/hour based on weight, etc.); Adolescent: 1 hour, no more than 4 hours | Infant/child: 19–21 ga; Adolescent: 18–20 ga (larger bores for rapid administration) | Straight; Y-type with filter or microaggregate recipient set (resolution of less than 40 microns) | Same as for whole blood |
| White blood cells (WBCs) leucocytes | Elevate leucocyte level; neutropenia, bone-marrow aplasia, severe granulocytopenia, infection unresponsive to antibiotics | Patient receiving amphotericin B (risk of severe pulmonary toxicity); admin-ister WBCs only in life-threat-ening situation | Yes (ABO and human leucocyte antigens) | Infant/child: as specifically ordered | Infant/child: 22–24 ga; Adolescent: 20–22 ga (20 ga in all for rapid administration) | Straight-line set with in-line blood filter; DO NOT use microag-gregate filter; transfuse within 24 hours of collection | Rash, pruritus, chills, fever, laryngeal edema, hypotension, cyanosis, respiratory distress, chest pain, hepatitis, cytomegalovirus, graft vs host disease |

| | | | | | | |
|---|---|---|---|---|---|---|
| Platelets | Elevate platelet count to improve hemostasis in thrombocytopenia; platelet count less than 20,000/mm³; active bleeding with count less than 50,000/mm³; thrombocytopenia related to decreased platelet production, increased platelet destruction, abnormal platelets, massive transfusions of stored blood | Post-transfusion purpura; thrombotic thrombocytopenic purpura; bleeding unrelated to decreased platelet count | No | As rapidly as possible regardless of age; within 2 hours | Infant/child: 22–24 ga; Adolescent: 20–22 ga | Syringe (pump) or nonwettable filter component drop set; roll syringe q30min to prevent platelet settling | Allergy, fever, hepatitis, fluid overload |
| Plasma, fresh or frozen (FFP) | Elevate low clotting factor level; expand blood volume; used in active bleeding, deficient coagulation factors (from hepatic disease or genetic bleeding disorders) | Availability of more specific therapy | Yes (ABO only) | If given for clotting factors (which rapidly deteriorate) give as quickly as possible; for volume expander, give up to 4 hours | Infant/child: 22–24 ga; Adolescent: 20–22 ga | Straight line set with standard clot filter | Allergy, fever, circulatory overload, hepatitis |

**Table 2.15**  Blood Products (continued)

| Product | Use | Contra-indications | Crossmatch | Usual Administration Rate | Recommended Needle Gauge | Equipment for Administration | Adverse Reactions |
|---|---|---|---|---|---|---|---|
| Factor VIII (cryoprecipitate: Factorate, Hemophil, Hamafac, Koate, Profilate) | Hemophilia A, classic hemophilia, factor VIII deficiency, von Willebrand's disease, hypofibrinogenemia, afibrinogenemia | Undefined coagulopathies. Use cautiously in patients with hepatic disease | No | 10–20 ml/3 minutes (as rapidly as possible) via drip; 1 ml/minute IV push | Infant/child: 22–24 ga; Adolescent: 20–22 ga | Syringe, straight or Y-type setup; clot filter; reconstitute by rolling vial between hands; do not shake | Allergy, hepatitis, AIDS, chills, fever, backache, flushing, constriction in chest, headache, leg pain, paresthesias, clouding or loss of consciousness, visual disturbances, tachycardia, hypotension, nausea, vomiting, erythema, possible intravascular hemolysis (blood types A, B, AB) |
| Factor IX (Proplex, Konyne [factors II, VII, IX, X complex]) | Hemophilia B (Christmas disease), hereditary factor IX deficiency; severe hemorrhage; | Fibrinolysis, hepatic disease, intravascular coagulation; use cautiously in neonates and infants | No | 1 vial in 5–10 minutes. DO NOT PUSH. | Infant/child: 22–24 ga Adolescent: 20–22 ga | Straight or Y-type setup; reconstitute by rolling vial between hands; do not shake; filter | Hepatitis (high risk), headache, transient fever, chills, flushing, tingling, hypersensitivity, thrombosis, |

| | | | | | | | |
|---|---|---|---|---|---|---|---|
| | anticoagulant overdose; stop bleeding, permit surgery | | | | | | possible intravascular hemolysis (in patients with blood types A, B, AB); intravascular clotting during administration may lead to emboli |
| Albumin, Albumin 5% (buffered saline), Albumin 25% (salt-poor), Albuconn, Albuspann, Albuminar, Albumisol, Buminate, Plasbumin | Restores blood volume and protein; volume or colloid deficiency, hypovolemic shock, burns, hypoalbuminemia, severe protein deficiencies; prevention of and therapy for cerebral edema (osmotic diuretic) | No | Severe anemia; congestive heart failure | Rapidly for shock; 5–10 ml/minute for hypoproteinemia (less rapidly in neonates) | Infant/child: 22–24 ga; Adolescent: 20–22 ga (larger bore for more rapid administration) | Filtering not necessary; may be pushed IV | Circulatory overload, microbial contamination, pyrogenic reaction, altered pulse rate, increased salivation, nausea, vomiting, urticaria, chills, fever, allergy |

**Table 2.15**  Blood Products (continued)

| Product | Use | Contra-indications | Crossmatch | Usual Adminis-tration Rate | Recommended Needle Gauge | Equipment for Administration | Adverse Reactions |
|---|---|---|---|---|---|---|---|
| Plasma protein fraction, Plasmanate, Plasmatein, Proteinate | Restore blood volume and protein; hypovolemic shock, protein deficiencies, shock (initial treatment in infants); initial treatment for children with electrolyte imbalance or dehydration | Clotting factor deficiency, severe anemia or heart failure, patients on cardiac bypass. Cautious use: hepatic or renal failure, low cardiac reserve, sodium-restricted patients | No | 5–10 ml/minute (small children and infants less rapidly) | Infant/child: 22–24 ga; Adolescent: 20–22 ga (larger bore for more rapid administration) | Standard straight-line set | Circulatory overload; hypotension |

(Masoorli & Piercy, 1984; Sporing, Walton, & Cady, 1984)

**Table 2.16**    Nursing Interventions to Assure a Safe Transfusion

- Before obtaining blood product from blood bank, assure that an adequately gauged, patent IV is in place.

NOTE: A 23-gauge butterfly is the smallest safe gauge for infants (a smaller gauge will damage erythrocytes). If a butterfly needle is used, a stopcock could be added to the line to flush the IV with normal saline periodically. Order infusion pump and obtain blood warmer if necessary.

- Check MD's orders: type of product, rate, volume, infusion duration, premedication (amount and type), adjustment of other fluid rates during transfusion, and necessity of irradiation (common in oncologic, transplant, and immunosuppressed patients).
- Stay with child for the first 15 minutes of the infusion. Administer blood product within 4 hours to preclude bacterial proliferation. Begin transfusion within 10 minutes of obtaining blood. Do not refrigerate blood product on unit if treatment is delayed; return to special blood refrigerator in lab. If full amount cannot be administered in 4 hours, notify MD and stop transfusion.
- Verify patient identify (ID band and verbal confirmation from child, family, or other staff member).
- Check records: blood bank record vs corresponding bag information. Two RNs (or MD) must simultaneously check the two sources for
  - donor number
  - donor and patient blood types (ABO and Rh)
  - product sent vs product ordered (e.g., packed RBCs vs whole blood)
- Filter all blood products. If a Harvard pump is used for administration, blood product must first be drawn up into syringe via a filtered administration set.
- Do not administer medications through an IV line in use for blood products. Flush line completely with normal saline before and after transfusion and/or interruption for medications.
- Record baseline vital signs (TPR and BP) immediately before beginning treatment. Take again 15 minutes after initiation, and as needed (hourly recommended) if there is no reason to suspect reaction. Continually assess for problems, including IV infiltration, sluggish IV line, and reactions.

(Masoorli; Sporing, Walton, & Cady).

**Table 2.17**    Undesirable Transfusion Sequelae

| Reaction | Cause | Symptoms | Possible Sequelae |
|---|---|---|---|
| Pyrogenic Reaction | Nonpathogenic bacteria | Chills/fever either during or after transfusion | Recovery usually uneventful |
| Febrile Reaction | Leucocyte, platelet, or other antigen agglutination | May begin any time (early in treatment to 1–2 hours after). Temperature increase of 1° C (1.8° F) or greater; chills, headache, back pain, nausea, vomiting, confusion, flushing; occurs in repeatedly transfused patients | Shock |

**Table 2.17**  Undesirable Transfusion Sequelae (continued)

| Reaction | Cause | Symptoms | Possible Sequelae |
|---|---|---|---|
| Allergic Reaction | Antigen/antibody reaction | Coughing, respiratory distress, hives, itching, facial edema, flushing, abdominal pain, nausea, vomiting, diarrhea, no fever; occurs after minimal amounts are infused | Reactive airway symptoms (bronchospasm) and anaphylactic shock, loss of consciousness, death |
| Hemolytic Reaction | Introduction of incompatible blood-type results in intravascular hemolysis | Fever is the only symptom in 50% of cases, others may experience flank pain, tightness in chest, breathlessness, apprehension, fear, nausea, vomiting, flushing, lower back and leg pain, jaundice, oliguria, anuria, tachycardia, bleeding from IV site | Hemoglobinuria, hemoglobinemia, hypotension, disseminated intravasulcar coagulation, acute renal failure, shock, death |
| Sepsis | Bacterial contamination (usually gram-negative rods) of donor blood (rare) | Begins shortly after transfusion start; fever greater than 38.4°C, chills, flushing, headache, substernal pain, vomiting, bloody diarrhea, hypotension; dry, flushed skin with shock symptoms; respiratory distress, rapid, thready pulse, coma | Circulatory collapse, disseminated intravascular coagulation, death |
| Circulatory Overload | Infants with congenital heart or renal disease at highest risk | Jugular venous distension, dyspnea, cough, chest pain, tachycardia, cyanosis, pulmonary edema (frothy, pink sputum), rales, headache, back pain, chills, fever, flushing | Congestive heart failure, fluid shifts |

**Table 2.17**   Undesirable Transfusion Sequelae (continued)

| Reaction | Cause | Symptoms | Possible Sequelae |
|---|---|---|---|
| Citrate Intoxication | Ionized calcium in patient's blood binds with citrate in blood-product preservatives | Usually occurs with massive volume replacement. Hypocalcemic symptoms: nervousness, cramps, circumoral and fingertip tingling, hyperactive reflexes, seizures, carpopedal spasms, hypotension | Laryngospasm, cardiac arrest |
| Hypothermia | Blood not warmed prior to transfusion | Chills, decreased body temperature, hypotension, cardiac dysrhythmias, labile blood pressure | Exacerbated acidosis, cardiac arrest |
| Vasospasm | Can occur with any infusion, particularly with cold blood | Pain along vein shortly after initiation of treatment, no evidence of phlebitis/infiltration | No long-term effects |
| Pulmonary Embolism | Air, clots, or foreign material infused into vein | Sudden chest pain, dyspnea, cough, hemoptysis, anxiety, rapid (weak), thready pulse | Death |
| Hyperkalemia | Migration of potassium from RCs into plasma; infants, cardiac, and renal patient at greatest risk | Nausea, muscle weakness, diarrhea, paresthesias (tongue and extremities), apprehensiveness, irregular bradycardia | Cardiac arrest related to flaccid paralysis of myocardium or respiratory muscles |

(Masoorli & Piercy; Sporing, Walton, & Cady)

**Table 2.18**    Nursing Interventions for Transfusion Complications

- Immediately discontinue transfusion. Disconnect the blood product and keep vein open with normal saline.
- Take vital signs.
- Notify physician immediately.
- Do not leave patient unattended. Alert other staff members to situation.
- Send blood bag and attached equipment to blood bank or lab immediately for analysis.
- Send full red-topped tube of patient's blood to lab with blood bag.
- Fill out a transfusion reaction form with the following information (also record fully in nurses' notes)
  - time and reason transfusion was stopped
  - pre-initiation vital signs
  - current vital signs
  - description of events
  - volume of blood infused
  - unit number on blood bag
  - blood type
  - child's wrist band and ID number
  - time of incident, response and name of physician notified
- Send first postreaction urine sample for stat urinalysis check for hemolysis.
- Implement medical interventions (determined by the physician) based on the patient's specific symptoms. (Examples: diphenhydramine for allergic reaction, 1:1,000 epinephrine subcutaneously for anaphylactic reactions, diuretics for circulatory overload)

(Masoorli; Kirkis & Etorre, 1983).

# References

Burroughs-Wellcome. (1982). *A compendium of medical tables.* Research Triangle Park, NC: Author.

IC & IM antibiotics: When giving. *RN, 44*(3), 47-51.

Kirkis, E., & Etorre, D. (1983). Seven sticky problems (and their solution) in blood transfusions. *RN, 46*(4), 58-62.

Malseed, R. (1982). *Pharmacology: Drug therapy and nursing considerations* Philadelphia: Lippincott.

Masoorli, S., & Piercy, S. (1984). A step-by-step guide to trouble free transfusions. *RN, 47*(5), 34-42.

Ross Laboratories. (1966). *Inservice Aids.* Columbus, OH: Author.

Schmidt, A., & Williams, D. (1982). The Hickman catheter—sending your patient home safely. *RN, 45*(2), 57-61.

Sporing, E., Walton, M., & Cady, C. (1984). *The Children's Hospital manual of pediatric nursing policies, procedures, and personnel.* Oradell, NJ: Medical Economics.

Whaley, L., & Wong, D. (1983). *Nursing care of infants and children.* (2nd ed.). St. Louis: Mosby.

# CHAPTER 3

# LEGAL CONSIDERATONS

An important aspect of health management in nursing of children is protecting the rights of the child under the law. Several legal concerns are of particular importance to the practicing pediatric nurse. These include informed consent, child abuse reporting and documentation, nursing responsibilities in the death of a child, professional liability and insurance, documentation, and incident reporting.

## Informed Consent

What constitutes rational, adult thinking and decision making? At what age can children reasonably be expected to make sound decisions regarding their own health care? The literature on this subject is confusing; the law, the laity, and the many concerned professional disciplines disagree. No position is absolutely right or wrong, and every opinion carries its own set of personal, legal, and ethical dilemmas.

The idea of informed consent stems from the principle of autonomy in classical ethics, which on the individual level encompasses independence, self-reliance, and the self-contained ability to decide. This concept has only recently been developed in nursing, biomedical, and legal literature, and has inspired a multistage process for protecting patient choice in medical care. By allowing parents or adolescents to choose freely and specifically among all care options, informed consent allows a greater sense of control over individual destiny and greater confidence in the overall direction of care.

General consensus in the literature as to what constitutes an informed consent is described by Kelly (1981). Informed consent is not simply a matter of

signing a consent form. It is a process that must contain the following six trans-
actions to be considered full disclosure:

1. An explanation of the condition
2. A fair explanation of the procedures to be used and the consequences
3. A description of alternative treatments or procedures
4. A description of the benefits to be expected
5. An offer to answer the patient's inquiries
6. Freedom from coercion, unfair persuasions, and inducements (p. 215)

The American Nurses' Association (ANA, 1976) places informed consent
first in its "Code for Nurses"

*1.1  Self-determination of clients.* Whenever possible, clients should be
fully involved in the planning and implementation of their own health
care. Each client has the moral right to determine what will be done with
his/her person; to be given information necessary for making informed
judgments; to be told the possible effects of care; and to accept, refuse, or
terminate treatment. These same rights apply to minors and others to the
fullest degree permissible under the law. The law in these areas may differ
from state to state; each nurse has an obligation to be knowledgeable about
and to protect and support the moral and legal rights of all clients under
state laws and applicable federal laws, such as the 1974 Privacy Act (p. 4).

**Developmental Considerations.**  Writers concerned about informed
consent in children have given numerous examples of adolescents making
responsible decisions about their own health. Their evidence indicates that,
excluding the psychologically or mentally incompetent teen (e.g., the retarded
or those who use psychotic defense mechanisms), most adolescents have
reached the age at which they are capable of abstract thinking and formal operations. An adolescent with formal operations is able to problem-solve, look at
many aspects of a situation, and draw conclusions as to the best logical decision.
Some behavioral examples of formal operations include the consideration of
philosophical points of view, abstract thinking, and resolution of some of the
world's paradoxes.

**Adolescent Consent.**  In the professional literature, ethical, moral, and
legal aspects of obtaining informed consent from adolescents are often considered together, because in real life these aspects are frequently intertwined.
      In most states, the legal age of majority is 18 years, whereas others establish
21 as the official start of adulthood. In special cases, younger adolescents may
be considered "emancipated." All these facts may bear directly on the adolescent's legal ability to offer informed consent.

**Emancipated Minor.**  Holder (1977) defines an emancipated minor as one who has been recognized as 'one who is not subject to parental control or regulation' in a wide variety of legal contexts for many years (p. 579).

Hoffman (1973) offers another definition—"a youth who by being away from home or by his maturity is managing his own affairs"—and elaborates with a discussion of the law, which

increasingly recognizes that under certain circumstances youths will not seek treatment unless their confidentiality is assured.... For the most part, current legislative trends tend to deal with limited specific circumstances and specific conditions such as emancipation, being married, pregnancy, or venereal disease (p. 35).

Any minor who is self-sufficient and living away from his parent(s) may be considered emancipated. Any minor female who has given birth to a child is usually considered emancipated. Some states have liberalized their laws to permit any minor to give consent to the diagnosis and treatment of

* Pregnancy
* Infectious disease
* Substance dependency
* Emergency care when life or health are threatened

Case laws for the state in question should be consulted when treating any minor without the parents' knowledge or consent.

Most legal cases to date have upheld the following principles:

* The right to abortion as an extension of constitutionally guaranteed personal freedoms
* Consultation of a minor's parents/guardians in nonemergency cases and at least an attempt to consult unless dealing with an emancipated minor

The law is only beginning to recognize the individuality and differing developmental capabilities of adolescents. Unless an adolescent is considered legally emancipated and can provide proof of that fact, you need to obtain consent signatures of both the patient and a parent. This satisfies both the legal requirement of parental consent and the thinking youngster's need to feel a part of crucial health decision making.

**Uncertain Consent.**    On realizing that a truly informed consent has not been obtained before a procedure, it is the nurse's responsibility to notify the attending physician. This is important *even if a consent form has already been signed.* The physician may not be too happy about this, but it is the duty of every health professional to provide the family with an in-depth picture of every clinical eventuality and not to force them to deal with an unexpected procedural outcome. Early explanations also leave patients and families the option of obtaining second opinions, particularly prior to surgical or invasive procedures. Many lay people are far too intimidated to exercise this right on their own. All of these measures may ultimately prevent costly and embarrassing lawsuits.

**Telephone Consent.**   The nurse may sometimes be asked to witness parental consent obtained by telephone. This is not advisable, for it can leave the witnessing nurse open to possible legal action should client/family expectations be unfulfilled. The nurse might be considered to be in collusion with the physician. Nonprofessional support staff can serve as equally valid witnesses at little or no personal risk.

**Consent for Research Participation.**   Many bioethicists today argue that children should never be used as human research subjects because they are not cognitively and developmentally capable of giving a truly informed consent. Even proxy consent from parents, they feel, is not good enough. Their objections are not grounded in the theoretical and empirical knowledge of development experts, however. An adolescent may consent and a child of younger years assent to participation in research. This position has been enjoined by the Department of Health and Human Services (HHS) in final regulations published in the March 3, 1983, *Federal Register* and effected June 6, 1983.

### *Nursing Considerations in Obtaining an Informed Consent*
1.  Obtain informed consent from the minor patient whenever possible to avoid violating his or her autonomy in decision making.
2.  Use these guidelines for determining patient ability to provide informed consent:
    a.  Is the patient competent and rational?
    b.  Has *every* alternative been discussed?
    c.  Have all the risks been disclosed and the patient reminded of his or her freedom to not take those chances?
    d.  Has a family-centered approach been attempted?
    e.  Are requests for confidentiality (e.g., the exclusion of a parent or child from the decision-making process) or for excluding the patient from determining his/her own care justifiable?
3.  Foster patient trust by respecting the adolescent's cognitive maturity. Refusal to acknowledge such maturity may be interpreted by the patient as denying his or her personhood.
4.  Know the consent laws in every area in which you practice. Be alert to the sometimes wide variations in such statutes among states.
5.  Do not witness a telephone consent. In cases of withdrawn consent and subsequent legal action, the nurse may be viewed as colluding with the physician to elicit permission from reluctant patients and families. When faced with such a request, politely refuse and suggest that a unit secretary take that responsibility.

**Consent for Autopsy.**   Obtaining consent for autopsy of a child is a sensitive subject and is solely the physician's responsibility. Nurses, however, frequently become involved in the process when asked to serve as witnesses. Some institutions do not allow nurses to witness any permission request for autopsy, feeling that a court of law may construe such collaboration between nursing and medicine as an act of "collusion" to "coerce" an unwilling family into granting permission.

### Guidelines for Pediatric Autopsy Consents

- Agreement of both parents is required in most instances of pediatric autopsy.
- Signature of one parent is acceptable only if he or she is the sole legal parent or if one of two consenting parents is unable to sign.
- Telephone permission is acceptable only if witnessed by the requesting physician and one other person.
- Certain nonprofessional personnel, including unit assistants (secretaries) or telephone operators, can witness telephone consents with relative impunity.

## Child Abuse Reporting and Documentation

Most states have child abuse reporting laws requiring the professional nurse to report any suspicious occurrences, specifically unexplained injuries, multiple injuries in various stages of healing, evidence of old fractures on a skeletal survey, or conflicting information. If it is later determined that the nurse possessed knowledge of such injuries and did not report them, the nurse would be liable for criminal prosecution.

Table 3.1 lists health professionals who must report suspected child abuse.

**Table 3.1**    Persons Required To Report Suspected Child Abuse

| | |
|---|---|
| Chiropractor | Mental health professional |
| Christian Science practitioner | Optometrist |
| Coroner | Osteopath |
| Dentist | Peace officer |
| Hospital personnel engaged in the admission, care, and treatment of patients | Podiatrist |
| Intern | Registered nurse |
| Law enforcement official | School administrator |
| Licensed physician | School nurse |
| Licensed practical nurse | Social services worker |
| Medical examiner | Teacher |

### Reporting Child Abuse

- Privileged communication between the professional person and patient or client does not apply in child abuse situations.
- Most states have toll-free hotlines for reporting suspected child abuse 24 hours a day.
- Factual documentation without extraneous judgmental information is very important.

- In some states, the law also includes a stipulation protecting anyone who reports child abuse or assists in a report. Should such an action be followed by discharge from employment or discrimination in compensation, hire, tenure, terms, conditions, or privileges of employment, the employee may file a cause of action in the court of common pleas.
- Each state's statutes vary, but in most the report is processed through the child protective services unit of the child welfare agency after the incident has been centrally reported to the state capital.

**Failure to Treat.**    Bills were introduced in the US House of Representatives and Senate to expand the definition of child neglect and abuse to include failure to provide medical treatment or nutrition to infants with life-threatening congenital impairments, and in 1983 the Child Abuse Prevention and Treatment Act was signed into law. One of the most controversial outgrowths of this act was the H.H.S.'s rule requiring hospitals to post notices of a toll-free hotline for reporting infractions of the "failure to treat" law.

By June 1984, a compromise statement on this issue had been drawn up and agreed on by the American Nurses' Association, American Academy of Pediatrics, American Hospital Association, College of Obstetricians and Gynecologists, American College of Physicians, Association of Retarded Citizens, American Coalition for Citizens with Disabilities, Spina Bifida Foundation, National Right to Life Committee, and American Life Lobby.

The statement, a proposed amendment to the Child Abuse Prevention and Treatment Act (ANA, 1984), requires states that participate in the (federally funded) state child abuse grant program to establish procedures for reporting medical neglect (withholding treatment from disabled infants). The key clause in the compromise is "withholding of medically indicated treatment," which includes nutrition, medication, and hydration that, in the treating physician's reasonable medical judgment, would improve or correct a handicapping condition. The clause continues,

> However, the term does not include the failure to provide treatment (other than appropriate nutrition, hydration, or medication) to an infant when . . . (a) the infant is chronically and irreversibly comatose . . . (b) the provision of such treatment would merely prolong dying or . . . (c) the provision of such treatment would be virtually futile in terms of the survival of the infant . . . and inhumane (pp. 1–2)

# Death of a Patient

As regards legal care requirements in the case of patient death, no rules have been addressed specifically to nurses. The court system tends to concentrate upon social policy in decisions involving dying persons (Cowles & Murphy, 1982). Some state legislatures have begun attempts to arrive at a legal definition of death.

The Uniform Determination of Death Act (1982) attempts to unify the law on patient death in all states. Those that have adopted it include California, Colorado, the District of Columbia, Georgia, Idaho, Maine, Maryland, Missouri, Mississippi, Montana, Ohio, Pennsylvania, Rhode Island, and Vermont. The act stipulates that in the determination of death, only an individual who has sustained either

- irreversible cessation of circulatory and respiratory functions or
- irreversible cessation of all functions of the entire brain, including the brain stem

is dead. A determination of death must be made according to accepted medical standards.

Cardiorespiratory death is determined by the physician. In brain death, electroencephalographic (EEG) readouts will have an isoelectric (flat) line. There must be complete absence of electrical activity in the brain for death to be declared.

**Medical Examiners' Cases.**    Various local and state laws govern deaths with circumstances that must be reported to the medical examiner (coroner). These include deaths with suspicious circumstances of any kind, particularly if a professional error or misjudgment contributed to the death. (See table 3.2 for a list of reportable deaths.)

**Table 3.2**    Reportable Deaths

Sudden Infant Death Syndrome (whether "dead on arrival" [DOA] or near miss with subsequent death)
Any unexpected death or DOA
Surgical death (any procedure from which a child did not recover in the expected pattern)
Aplastic anemia
Injury from therapeutic or diagnostic procedures (unusual or unexpected events such as anaphylactic or allergic reactions)
Anesthetic death
Complications of blood product transfusion
Trauma (falls or injuries in the hospital or at home, battering, stabbing, gunshot wound, beating, auto accident, or drowning)
Biologic injury (allergy, anaphylaxis, idiosyncratic reactions, overdoses, or medication errors)
Thermal injuries (fire, hot water, hot or freezing temperatures, exposure)
Chemical injuries
Radiation injuries

Note: From unpublished policy "Outline for House Staff in the Event of a Death," St. Christopher's Hospital for Children, Philadelphia. Adapted by permission.

## Patient Identification

The nurse is responsible for administering medications, performing and preparing children for a variety of medical procedures, even transporting infants to and from various departments. Under any of these circumstances, the consequences of mistaken identity can range from mere embarrassment to personal and professional tragedy. Double-checking the child's identity is a vital part of every nursing procedure, particularly when dealing with preverbal infants or with children whose communicative abilities have been impaired by illness or medical treatment.

---

**NURSING TIPS**
- **Always check the child's name band before performing any nursing procedure.**
- **Identify and double-check the organ or extremity to be treated.**
- **Double-check crib and wrist tags before removing or replacing infants.**
- **Be aware of more than one child with the same name.**
- **Be aware of child's whereabouts on or off the unit.**

---

## Visitor Identification and Management

Regardless of how busy the unit may become, the nurse should be aware of every individual on the premises, as well as of visitors' or callers' relationships to specific patients. The possibility of unauthorized adults trying to obtain information about a child's condition, or even of kidnapping, is very real, the latter especially in large urban hospitals where visitor flow is more difficult to control.

In addition, situations in which children are sick or injured can trigger bizarre, disruptive, or even combative behavior in overstressed relatives or friends. Whether or not such behavior is aimed directly at the nurse, it is the nurse's responsibility to contain the disruption before it disturbs patients, other visitors, or the work of other nursing and medical personnel.

## Documentation

Accurate and complete documentation is of paramount importance to the health maintenance and safety of hospitalized children. It enables nurses to explicate their role to other disciplines and protect themselves, their patients, and their institutions. The progress of the teaching plan is as important as information about the patient's physical condition. Nurses must document patient teaching needs explicitly (how much patients and their parents learned so they may take responsibility for their own care and their remaining nursing needs).

**NURSING TIPS**
- Know hospital policy on release of information. Generally, information about a pediatric patient's status may be released to parents or legal guardians only. They may then reveal what they wish to relatives and friends.
- Carefully identify telephone contacts. It is not uncommon for a nurse to receive two or three phone calls in a day requesting condition reports from a child's "mother," yet detectives, representatives of law offices, and news media reporters have all been known to make similar calls in search of confidential information.
- Be aware of the subtle behavioral cues (e.g., inappropriate remarks) that often precede disruptive behavior, and intercede before the situation becomes unmanageable.
- Disclose devastating information in a private conference room rather than a crowded hallway or waiting area. The family may then emote in private, lessening the possibility of panic.
- Know when to call security and where to redirect individuals who are behaving inappropriately.
- Redirect the attention of distraught family members who wander into inappropriate areas of the hospital or request information concerning other patients. Be careful not to use a harsh, punitive manner, which may agitate them.
- Notify security and arrange for an interdisciplinary behavior management conference to determine approach strategies if you suspect theft by a family member. Occasionally, family members respond to an illness by stealing. *Do not* attempt to manage theft or other crime situations without help.

**Documentation and the Law.**    Although charts and records are considered to be the property of the institution, they may be subpoenaed and are admissible evidence in court. Records are considered more reliable than memory. In many states, new laws have been passed granting the patient or family the right to read the patient's chart. Most institutions monitor this by requiring that a physician be present when a chart is perused.

*Nursing Actions for Documentation*
- Keep good records—they are a potent defense against malpractice.
- Be sure each page has the correct child's name stamped at the top.
- Record legibly. Unintelligible and incomplete records may be grounds for negligence in the eyes of some attorneys (Kempe & Helfer, 1972).

- Chart all observations and actions. Information that is not charted is considered undone, as in the case of a high-risk patient who needed frequent vital signs that were not charted.
- Write the doctor's name in the nurses' notes when reporting a change in a child's condition to the physician, e.g., "Dr. Swain notified of temperature elevation to 38.5° C at 4 P.M.," not, "MD aware."
- Avoid taking verbal orders when possible.
- Abbreviate infrequently and use only those approved by a committee that represents all patient care disciplines in the hospital. An example of an unclear abbreviation would be BS. Does this mean breath sounds, bowel sounds, or blood sugar? (Kempe & Helfer).
- Describe patient behaviors rather than making evaluative comments such as "appropriate," "inappropriate," "manipulative," or "obnoxious" (Kempe & Helfer). An example of descriptive charting is "The patient's mother was seen wandering into the intensive care unit down the hall. She was redirected to the parent services lounge, and the head nurse was able to spend some time with her . . ."
- Include behaviors that evaluate the objectives of the teaching plan, such as "Mother was able to demonstrate drawing up the accurate dose [name the amount] of digoxin in a tuberculin syringe." This will exonerate the nurse from claims by malpractice attorneys that discharge teaching was inadequate. This type of charting will also document the amount of nursing time needed for patient/parent teaching, which will be useful when Medicaid prospective payment systems (diagnosis related groups— DRGs) or other cost-containment strategies are in effect.

**Table 3.3**   System-by-System Documentation of Physical Condition

| System | Observations |
| --- | --- |
| Neurologic | Level of consciousness, mood, affect |
| Cardiovascular | Monitor; murmurs; indwelling central, umbilical, or arterial lines; IV sites and their condition; core temperature; heart rate and rhythm; blood pressure and any medications or infusions that influence it; capillary refill, peripheral pulses |
| Respiratory | Dyspnea, presence/absence of retractions, rate, color (cyanosis or pallor), breath sounds (equality, excursion-expansion), respiratory equipment from mask to ventilator, child's tolerance of the equipment |
| Gastrointestinal | Bowel sounds, tolerance of feedings, lack thereof, route of feedings, number of stools: color, consistency, frequency, odor |
| Urinary/Renal | Kidney function and voiding patterns, urine specific gravity, amount of urine/kilogram/hour (normal is 1 ml/kg/hr), route of voiding (via catheter or spontaneously) specific gravity and dipstick |
| Integumentary | Any tubes, drains, or wires exiting the child's body; incision site and condition; areas of bruising or abrasion; color, temperature, turgor |

When going through each system, record the information you take in with your senses

**Table 3.3**    System-by-System Documentation of Physical Condition (continued)

| | |
|---|---|
| Sight | Bleeding: color, amounts |
| Hearing | Speech and verbal patterns |
| Smell | Characteristic odor of a specific infection |
| Touch | Heat or edema in a specific area |

**SOAPE Charting.**    Table 3.4 is a sample of SOAPE (Subjective Objective Assessment Planning Evaluation) charting. Although the identified nursing problem of this SOAPE note is "alteration in cardiac output," this note includes all information needed to document the patient's well-being and general recovery postoperatively.

**Table 3.4**    Sample SOAPE Note

| | |
|---|---|
| Problem 1: | Alteration in cardiac output related to cardiac surgery |
| S: | "How long will Sherry have a sore throat?"—Mom. "Will she have to have another transfusion?"—Dad. "I can't cough! My throat hurts!"—Sherry. |
| O: | *Sherry* (10 years old, weight 36.0 kg). Arrived on the surgical floor on her first post-op day after repair of an atrial septal defect. Cardiac oscilloscope shows sinus tachycardia to 110. A routine EKG was done. Breath sounds equal to auscultation bilaterally in all lobes. No dyspnea. Reported postintubation throat discomfort and relief with ice chips. Capillary refill 1 sec. Blood pressures by cuff WNL. Nailbeds pink. Humidified $O_2$ by ventimask at 0.3 $FIO_2$ (fractional inspired oxygen concentration). Heparin lock intact in right dorsal forearm. IV fluids and meds infusing via peripheral IV in dorsum of left hand. Normothermic. Bowel sounds present. Tolerating ice chips. No stools post-op. Foley to straight drainage draining clear, amber urine with a specific gravity of 1.018, pH of 6, and dipstix negative. Sternal midline thoracotomy incision; dressing dry and intact. Mediastinal and left lateral chest tube insertion wounds healing normally. Received 3.6 mg morphine sulfate IM RUQ at 2 P.M. Reported good relief. |
| A: | Stable post-op. Alteration in cardiac output. |
| P: | Evaluate for need of ongoing post-op analgesia and give 1.0 mg/kg morphine sulfate as ordered by Dr. Coeur. Support Sherry and parents. Assist to cough and deep breathe every two hours. |
| E: | (Evaluation can be written as a follow-up later by a nurse on another shift to document the effectiveness of the nursing care plan related to Sherry.) |

Fidelity to the Weed method (problem-oriented medical records) is sometimes superficial in content, because practitioners tend to leave out information not directly related to a medical subsystem. For example, how the patient tolerates a diet postoperatively is related to surgical outcome because circulation will be shunted away from the periphery (GI tract) if post-op recovery is compromised. Pulmonary function, skin integrity, and capillary refill are similarly related to surgical outcome, and are part of complete disclosure in record keeping. A short but informational sentence in the subjective section from each parent helps indicate their anxiety level. A sentence from the child demonstrates his or her level of consciousness. The note explains nursing care being administered, confirms the presence and level of functioning of each tube or wire, describes the incision condition, and offers a system-by-system assessment of level of functioning. Avoid such clichés as "patient received" or "no complaints." Assess each body system to determine whether there is anything relevant about that system.

## Professional Liability

Working in an acute care setting with ill children places the pediatric nurse in a very vulnerable position regarding the possibility of legal actions brought by parents who feel their child was injured by hospital treatment. Children, because of their metabolism, size, and developmental status are highly susceptible to drug interactions and reactions, drug dosage and administration errors, and accidental injury. If a nurse deviates from sound, reasonable professional care, malpractice exists. Parents or legal guardians have a legal right to sue and recover damages if the child is injured by malpractice. The standard of reasonable care in any particular case is that of the surrounding geographic community; therefore, for example, that standard for a large metropolitan area would be higher than in a rural community without access to any teaching, research, or other sophisticated medical institution. The statute of limitations for malpractice action differs from state to state.

**Reasonable Care.**    It is important to recognize that this legal standard—i.e., reasonable care—does not make the medical profession or its personnel (e.g., physicians, nurses, and hospitals) guarantors of patient health. No one would suggest that anyone entering a hospital has a legal right to emerge from that institution free from all pre-existing aches and pains. In fact, reasonable "mistakes" in judgment do not constitute malpractice. A health care provider may decide on a particular course of action that seems reasonable at the time it is instituted without being vulnerable to a valid malpractice claim.

Take, for example, the situation of an emergency room nurse faced with two or three patients seriously injured in an auto accident. While waiting for a physician to arrive, this nurse will have to decide which injured person most urgently needs attention. The decision of whom to treat first, so long as it does not encompass a failure to notice a patient who is clearly more in need of immediate care, is not susceptible to later legal action.

The standard remains *reasonable* care. Only when a nurse deviates from sound nursing practice, thus potentially endangering patient health, may the nurse be sued. In addition, practitioners protect themselves against lawsuits by maintaining a good relationship and keeping parents informed.

**Captain-of-the-Ship.**    From a practical standpoint, however, nurses are rarely named as malpractice defendants because of the so-called "captain-of-the-ship" doctrine. This doctrine arose from a 1949 case, *McConnell v. Williams*, in which an operating surgeon was held responsible not only for his own actions, but for the performance of those working under him during the period of the operation. This same doctrine (*respondeat superior*) is also frequently applied to hold the hospital liable for its employees, nurses, and physicians.

This is not to say that nurses are never sued. An attorney certainly has the option to file a suit against an individual nurse who provides improper treatment to a patient in addition to the hospital. There is no particular "type" of nursing malpractice most susceptible to personal suit.

### Examples of Nursing Malpractice
- Carelessness in triage and admission (e.g., failure to identify a serious problem, provide prompt treatment, or notify a physician)
- Omission in taking a patient history (e.g., failure to detect and note drug allergies, previous illnesses)
- Carrying out the orders of the attending physician improperly (e.g., not monitoring vital signs, not checking a questionable dosage)

**Malpractice Insurance.**    Do nurses need malpractice insurance? Although nurses are rarely sued personally, a nursing mistake can certainly become the basis of a malpractice claim. Ironically, however, the acquisition of malpractice insurance may actually lead to involvement in a suit; the attorney may see a deep pocket (the insurance company) where there would not have been one otherwise.

Individual malpractice insurance is sound professional policy for all nurses, despite possible involvement. Maximum coverage, even for educators supervising undergraduate nursing students, can still be purchased for a reasonable amount. And nurses *are* being named in suits more and more frequently.

**Incident Reporting.**    When a safety infraction occurs, it is the responsibility of the nurse to notify the authorities in the appropriate chain of command. As unpalatable as incident reporting may be to many nurses and others, it can prevent a great deal of anguish later.

A report should be filed not only when someone from nursing is responsible for a mistake or accident, but also when someone from another discipline (e.g., medicine, pharmacy, dietary) is involved.

The objective of an incident report is not to place blame on an individual, but to describe an occurrence as accurately as possible without undue emotionalism. The report is used by the hospital's risk management office (insurance company) to keep a clear record.

The head nurse or supervisor is responsible for filling out a detailed analysis and follow-up action report.

### An "Incident"
- A circumstance that occurs out of the realm of the ordinary
- An act that endangers or injures an individual on the hospital premises
- A medication error
- Unusual data collection by a patient or his/her family
- A fall (even in a situation in which all reasonable precautions have been taken)

- Theft of a patient's personal belongings
- Injuries to staff and visitors

### Guidelines for Writing an Incident Report

- Document all occurrences of an incident in which a patient is injured, although some risk management offices advise avoiding this. It looks very strange to malpractice attorneys when there is a reference to a patient's "IV slough site of two days ago" and there is no documentation that an infiltration even occurred on the day identified.
- Chart ongoing notations about resolving injuries shift by shift.
- Write a narrative on a piece of paper before writing in the chart; go over it with the nursing supervisor.
- Notify the appropriate physician and the nursing supervisor of an incident, but do not obtain a signature from a reluctant physician although many institutions request that a physician sign an incident report. Document the names of individuals notified.
- Direct the report promptly (within 24 hours) to the risk management office with or without the physician's signature.

To summarize, in most cases incident reporting protects the nurse. Nurses are perceived as professionals by the courts, and may be held liable for actions that they did or did not take. Therefore, the nurse requires *both* accurate documentation and strong malpractice insurance in order to be fully protected. Table 3.5 lists information that should be included in an incident report.

**Table 3.5**    Information for Incident Reports

| |
|---|
| Identification of injured party |
|   If a patient: |
|    –  number of medical record |
|    –  condition for which she/he was admitted |
| Date, time, location of incident |
| Specific description of incident |
| Obvious injuries |
| Complaints registered by injured party |
| Name of examining physician |
| Date and time of physician's examination |
| X-rays or diagnostic tests ordered, and results |

# References

American Nurses' Association. (1984). *Capitol update*. 2(6), 1-2.

American Nurses' Association. (1985). *Code for nurses with interpretive statements*. Kansas City, MO: Author.

Cowles, K., & Murphy, E. (1982). *Nursing practice in the care of the dying*. Kansas City. MO: American Nurses' Association.

Hoffman, A. (1973). Consent, confidentiality, the law, and adolescents. *Delaware Medical Journal*, February, 35.

Holder, A. (1977). The minor's right to consent to medical treatment. *Connecticut Medicine*, 41, 579-582.

Kelly, L. Y. (1981). Legal aspects of patients' rights and unethical practice. In J.E. Thompson & H.O. Thompson, Eds. *Ethics in nursing.* (pp. 211-232). NY: Macmillan.

Kempe, C., & Helfer, R. (1972). *Helping the battered child and his family.* Philadelphia: Lippincott.

# SECTION II

# FUNCTIONAL HEALTH PATTERNS

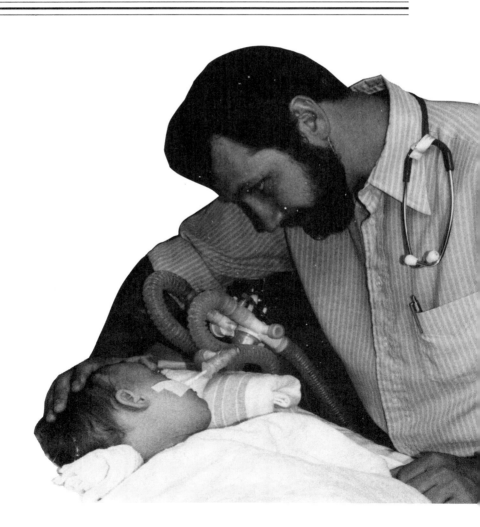

# CHAPTER 4

# HEALTH PERCEPTION— HEALTH MANAGEMENT
## FUNCTIONAL HEALTH PATTERN

C hildren comprise a significant percentage of the emergency patients at most hospitals. A major reason for this generally high treatment rate is the anxiety of parents unable to differentiate between a minor illness or injury and a serious health problem. Addressing the concerns of the parents is therefore as much a part of nursing care and health promotion as treating the child.

Another important consideration in pediatric nursing is the unique nature of the young patient; a child is *not* just a small adult. Although many pediatric problems are similar to those of adults, it must be remembered that children differ emotionally, anatomically, and physiologically from adults. Care must be provided accordingly. Knowledge of the normal growth and development stages is crucial to proper nursing assessment and care of a child.

Most children are less fearful and more amenable to treatment if allowed to remain with their parents. However, each family must be assessed individually. The desire of parents to stay with their child is a prime consideration; under certain circumstances, parents may prefer to leave the room, and the nurse must be sensitive to this feeling. Also, older children may offer a more complete and honest health history when parents are not present.

Maintaining the health and safety of well children and promoting the optimum health of children with chronic illness are vital issues in pediatric health maintenance and the major concern of this chapter. This chapter covers the area of health maintenance in a pediatric setting.

## GENERIC CARE PLAN FOR THE NURSING DIAGNOSIS
## ALTERATION IN HEALTH MAINTENANCE

### 1.  General Information

a.  **Etiology**
- Unachieved developmental tasks
- Perceptual or cognitive impairment
- Ineffective family coping
- Lack of materials or money to meet health care needs

b.  **Clinical Manifestations**
- Poor hygiene (oral and body)
- Frequent infections
- Lack of knowledge of health care practices

c.  **Multidisciplinary Approaches**
- Community support agencies
- Social services
- Dietary
- Hospice service if appropriate
- Legal assistance if needed
- Spiritual advice

### 2.  Nursing Process

a.  **Assessment**
- Communication skills of child and/or parents
- Motor skills of child and/or parents
- Growth and development, including cognitive skills
- Financial status of family
- Parental support systems
- Level of independence

b.  **Goals**
Child and family
- will maintain an adequate level of basic health care.
- will communicate their needs to appropriate health care providers.
Family will be able to care for child adequately.

c.  **Interventions**
• Determine cause of health maintenance deficit.

- Coordinate plan for obtaining needed health care with child, family, hospital, and home care staff.
- Arrange for respite care for family as needed.
- Teach child and family appropriate health care practices.

**d.  Evaluation**
- Parents maintain child's health schedule (e.g., well-baby visits, immunizations, vision, hearing, and speech screening).
- Child and/or family identify and use health care resources.
- Child is kept safe from infection and other injuries.

**e.  Possible Related Nursing Diagnoses**
Ineffective family/individual coping
Knowledge deficit

## GENERIC CARE PLAN FOR THE NURSING DIAGNOSIS
## POTENTIAL FOR INJURY (*Temperature Instability*)

## 1.  General Information

Fever is an oral temperature of over 100°F (37.8°C) or rectal temperature over 101°F (38.8°C). It is the most common symptom of illness in children, accounting for a significant proportion of pediatric ER visits. Most fevers are of brief duration, self-limiting, and of viral origin.

Moderate hypothermia occurs when the surface of the body is cooled from 71.4°–89.6°F (23°–32°C). Profound hypothermia occurs with a body temperature of 53.6°–68°F (12°–20°C). This can occur accidentally (near-drowning in cold water) or deliberately (cardiopulmonary bypass). Loss of body heat can cause a decrease in body functioning as peripheral circulation diminishes to preserve central circulation.

**a.  Etiology**
- Infection
- Newborn status
- Dehydration

**b.  Clinical Manifestations**
- *Elevated* temperature, pulse, respiration
  - irritability
  - altered level of consciousness
  - flushed skin
- *Decreased* temperature, pulse, respiration
  - altered level of consciousness
  - acrocyanosis
  - mottling

c. **Multidisciplinary Approaches**
  - Antipyretics as needed
    • low-grade fevers (less than 102°F [38.9°C] orally) do not require specific treatment beyond that required for the underlying cause, if known
    • fevers over 102°F (38.9°C) may be treated with aspirin or acetaminophen
    • children with a history of febrile seizures may require treatment of fever less than 102°F (38.9°C)
    • children with fever over 104° (40°C) not responsive to antipyretic medication will usually respond to a sponge bath
  - Hypo/hyperthermia blanket

## 2. Nursing Process

a. **Assessment**
  - Vital signs, especially temperature and pulse
  - Skin turgor and color
  - Changes in behavior (e.g., irritability, lethargy)

b. **Goals**
  Child will
  - remain free of seizures (elevated temperature).
  - be free from decreased metabolic function owing to heat loss (decreased temperature).

c. **Interventions**
  • Allow 30 minutes for the antipyretic to work before resorting to a bath.
  • Use tepid water (98.6°F [37°C]) if sponging is indicated.
  • Immerse or rinse all body areas for 20–30 minutes.
  • Alternatively, wet towels or sheets can be placed around each extremity and the trunk and replaced as they become warm.
  • Observe the child carefully for chilling or shivering; stop the bath if these occur.
  • Recheck the temperature 30 minutes after sponging.
  • Use cooling blanket if other methods fail for children with prolonged hyperpyrexia greater than 102.2°F (39°C):
    - set blanket temperature at 41°F (5°C)
    - turn off the blanket when the child defervesces to a temperature of 100.4°F (38°C)
    - set blanket temperature to 104°F (40°C) if the child has problems with hypothermia, such as post-op cardiothoracic surgery
    - place the child directly on the blanket or have only one sheet thickness between the child and the blanket

- place blanket rolls used for positioning under the blanket so that more of the child's skin surface is in contact with the blanket
- place one or more blankets on top of the child if necessary
- monitor vital signs every 15 minutes for 1 hour; if stable, monitor every 30 minutes for 2 hours, then hourly
- turn off the cooling blanket if shivering occurs, take vital signs, and notify the physician (shivering increases the metabolic rate, which is the mechanism of a fever, and is therefore counterproductive to therapy)

---

**NURSING TIP: Warming/cooling therapy may not be helpful for patients who have neurogenic temperature drift, since their thermoregulatory problems are related to damage in the central nervous system.**

---

  d. **Evaluation**
- Child's temperature, pulse, and respiration remain within normal limits for age (see table 1.3).
- Child manifests no behavioral alterations related to temperature instability.
- Child's skin color and condition remain within normal limits.

  e. **Possible Related Nursing Diagnoses**
   Alteration in comfort
   Fluid volume deficit
   Ineffective breathing patterns
   Parental anxiety
   Sensory-perceptual alteration

## Selected Health Problem Frequently Associated with the Nursing Diagnosis
## POTENTIAL FOR INJURY (*Temperature Instability*)

---

## Ineffective Temperature Regulation in the Newborn

  a. **Definition/Discussion:**  Newborns have difficulty maintaining a normal body temperature because their proportionately large body surface area rapidly loses heat to the atmosphere and their metabolic activities cannot generate enough heat to keep up with undue loss of heat to the environment.

b. **Multidisciplinary Approach**
   – Isolette/radiant warmer

# Additional Nursing Care That Can Be Incorporated into the Generic Care Plan

a. **Assessment**
Axillary temperatures (suggested time is during feedings)

b. **Goals**
Child's temperature will be within the range of 96.8°–98.6°F (36°–37°C).
Child will be weaned from Isolette/radiant warmer as tolerated (after temperature has remained between 96.8°–98.6°F [36°–37°C] with the servo control set point between 96.8°–97.7°F [36°–36.5°C] for at least 48 hours).
Parents will
   – state how heat is lost.
   – describe strategies for preventing heat loss.

c. **Interventions**
   • Place infant in neutral thermal environment immediately following birth and avoid exposure to cold.
   • If artificial source of heat (such as radiant overbed warmer or Isolette) is used
      – observe position of heat-sensing probe to prevent false high reading
      – compare infant's temperature with that of the heat source
      – if heat source is on manual control rather than servo control, take temperatures hourly
      – if servo control is being used, monitor temperatures every 2–4 hours
   • Keep infant undressed if in incubator.
   • Clothe and wrap infant in blankets if taken out for feeding; place stockinette or knitted cap on head.
   • Avoid using face or bony prominences as sites for thermal probes (abdominal area is generally acceptable).
   • In open units, keep probe covered with foam or a felt disk.
   • Use plastic "bubble wrap" (sheet of clear plastic or Saran wrap placed like a blanket) to prevent heat and fluid loss, especially if infant is under a radiant warmer.
   • Avoid cold stress episodes by doing procedures (e.g., drawing blood, IV stick, or lumbar punctures) under a radiant warmer.
   • Keep infant out of drafts.
   • Maintain room temperature between 75° and 78°F (24°–25.5°C).
   • Postpone bath if heat loss is a problem.

- If Isolette is not available, use K-pads, rubber gloves filled with warm water, or goose-necked lamp, but exercise extreme caution to avoid burns.
- Wean infant slowly from the Isolette; term or small-for-gestational-age infants can be weaned faster than premature infants.

**d. Evaluation**
- Infant
    - remains euthermic.
    - is weaned gradually but steadily and only when other subsystems (such as respiratory or digestive) are functioning well.
    - gains weight.
- Parents
    - state four major methods of heat loss (convection, radiation, evaporation, and conduction) and give examples of each.
    - demonstrate strategies for retaining heat in infant (e.g., "bundling" in heat-retaining blankets, dressing appropriately when away from heat source, placing cap over head).

## Other Possible Nursing Diagnoses

Alteration in parenting
Fluid volume deficit

## GENERIC CARE PLAN FOR THE NURSING DIAGNOSIS
## POTENTIAL FOR INJURY: *Trauma (Inpatient Prevention)*

## 1. General Information

An important aspect of the health management role of the pediatric nurse is to meet the safety needs of patients, their families, visitors, and those who work in the hospital setting. Florence Nightingale (reprint, 1965) recognized this when she wrote, "In the great majority of instances, when sudden death befalls the infant or young child, it is an accident; it is not a necessary, inevitable result of any disease from which it is suffering" (p. 72).

At the physiologic level, safety may be promoted by assuring proper nutrition, oxygenation, and fluid replacement.

Siderails are of great importance in any of the pediatric age groups, even though some adolescent patients find them embarrassing. Other patients find siderails reassuring, and some may be saved from serious injury. Many newborns have been found at the edge of cribs with arms or legs hanging over the side, and it is not unheard of for a small infant to slip out of an Isolette porthole inadvertently left open. Siderails can also be important if an unconscious child regains consciousness or has seizures when the nurse is away from the bedside. The use of siderails should become automatic. Always elevate them when leaving the bedside, even if only for a moment. However, if a child wants to get out of bed and is physically capable of doing so, siderails are not likely to stop him or her.

Restraints should never be used as a punishment, since such use is often perceived as a personal assault. If a child suffers injury or death related to prolonged use of restraints, it is reportable to the district attorney or medical examiner. The use of restraints becomes more emotionally laden as children become older. It may constitute "imprisonment" in some situations, and the burden of proof for the necessity of restraints falls on the provider who applies them. The use of restraints for older adolescents requires a written physician's order in many states.

The use of limb restraints should be restricted to incidences when the patient is a danger to self or others. In many cases, limb restraints are used to prevent injury or interruption of therapy, such as administration of oxygen and ventilation via endotracheal tube, to prevent a preverbal child from scratching infected eczema, or self-extubation by a child with post-pump intensive care psychosis. Table 4.1 lists some common restraints.

**Table 4.1**    Common Types of Restraints

Elbow restraints (cleft palate tubes)
Jacket
Limb
Mitts (prevent scratches, rumination; permit limb movement)
Mummy (to immobilize during procedures)
Nets
Papoose or "circ" board
Plexiglass domes
Safety belts
Siderails
Total body restraint (tie on screen, a sheet with ties at four limb sites)

Microshock (100 mu or less) is particularly dangerous to the electrically sensitive patient (e.g., children in cardiac and intensive care units; children who have exposed pacemaker wires or indwelling catheters such as central or Swan-Ganz lines). The act of turning on a piece of equipment may send flashes of current to the child. This current may not be perceived by sensory organs but may be life threatening nonetheless; the electrical conduction system of the heart can be disrupted by the current, and ventricular fibrillation may ensue.

a.  **Etiology**
    − Thermal trauma
       • heat lamps
       • k-pads

- hair dryers
- compressors
- hot soaks
- hypo- or hyperthermia units
- radiant overbed warmers
- overheated food or formula (especially if heated in a microwave)
- Chemical trauma
  - incorrect administration of medications
  - ingestion of toxic treatment agents (e.g., Betadine, Clinitest tablets)
  - unsupervised play with caustic substances
  - oxygen toxicity (injures the retinas of premature infants or the basement membranes of the alveoli)
  - caustics (e.g., institutional cleaning agents) in the environment
- Mechanical trauma and falls
  - slippery floors in corridors and staircases
  - slippery tubs and no railings in halls and bathrooms
  - lack of or improper use of restraints and/or siderails
- Electrical trauma
  - loose or defective control knobs or switches
  - burned-out pilot lamps
  - frayed or cut power cords
  - bent or broken plug pins
  - loose strain reliefs or outlets
  - two-wire power cords
  - "cheater" adapters without ground wires
  - improperly used extension cords
- Microshock

b. **Clinical Manifestations**
   - Burns
   - Sprains
   - Fractures
   - Bruises
   - Cuts
   - Contusions

c. **Multidisciplinary Approaches**
   - Sutures, reduction of fractures, casting, traction
   - See *burns*, page 178
   - See *accidental poisoning*, page 113

# 2. Nursing Process

a. **Assessment**
   - Age: independence-seeking toddlers and thrill-seeking adolescents are especially vulnerable to accidents

- Orientation and level of consciousness: neurologic impairments may alter perceptions of heat, pain, or discomfort
- Alterations in communication (e.g., expressive aphasias): children may be unable to convey their perceptions to others
- Paralysis: both perception and communication may be blocked
- Absence of the protective reflexes, such as cough, gag, or blink
- Drug-induced states: postanesthesia, street drug narcosis, or medication overdose
- High anxiety: narrows perception and dims awareness of peripheral activities
- Progressive change in level of functioning
- Unfamiliar environment (e.g., smoking in an environment where oxygen is being administered may produce an explosion)

**b. Goals**

Child will be
- protected from environmental hazards in the hospital.
- free from injury.

**c. Interventions**
- Place the bedside and overbed tables within reach.
- Use locks on wheelchairs, stretchers, and beds when appropriate.
- Advise post-op patients, sedated patients, and those on prolonged bedrest to call for assistance when first getting out of bed.
- Wipe up spills immediately.
- Ensure halls, stairs, and tubs have nonslip surfaces.
- Keep environment tidy: remove cords, toys, and extra furniture when not in use.
- Send faulty equipment to maintenance for repair.
- Institute safety measures in the use of restraints.
  - allow as much movement as possible
  - avoid occlusion of circulation (check neurovascular status of extremities frequently to determine obstructions in blood flow)
  - loosen restraints and exercise each limb every four hours and at the first indication of occluded peripheral circulation (the 5 *P*s: *p*allor, *p*ulselessness, *p*ain, *p*aresthesias, *p*aralysis)
  - pad bony prominences well to avoid abrasions
  - permit the body to assume its normal position when restrained (slight flexion of arms)
  - use the least conspicuous type of restraint possible (visitors find them disturbing); a crossover jacket is much less conspicuous than four-point arm and leg restraints
  - never restrain a person with a decreased level of consciousness in a spread-eagle position; vomiting, aspiration, and airway obstruction may ensue

- Promote electrical safety.
  - do not use defective equipment (e.g., cords that are frayed or produce a shock; intermittently functioning equipment)
  - know where circuit breakers are on the unit and have them labeled according to outlets they serve
  - discourage parents from bringing in personal appliances such as TVs, radios, hair dryers, curlers, or items that must be plugged in (battery-operated items are more acceptable; home appliances may be in questionable repair or condition and rarely have a ground wire to direct stray current safely)
  - disconnect electrical devices by the plug, not by the cord
  - do not place liquids, jellies, or creams on electrical appliances
  - do not place power cords where wheels may roll over them
  - send adjustment or repair work to appropriate department to be done; if you *must* do work, such as exchanging monitor modules, unplug the equipment first
- Prevent microshock (Children's Hospital of Philadelphia)
  - turn on equipment before connecting it to child
  - disconnect child from equipment before turning it off
  - do not place equipment, such as electrically driven infusion pumps, on the child's bed
  - do not touch child and equipment simultaneously
  - make a habit of touching a grounded surface before touching the child to discharge static electricity; this is especially important during the winter months
  - wear rubber gloves when handling pacemaker wires, the ends of central catheters, metal stopcocks, or conductive connections
  - if you experience a tingling sensation when using a piece of equipment, unplug it and remove it from service immediately
  - if a piece of equipment is dropped, has had fluids spilled on it, or is malfunctioning, remove it from service until it can be checked
  - a wide baseline on a cardiac monitor scope may reflect interference with other equipment in the vicinity (rather than a conduction problem in the child's myocardium)
    * replace/reposition electrodes
    * replace wires and/or cable
- If any child reports a sensation of mild current or shock
  - remove the equipment and disconnect it from the power source at once
  - remove the current source with a wooden, nonconductive, object (e.g., a broom handle) without touching the equipment and *after* breaking the circuit
  - institute cardiopulmonary resuscitation (CPR) if the child begins to fibrillate

    d.  **Evaluation**
- Child is free from burns, chemical injuries, or orthopedic injuries occurring during hospitalization.

    e.  **Possible Related Nursing Diagnoses**
Alteration in cardiac output
Sensory-perceptual alteration (specify)

**Table 4.2**   General Safety Precautions by Developmental Stage

**Infants**
Provide rails with small distance between slats (to prevent rolling and falling accidents).
Avoid tiny objects and pins.
Place infant in safe feeding and postfeeding positions
Cover electric outlets (plastic safety plugs when not in use).
Do not leave infant unattended in or near containers of water.
Check water temperature (120°–130°F [49°–54.5°C]).
Enforce child car and ambulance safety restrictions

**Toddlers**
Avoid knives, sharp tools, scissors, matches.
Keep stove-top pots or bottle warmers on back burners.
Lock away cleaning solutions, chemicals, insecticides, medicines. Never say medicine is candy.
Establish a safe play area.
Do not leave swimming pools, even "baby-style," unattended.
Use "No" and "Don't" with discretion.
Use child car and ambulance safety restraints.
Keep an eye on inquisitive walkers and climbers.

**Preschoolers**
Teach them to expect falls.
Stress importance of sidewalk play versus street play.
Provide swimming lessons.
Prevent children from running while carrying sharp utensils.
Teach children not to accept rides or gifts from strangers.
Teach children to use regular safety belts in cars.

**School Age**
Teach safe use of play and sports equipment.
Teach traffic and bicycle rules.
Use seat belts.
Teach children to handle animals safely.
Provide swimming and first-aid instruction.
Reinforce need for caution with strangers.

**Adolescents**
Provide constructive diversional activities.
Promote development of inner discipline.
Provide with appropriate safety gear (e.g., helmets) and instruction for avoiding sports accidents.
Instruct in the dangers of alcohol and drug abuse.
Remind the teenager that "it won't happen to me" too often does.
Stress use of seat belts.
Teach first aid and CPR.
Reinforce need for caution with strangers.

## GENERIC CARE PLAN FOR THE NURSING DIAGNOSIS
# POTENTIAL FOR INJURY *(Infection)*

## 1. General Information

Infants and children are at special risk of certain infections owing in part to their still-developing immune systems. Infections in young hospitalized children pose many problems for a variety of reasons:
- Symptoms may be diffuse or nonspecific, especially in very young children.
- Preverbal children may not be able to tell you "where it hurts."
- High fevers in children may be accompanied by febrile seizures.
- Vomiting and diarrhea can cause profound fluid and electrolyte imbalances very rapidly in young children.
- Children who are immunosuppressed may not show the usual symptoms of infection.

Viral upper respiratory infections (URI) and bacterial otitis media are the most frequently identified infections in children. Whereas URIs are usually self-limiting, otitis media requires antibiotics.

Prevention of infections in children includes not exposing the child to others who are ill (school-age children and children in day care situations may be at high risk).

Prevention of nosocomial infections in hospitalized children includes
- Handwashing between patient contacts
- Isolating children with contagious diseases
- Monitoring staff and visitors for contagious diseases
- Maintaining sterile technique for dressing changes

Any potentially serious or life-threatening infections can be prevented with appropriate immunizations.

Guidelines as stipulated by the Hospital Infections Program, Centers for Disease Control (CDC, 1983) have been used to develop table 4.3.

The CDC does not stipulate guidelines for protective isolation; however, some institutions with severely immunocompromised patients, such as those receiving transplants or chemotherapy, do maintain guidelines such as those in table 4.4.

### a. Etiology
- Contact with infectious agents
- Inadequate personal hygiene
- Open wounds
- Treatments and therapies
  - surgery
  - IVs, Foley catheters
  - chemotherapy
- Immunosuppressed system
- Chronic diseases

**Table 4.3**    Guidelines for Isolation Precautions

| Strict | Contact | Respiratory |
|---|---|---|
| *Common Indications* | | |
| Smallpox, pharyngeal diphtheria, herpes zoster varicella (localized in immunosuppressed child or disseminated), bubonic plague, lassa fever and other viral hemorrhagic fevers | Acute respiratory infections caused by respiratory syncytial virus, adenovirus, coronavirus, influenza viruses, parainfluenza viruses, rhinoviruses; gonococcal conjunctivitis in newborns; multiple resistant bacterial colonization with gram-negative bacilli resistant to aminoglycosides; *S. aureus* resistant to methicillin; pneumococcus resistant to penicillin; *H. influenza* resistant to ampicillin and chloramphenicol; pediculosis; viral pneumonia in infants and young children; *S. aureus* or group A streptococcus pneumonia; rubella; scabies; major skin wound or burn infection; vaccinia; rabies | Measles; mumps; pertussis; meningococcal meningitis (all cases of meningitis until 24 hours on antibiotics); pseudomonas pneumonia; *H. influenza* epiglottitis or pneumonia; erythema infectiosum |
| *Defined as Contaminated* | | |
| Air, *all* equipment and supplies in room, furniture, exposed surfaces | Dressings, linen, patient clothing, stuffed and other toys | Air only |
| *Room* | | |
| Private essential, with door closed, special ventilation needed for smallpox and Marburg virus diseases | Private desirable, bedside acceptable | Private essential, with door closed. Patients infected with the same organism may share a room. |
| *Mask* | | |
| Wear when entering | Wear for dressing changes | Wear when close to patient |
| *Gown* | | |
| Wear when entering | Wear for direct contact with patient or linens | Not indicated |
| *Gloves* | | |
| Wear when entering | Wear for direct contact | Not indicated |

| AFB (Acid-fast bacilli) | Enteric | Drainage/ Secretion | Blood/Body Fluid |
|---|---|---|---|
| Current pulmonary or laryngeal TB with a positive sputum smear or chest x-ray appearance that strongly suggests current active TB | Diarrhea (especially bacterial, such as salmonella or shigella); cholera; E. coli or giardia lamblia gastroenteritis enteritis; amoebic dysentery; coxsackie virus disease; echo virus disease; hepatitis A; viral meningitis unless known not to be caused by enteroviruses | Minor abscess; conjunctivitis; viral diseases; minor skin or wound infections; minor burn infection; decubitis ulcer (minor infection) | Hepatitis: B, non-A, non-B; malaria; Rocky Mountain spotted fever; syphilis, primary and secondary with skin and mucous membrane lesions; AIDS; any disease transmitted by arthropod vectors; leptospirosis |
| Articles contaminated with respiratory secretions | Fecal matter | Dressings, tissues, equipment | Blood/body fluids |
| Private room not necessary for infants and children with pulmonary TB because they rarely cough and their bronchial secretions contain few AFB | Private for children; private not necessary for cooperative adolescents; patients with same organism may share room | Private unnecessary | Private unnecessary unless patient hygiene is poor; patients with same organism may share room |
| If child is coughing and does not cover mouth | Not indicated | Not indicated | Not indicated |
| Only if contamination is likely | Wear if soiling is likely | If soiling is likely | If soiling with blood or body fluids is likely |
| Not indicated | Wear to touch bedpan, urinal, toilet, diapers | For touching infective material | For touching blood or body fluids |

**Table 4.3**   Guidelines for Isolation Precautions (continued)

| Strict | Contact | Respiratory |
|---|---|---|
| *Equipment* | | |
| Double bag, wash toys | No special care unless purulent drainage; wash toys | If contaminated with infective material, double bag and send for decontamination and reprocessing |
| *Linen* | | |
| Double bag | Double bag | No special care |
| *Dishes* | | |
| Disposable | Disposable | Disposable |
| *Dressings/Tissues* | | |
| Double bag | Double bag | Gloves/double bag |
| *Urine/Feces* | | |
| Flush immediately | No special care | No special care |
| *Other* | | |
| | | Blood spills should be promptly cleaned with a solution of 5.25% sodium hypochlorite diluted 1:10 with water. |

Note: *CDC guidelines for isolation precautions in hospitals.* by J. Garner and B. Simmons, 1983, Atlanta, GA: US Department of Health and Human Services, Public Health Service. Adapted with permission.

**b.   Clinical Manifestations**
   - Altered white blood cell count
   - Altered immune system
   - Altered circulation
   - History of infections
   - Fever, pain

**c.   Multidisciplinary Approaches**
   - Antibiotics
   - Isolation

# 2.   Nursing Process

**a.   Assessment**
   - Vital signs
   - Nutrition
   - Health history
   - Exposure to infectious agents

| AFB (Acid-fast bacilli) | Enteric | Drainage/ Secretion | Blood/Body Fluid |
|---|---|---|---|
| Discard, clean, or send for decontamination and reprocessing | Bag, label, and send for decontamination if contaminated with fecal material. | Double bag if contaminated. | Syringes and needles (unbent) in separate containers. DO NOT recycle "reusable" syringes and needles. |
| No special care | Double bag | Double bag | Double bag |
| Disposable | Disposable | Disposable | Disposable |
| Double bag | Double bag | Double bag | Double bag |
| No special care | Flush immediately | Sanitary disposal | Hepatitis urine and feces should be double bagged and incinerated. |

    — Medications
    — Immunization history

  **b. Goal**
    Child will be protected from contracting infections.

  **c. Interventions**
    • Isolation and restriction.
      — serve food on disposable dishes to all children with infectious diseases
      — wash toys that have come into contact with contaminants before use by another child
      — double-bag and label contaminated materials for disposal
      — educate all individuals involved with the child to carry out isolation measures
      — be a role model of proper isolation techniques for family members and other health care providers
      — institute protective measures as well as routine isolation precautions for children who may be in isolation because of

**Table 4.4**    Elements of Protective (Reverse) Isolation

**All Cases**

    All objects disinfected or sterilized before use (may include linens).

    Sterile gowns and gloves donned by all entering room. Masks worn by all entering room.

**Selected Cases**

    Hats and shoe coverings may be used.

    Food may be irradiated and dishes sterilized.

    All blood products may be irradiated.

    Laminar flow room may be used to remove ambient airborne organisms.

    Plastic "bubble" room may be used.

**Table 4.5**    TORCH Infections*

| Name | Type | Transmission and Precautions | Comments |
|------|------|------------------------------|----------|
| Toxoplasmosis | Parasitic | Hand to mouth transfer of oocysts from cat feces, soil or contaminated meat | |
| Other: Hepatitis B | Viral | Serum to serum, contact with contaminated or infected urine, bile, saliva, feces, vaginal secretions, semen, tears, synovial fluid, perspiration, amniotic fluid, stool, and blood across a mucous membrane (including sclera) | The National Center for Disease Control (CDC) in Atlanta has determined that it is clinically impossible to distinguish between serum and infectious hepatitis. |
| | | Enteric, blood, and secretion precautions | Over 90% of hemophiliacs carry hepatitis B. |
| Rubella | Virus | Air droplet | May be shed for up to two years in tears or urine. |
| | | Respiratory precautions | |
| Cytomegalovirus (CMV) or Cytomegalic Inclusion Disease (CID) | Virus | Blood transfusions, organ transplants, contact with contaminated body fluids (such as saliva, nasopharyngeal secretions, urine, feces, semen, or blood) | May be shed in urine for up to two years. |
| | | Enteric, blood, and secretion precautions | |
| Herpes | Virus | Mucous membrane to mucous membrane (sexual contact) | |
| | | Secretion precautions | |

*"TORCH" (Toxoplasmosis, Other, Rubella, Cytomegalovirus, Herpes) infections are especially important to pediatric nurses because they are dangerous not only to the child but to the fetus as well.

overwhelming infections (e.g., systemic candidiasis, purulent draining wounds, viral or bacterial sepsis)
  – place children who are immunosuppressed for any reason (e.g., chronic steroid therapy, congenital immunodeficiency, hypoplastic or aplastic anemia, or other immunosuppression phenomena) in private rooms
• Implement TORCH precautions when appropriate (see table 4.5)
  – place sign indicating "Pregnant Woman Precautions" on the child's bed or crib and in the kardex
  – consider children with anomalies of undetected origin infected even if a physician has not ordered isolation precautions
  – do not ask a woman who is pregnant or suspects that she is to provide care to someone with any of the TORCH infections
  – discourage visitors to the hospital, especially pregnant women, from touching or playing with children other than their own

**d.  Evaluation**
  • Child's
    – vital signs are within normal limits.
    – white blood cell count is within normal limits.

**e.  Possible Related Nursing Diagnoses**
  Social isolation
  Diversional activity deficit
  Alteration in parenting

## GENERIC CARE PLAN FOR THE NURSING DIAGNOSIS
## POTENTIAL FOR INJURY: *Poisoning*

## 1.  General Information

Accidental poisoning is the major cause of death in children 1–5 years old. Natural childhood curiosity and a tendency to put everything into the mouth place toddlers and preschoolers at high risk for poisoning. Aspirin is the most common accidentally ingested drug among children. Episodes are usually acute (although chronic ingestion can lead to the same symptoms). Toxic dose of aspirin is 4.4 grains/kg; 6.6–8.8 grains/kg is lethal (Rumack, 1979). For the average 2-year-old (12 kg), a toxic dose is 10–11 adult aspirin or 40 baby aspirin. Overdose of acetaminophen can lead to hepatic necrosis. The exact lethal dose is uncertain (Whaley & Wong, 1983). If the child survives the acute liver failure, recovery is likely.

The current proliferation of vitamins in the home makes iron ingestion one of the most common pediatric poisonings. Mortality varies greatly with the amount ingested and time elapsed between ingestion and initiation of treatment. The toxic dose has not been determined.

Hydrocarbon/petroleum distillates have a lethal dose as small as 1 oz. Low-viscosity hydrocarbons (e.g., mineral oil, furniture polish) have minimal effects when absorbed via the gastrointestinal tract. Generally, this ingestion is not treated unless pulmonary complications occur. The greatest danger is aspiration leading to severe chemical pneumonitis. Be aware of the most dangerous ingestible hydrocarbons—CHAMP (camphor, halogenated hydrocarbons, aromatics, heavy metals, pesticides) (Geebr, 1979).

Most poisonings of young children are not serious, and more than 80% do not require hospitalization. However, every poisoning should be a reminder to parents and health professionals of the importance of prevention; special emphasis must be placed on the recognition of poisonous plants (e.g., poinsettia, oleander, dieffenbachia), since most parents do not know that many common house and garden plants are toxic.

Most ingestion or injection of toxic substances by older children is not accidental, although an overdose may be. Given the steadily rising adolescent suicide rate, this should be strongly suspected in any such case. Most frequently abused substances are alcohol, tranquilizers, barbiturates, and psychotrophics. Treatment is symptomatic and substance specific. Follow-up with a psychotherapist is mandatory.

**Table 4.6**    Common Poisonings

| Substance | Symptoms | Medical Treatment |
|---|---|---|
| Salicylates | Tinnitus<br>Dizziness<br>Diaphoresis<br>Nausea, vomiting<br>4–6 hours after ingestion: hyperventilation, respiratory alkalosis, hyperpyrexia | Blood salicylate levels<br>Emesis or gastric lavage<br>Correction of respiratory alkalosis and/or metabolic acidosis<br>Peritoneal dialysis in severe cases |
| Acetaminophen | 36-hour symptom-free period<br>Anorexia, diaphoresis<br>Nausea, vomiting<br>RUQ pain, mental changes, poor coordination | Serum acetaminophen levels<br>Emesis or lavage<br>Mucomyst (acetylcysteine) orally or NG tube |
| Iron | Nausea, vomiting<br>Diarrhea<br>Abdominal pain | Asymptomatic: Induce vomiting with ipecac<br>GI symptoms: ipecac, gastric lavage, instillation with bicarbonate<br>Definitive: chelation with desferoxamine (DFOM) |
| Hydrocarbon/<br>petroleum<br>distillate | Altered mental status<br>Lethargy<br>Seizures, coma<br>Pulmonary toxicity: coughing, gagging, dyspnea, cyanosis, fever, intercostal retractions | Chest x-ray<br>Treat pulmonary dysfunction<br>No emesis or lavage |

a. **Etiology**
   - Drugs, medications
   - Alcohol
   - Poisons (e.g., plants, cleaning agents, insecticides)
   - Toxic chemicals

b. **Clinical Manifestations**
   - Dependent on substance ingested
   - See table 4.6.

c. **Multidisciplinary Approaches**
   - See table 4.6
   - Life-saving drugs, antidotes; CPR as needed
   - Induce vomiting with syrup of ipecac

---

**NURSING TIP: Do not induce vomiting if the child is unconscious or having seizures or if a caustic or a hydrocarbon/petroleum distillate material is ingested.**

---

   - • 15 ml followed by 200–400 ml water
   - • repeat syrup of ipecac once if vomiting does not occur in 20 minutes
   - • use in infants less than 1 year of age is controversial, and dose must be prescribed by a physician
   - Gastric lavage in the following children:
     - • any child who does not vomit following second dose of ipecac (e.g., children who ingest antiemetics such as Compazine or Thorazine may not respond to ipecac)
     - • unconscious children
     - • young infants
     - • when the ingested substance is a hydrocarbon in combination with a more toxic substance
   - Follow gastric lavage with activated charcoal (oral or NG) and a cathartic.

## 2. Nursing Process

a. **Assessment**
   - Nature, amount, and time of substance ingested
   - Burning in the mouth, esophagus, and stomach
   - Edema of the lips and tongue
   - Respiratory obstruction
   - Vomiting and agitation (indicate the presence of a caustic poison)
   - Shock

          – Cerebral edema
          – Seizures (can occur several hours postingestion)

**b. Goals**

Child will remain free from accidental poisoning.
Parents will
    – identify hazards in child's normal environments (e.g., home, day care, school, yard, car).
    – describe steps they plan to take to childproof environment.

**c. Interventions**

- Educate parents how to childproof home.
- Review with parents possible sources of contamination.
- Encourage parents to repair unsafe household items (e.g., medicine cabinets without locks, walls or furniture with peeling paint).
- Discuss with parents use of safety caps for bottles and need to lock up supplies.
- Educate parents to accidental poisoning first aid that can be done at home:
  - call poison control center and ask whether to induce vomiting
  - induce vomiting if instructed and if child is alert; if no syrup of ipecac available, give a glass of milk or water; save all emesis and bring to the emergency room
  - irrigate eye or exposed skin areas with tap water for 15 minutes
  - for inhalation poisoning, move child to fresh air; transport as quickly as possible
- Emotionally support child and family during initiation of vomiting or lavage procedure.
- Calculate the total amount of aspirin and acetaminophen ingested with cough/cold/allergy medications.
- Bathe child if ingestion occurs through the skin (pesticides).

**d. Evaluation**

- Child's physiologic parameters are within normal range (state highs and lows).
- Parents describe potential poisoning hazards in child's environment and describe measures to prevent accidental poisoning.

**e. Possible Related Nursing Diagnoses**

Alteration in oral mucous membranes
Ineffective airway clearance
Fluid volume deficit
Knowledge deficit

# References

Centers for Disease Control. (1983). *Guidelines, Hospital Infections Program*. Atlanta: Author.

Children's Hospital of Philadelphia. *Fire and safety*. Philadelphia: Author.

Greebr, E. (1979) Management of hydrocarbon ingestions. *Topics in Emergency Medicine,* *1*(3), 97–110.

Nightingale, F. (1965). *Notes on nursing* (facsimile reprint). Philadelphia: University of Pennsylvania Press.

Rumack, B. (1979). Aspirin and acetaminophen. *Clinical Toxicology, 15,* 1979.

Whaley, L., & Wong, D. (1983). *Nursing care of infants and children.* (2nd ed.). St. Louis: Mosby.

# CHAPTER 5

# NUTRITIONAL-METABOLIC
## FUNCTIONAL HEALTH PATTERN

T he nutritional-metabolic functional health pattern describes the intake of food and fluids in meeting the body's metabolic needs. This includes the feeding patterns and nutritional needs of infants and children as they grow and develop. The fluid and electrolyte needs and problems that occur in childhood because of the differences in children's metabolism are discussed and related to specific nursing measures necessary for fluid and electrolyte maintenance in childhood.

## Nutrition and Feeding of Children

Nutrition is of the utmost concern to pediatric nurses who must balance their patients' disease-specific nutrient needs with the ongoing dietary demands of growth. Satisfying these dual nutritional criteria is a major clinical challenge, particularly with seriously ill children. This section provides the pediatric nurse with useful information regarding the nutritional functional health pattern in childhood.

## Nutritional Assessment

The pediatric nurse can develop a more thorough understanding of nutritional problems by utilizing information collected by others in conjunction with information collected by nursing history and observation (see table 5.1).

**Table 5.1**    Nutritional Assessment

| Source of Data | Procedure | Interpretation |
|---|---|---|
| *Nursing History* | Interview parent and/or child to obtain the following data:<br>1. Child's age<br>2. Present diet<br>  • formula<br>  • breast/whole milk (type and amount)<br>  • infant foods<br>3. Present eating pattern or schedule<br>  • meals, snacks<br>  • who feeds<br>4. Utensils<br>  • bottle and nipple-type<br>  • cup<br>  • special utensils and techniques<br>5. Medical problems<br>  • treatments<br>  • medications<br>6. Food allergies<br>7. Nausea, vomiting, diarrhea<br>  • present?<br>  • frequency and onset<br>8. Symptons depressing intake<br>  • anorexia nervosa<br>  • decreased appetite<br>  • altered taste<br>  • sore mouth<br>  • loose teeth<br>  • trouble swallowing<br>  • reaction to medication<br>  • medical treatment<br>9. Excessive appetite<br>10. History of fever?<br>11. Activity level | • Determine if present diet meets age-appropriate needs and medical needs.<br>• Determine if there are any interferences with obtaining, ingesting, or absorbing nutrients.<br>• Determine if there are excess demands for nutrients. |
| *Anthropomorphic Measures*<br><br>Height | <br><br>0–4 years<br>• measure supine in special tray/table<br>• two people holding child flat, head against top board<br>• measure to heel with foot flexed<br>4 years–adolescent<br>• have child stand with back against a wall, heels flat on floor<br>• measure at mark perpendicular to top of head | <br><br>• Determine percentile rank.<br>• Use serial measurements to plot growth along a curve. |

**Table 5.1**   Nutritional Assessment (continued)

| Source of Data | Procedure | Interpretation |
|---|---|---|
| Weight | Use infant scale or adult scale as appropriate, with least amount of clothing possible.<br>Use same scale with same amount of clothing for later measurements.<br>Subtract weight of IV armboard or other equipment. | • Determine percentile rank.<br>• Use serial measurements to determine weight loss or gain pattern. |
| Weight for Height | Use above measures to calculate frame classification. | • Determine whether child is over-weight or underweight. |
| Sex | Observation | • Determine gender-specific nutri-tional requirements. |
| Head circum-ference (0–2 years) | Use paper tape to measure greatest circumference (from occipital process, over ears, on forehead). | • Evaluate brain growth.<br>• Compare to percentile rank and growth curve. |
| Mid-upper arm circumference (MUAC) | Measure from tip of bony process at shoulder to tip of bony process at elbow.<br>Mark midpoint.<br>Measure circumference of arm at midpoint using a tape measure. | • Compare to chart of standards for age (Malasanos, 1981).<br>• Determine available fat and protein stores. |
| Triceps Skinfold (TSF) | At MUAC mark, pinch up skin.<br>Measure with calipers 1 cm below fingers pinching up skin. | • Compare to chart of standards for age (Malasanos).<br>• Evaluate caloric reserves. |
| Arm-muscle circumference (AMC) | Calculate using above measures:<br>$AMC = MUAC - (0.314)(TSF)$ | • Compare to chart of standards for age (Malasanos).<br>• Determine degree of protein malnutrition (if any). |

*Laboratory Tests*

| | | |
|---|---|---|
| Serum albumin | Test Blood<br>Norms: gm/100 ml<br>Premature: 3.1–4.2<br>Newborn:  3.6–5.4<br>Infant:      4.4–5.3<br>Child:       3.5–4.7 | • Low value signals rate of protein catabolism greater than rate of protein synthesis.<br>• Determine ratio of protein catabo-lism/protein synthesis. |
| Serum trans-ferrin or Total Iron Binding Capacity (TIBC) | Test Blood<br><br><br><br>Child's Norm: 200–400 mg/dl | • Measures amount of iron present in the blood after transferrin is exposed to excess iron.<br>• Low values indicate decreased protein store in the body.<br>• Evaluate protein reserves, amount of iron in the blood. |
| Urine Urea Nitrogen | Test 24-hour urine specimen<br>Norm: 6/17 gm/24 hr | • Index of amount of nitrogen excreted as a result of body catabolism.<br>• Increases with protein wasting. |

**Table 5.1**    Nutritional Assessment (continued)

| Source of Data | Procedure | Interpretation |
|---|---|---|
| Blood Urea Nitrogen (BUN) | Test Blood<br>Norms: mg/dl<br>Premature: 3–25<br>Newborn:  4–18<br>Infant:    5–18<br>Child:     7–18 | • Elevated with increased protein metabolism (catabolic diseases).<br>• Decreased when protein metabolism inhibited, i.e., in negative nitrogen balance when protein breakdown is greater than intake.<br>• Check for catabolic disease, poor protein metabolism.<br>• Measures kidney function. |
| Urinary Creatinine | Test 24-hour urine specimen<br>Norms: mg/kg/24 hour<br>Infant: 8–20<br>Child: 8–22<br>Adolescent: 8–30 | • Compare 24-hour urine creatinine with standard.<br>• Estimates change in body muscle mass/catabolism of skeletal muscle. |
| Creatinine Height Index (CHI) | Norm: more than 60%<br>Marginal nutritional depletion: 40%–60%<br>Severe nutritional depletion: less than 40% | • CHI decreases with decrease in muscle mass. |
| White Blood Cell Count/ Lymphocyte Count | Norm<br>Newborn: WBC 9,000–30,000<br>          31% lymphs<br>6–12 months: WBC 6,000–17,500<br>          61% lymphs<br>2 years:   WBC 6,200–17,000<br>          59% lymphs<br>Child:     WBC 4,800–10,800<br>          30% lymphs | • Peripheral lymphocytes decrease with protein.<br>• Check for protein malnutrition. |
| Hematocrit | Test Blood<br>Norms:    %<br>Newborn: 53–65<br>Infant:    30–40<br>Child:     31–43 | • Percent of red cells in total volume of blood; decreases with blood loss: anemia, leukemia, excessive IV fluid replacement.<br>• Check for blood loss/disease/dilution by excessive IV fluid replacement. |
| Hemoglobin | Test Blood<br>Norms:        gm/dl<br>Newborn: 15–22 gm/dl<br>Infant:    10–15 gm/dl<br>Child:     11–16 gm/dl | • Measures oxygen-carrying capacity of blood.<br>• Decreases with iron deficiency. |
| Mean Corpuscular Volume (MCV) | Test Blood<br>Norms:    cubic microns<br>Newborn: 96–108<br>Male:     80–94<br>Female:  81–99 | • Describes individual red cell size: a ratio of *volume* of packed cells to the red cell *count*.<br>• Decreases with iron deficiency anemia.<br>• Increases with folate and vitamin $B_{12}$ deficiency.<br>• Check for adequate levels of iron, folate, $B_{12}$ |

## Age-appropriate Diets

The American Academy of Pediatrics (AAP) (1979) has recommended specific nutrition requirements for children at all age levels (table 5.2).

**Table 5.2**    Nutritional Requirements in Childhood

| Age | Calories Recommended cal/kg/day | Protein gm/day |
| --- | --- | --- |
| under 6 months | 117 | |
| 6–12 months | 108 | |
| 1–3 years | 1,300 | 23 |
| 4–6 years | 1,800 | 30 |
| 7–10 years | 2,400 | 36 |
| 11–14 years | | |
| girls | 2,400 | 44 |
| boys | 2,800 | 44 |
| 15–18 years | | |
| girls | 2,100 | 48 |
| boys | 3,000 | 54 |

**Breast-feeding.**    Infants can obtain most essential nutrients from breast milk or modified cow's milk formulas, although iron and fluoride supplements may be required by the breast-fed infant (Howard, 1982). Breast-feeding is highly recommended by the AAP for the first 6 months. Advantages of breast milk are:

- contains optimum percentages of carbohydrates, protein, and fat
- has a low renal solute load (determined by concentration of protein and electrolytes)
- has an easily digestible protein component (whey to casein ratio of 60:40 compared to 18:82 in pure cow's milk)
- contains an easily digested carbohydrate (lactose) in a higher concentration than that of cow's milk
- is a rich source of linoleic acid, an essential fatty acid

In addition, human milk contains protective factors against infection and may contain a "mucosal growth factor", which facilitates early maturation of the gastrointestinal system (Walker, 1977).

**Cow's Milk Formulas.**    If breast-feeding is not possible or is not desired by the parents, modified cow's milk formulas can be used. When choosing a formula, particularly for an infant whose metabolism has been altered by illness, consider several factors:

- digestibility and absorption of carbohydrate, protein, and fat
- percentage of calories from carbohydrate, protein, and fat
- renal solute load (concentration of protein and electrolytes)

Pure cow's milk should be avoided during the entire first year of life because it

- is a poor source of iron
- is associated with gastrointestinal bleeding
- contains excessive proteins and minerals, which increase the renal solute load (Bonner, 1981; Moore, 1981)

**Dietary Management of Premature Infants.**    Premature infants are born with immature systems, yet have tremendous nutritional needs. Premature infants lack

- lipases and bile salts needed for the breakdown of fat
- adequate amounts of lactase for the breakdown of milk sugar
- certain enzymes for the conversion of amino acids to proteins.

Because of immaturity of systems, poor absorption, and low intake, premies are prone to hypoglycemia, metabolic acidosis (secondary to increased renal solute load), and vitamin and mineral deficiences (particularly vitamins D and E, folate, and iron). Breast milk pumped by the mother or obtained from breast milk banks or specially tailored formulas (see table 5.3) contains the appropriate forms of nutrients for premature infants—a decreased percentage of lactose, a whey to casein ratio of 60:40, medium-chain triglycerides, low renal solute load, and increased calories per volume.

**Oral Feedings.**    Oral feedings are indicated when the child's mouth, esophagus, and entire GI system are intact and functioning well. Infants must be alert with an adequate suck and a coordinated suck-swallow reflex. Older children should be alert, able to chew, and have a coordinated chew-swallow movement. Whether the child can feed self or not is NOT a factor; oral feedings should not be avoided just because it takes a long time to feed a child.

### Bottle Feeding
- Bottles can be glass or plastic and come in 4 oz and 8 oz sizes.
- Playtex nursers have plastic sacs that fit into plastic frames.
- Volu-Feed nursers hold only 60 cc and may be used for very small feedings.
- Measure any feeding that must be accurately measured with a syringe before placing it in a bottle.
- Measure any residual after the feeding.
- Tighten caps and check for fit before feeding.
- *Never* leave children who can hold their own bottles alone with a bottle of fluid.
- Always use clean technique when handling nipples and bottles. *Never* place them in a hospital sink to warm them!

### Special Implements for Oral Feeding
- Use syringe with latex tubing or medicine dropper for children with
  - a post-op cleft lip/palate repair to prevent injury to the suture line
  - plastic surgery or fractures where the jaw is wired
  - a mental or neurologic deficiency who can swallow but who cannot get fluid into their mouths using a regular cup

**Table 5.3**  Comparison of Milk and Infant Formulas

| Formula | Cal/Oz | Indication | Source Of CHO/Pro/Fat | Gm/L | % Total Calories | Osmolality per liter | Potential Renal Solute Load | Na mOsm/L |
|---|---|---|---|---|---|---|---|---|
| *Normal Infant Formulas and Milk* | | | | | | | | |
| Human Breast Milk | 22 | *Recommended Infant Feeding | C: Lactose | 71 | 39 | 300 | 77 | 180 |
| | | | P: Mature human milk proteins | 11 | 6 | | | |
| | | | F: Mature human milk fat | 45 | 55 | | | |
| Whole Cow's Milk | 20 | Not indicated for infants up to 12 mos | C: Lactose | 48 | 29 | 290 | 226 | 500 |
| | | | P: Cow's milk whey/casein ratio = 18/82 | 33.8 | 20 | | | |
| | | | F: Butterfat | 37.7 | 51 | | | |
| 2% Lowfat Milk | 15–16 | Not indicated for infants or children due to decreased calories and decreased fat content | C: Lactose | 38 | 49.5 | Not available | 231 | 520 |
| | | | P: Cow's milk | 27 | 34.3 | | | |
| | | | F: Butterfat | 20 | 35 | | | |
| Skim Milk | 10–11 | Not indicated for infants or children due to decreased calories and decreased fat content | C: Lactose | 50.2 | 56 | 300 | 240 | 540 |
| | | | P: Cow's milk | 35.3 | 39 | | | |
| | | | F: Butterfat | 1.9 | 5 | | | |
| Advance (Ross) | 16 | Supplement for older infants and toddlers in place of whole cow's milk | C: Corn syrup and lactose | 55 | 40 | 200 | 128 | 200 |
| | | | P: Cow's milk and soy protein isolate | 20 | 15 | | | |
| | | | F: Soy and corn oils | 27 | 45 | | | |
| Enfamil Enfamil with Iron (Mead Johnson) | 20 | Normal Newborn Formula | C: Lactose | 69 | 41 | 300 | 98 | 181 |
| | | | P: Cow's milk 60% whey 40% casein | 15 | 9 | | | |
| | | | F: Coconut and soy oil | 38 | 50 | | | |

**Table 5.3** Comparison of Milk and Infant Formulas (continued)

| Formula | Cal/Oz | Indication | Source Of CHO/Pro/Fat | Gm/L | % Total Calories | Osmolality per liter | Potential Renal Solute Load | Na mOsm/L |
|---|---|---|---|---|---|---|---|---|
| Similac Similac with Iron (Ross) | 20 | Normal Newborn Formula | C: Lactose<br>P: Cow's milk<br>F: Coconut and soy oil | 72.3<br>15<br>36.3 | 43<br>9<br>48 | 290 | 105 | 220 |
| Similac with Whey and Iron | 20 | Normal Newborn (whey dominant) | C: Lactose<br>P: Cow's milk and whey<br>F: Coconut and soy oil | 72.3<br>15<br>36.3 | 43<br>9<br>48 | 300 | 101 | 230 |
| SMA Iron fort, SMA Lo-Iron (Wyeth) | 20 | Normal Newborn or when low renal solute load and low Na necessary (whey dominant) | C: Lactose<br>P: Cow's milk and whey 60/40<br>F: Oleo, coconut, safflower and soy oils | 72<br>15<br>36 | 43<br>9<br>48 | 300 | 91 | 150 |
| *Low Na/Low Renal Solute Load* | | | | | | | | |
| Similac PM 60/40 (Ross) | 20 | For renal, digestive, or cardiovascular disorders requiring low renal solute load and low Na | C: Lactose<br>P: Whey and Casein 60/40<br>F: Coconut and corn oils | 69<br>15<br>37.8 | 41<br>9<br>50 | 260 | 95 | 160 |
| *Soy Formulas* | | | | | | | | |
| Isomil (Ross) | 20 | For lactose intolerance | C: Corn syrup and sucrose<br>P: Soy protein isolate<br>F: Soy and coconut oils | 68.3<br>18<br>36.9 | 40<br>11<br>49 | 250 | 122 | 320 |
| Isomil SF (Sucrose-free) (Ross) | 20 | For lactose and sucrose intolerance | C: Polycose glucose polymers<br>P: Soy protein isolate<br>F: Soy and coconut oils | 68.3<br>20<br>36 | 40<br>12<br>48 | 150 | 131 | 320 |
| Prosobee (Mead Johnson) | 20 | For lactose and sucrose intolerance; gluten sensitivity | C: Corn syrup solids<br>P: Soy protein isolate<br>F: Soy and coconut oils | 67.6<br>20.3<br>35.9 | 40<br>12<br>48 | 200 | 127 | 240 |
| Nursoy (Wyeth) | 20 | For lactose and/or corn syrup solid sensitivity | C: Sucrose<br>P: Soy protein isolate<br>F: Oleo, coconut, safflower and soy oils | 69<br>21<br>36 | 40<br>12<br>48 | 291 | 122 | 200 |

| Product | cal/oz | Indications | Composition | g | % | | | |
|---|---|---|---|---|---|---|---|---|
| L-Soyalac (Loma Linda) | 20 | For lactose and/or corn allergy | C: Sucrose and tapioca dextrins | 66 | 39 | 270 | 134 | 340 |
| | | | P: Soy protein isolate | 21 | 12 | | | |
| | | | F: Soy oil | 37 | 49 | | | |
| Soyalac (Loma Linda) | 20 | Lactose intolerance | C: Corn syrup and sucrose | 66 | 39 | 240 | 138 | 350 |
| | | | P: Soybean solids | 21 | 12 | | | |
| | | | F: Soy oil | 37 | 49 | | | |
| *High-Calorie Formulas* | | | | | | | | |
| Similac 24 (and with Iron) (Ross) | 24 | increased calories/volume. Used with fluid restrictions or to increase caloric intake | C: Lactose | 85.3 | 42 | 360 | 152 | 350 |
| | | | P: Cow's milk | 22 | 11 | | | |
| | | | F: Soy and coconut oil | 42.8 | 47 | | | |
| Enfamil with Iron 24 (Mead Johnson) | 24 | | C: Lactose | 83 | 41 | 340 | 118 | 217 |
| | | | P: Cow's milk and whey | 18 | 9 | | | |
| | | | F: Soy and coconut oil | 45.6 | 50 | | | |
| SMA 24 Iron fort, SMA 24 Lo-Iron (Wyeth) | 24 | | C: Lactose | 86.4 | 43 | 360 | 110 | 180 |
| | | | P: Cow's milk and whey | 18 | 9 | | | |
| | | | F: Oleo, coconut, safflower, and soy oils | 43.2 | 48 | | | |
| Similac 27 (Ross) | 27 | | C: Lactose | 95.9 | 42 | 410 | 170 | 390 |
| | | | P: Cow's milk | 24.7 | 11 | | | |
| | | | F: Soy and coconut oils | 48.1 | 47 | | | |
| SMA 27 Iron fort, SMA 27 Lo-Iron (Wyeth) | 27 | | C: Lactose | 97 | 43 | 420 | 123 | 200 |
| | | | P: Cow's milk and whey 60/40 | 20.3 | 9 | | | |
| | | | F: Oleo, coconut, safflower, and soy oils | 48.6 | 48 | | | |

**Table 5.3**  Comparison of Milk and Infant Formulas (continued)

| Formula | Cal/Oz | Indication | Source Of CHO/Pro/Fat | Gm/L | % Total Calories | Osmolality per liter | Potential Renal Solute Load | Na mOsm/L |
|---|---|---|---|---|---|---|---|---|
| *Premature Infant Formulas* | | | | | | | | |
| Similac Special Care 20 (Ross) | 20 | Premature GI function | C: Lactose and polycose glucose polymers | 71.7 | 42 | 250 | 129 | 340 |
| | | | P: Cow's milk and whey 60/40 | 18.3 | 11 | | | |
| | | | F: Medium chain triglycerides (MCT), corn and coconut oils | 36.7 | 47 | | | |
| Enfamil Premature Formula 20 (Mead Johnson) | 20 | Premature GI function | C: Lactose and corn syrup solids | 74 | 44 | 244 | 181 | 260 |
| | | | P: Cow's milk and whey 60/40 | 20 | 12 | | | |
| | | | F: MCT, corn and coconut oils | 34 | 44 | | | |
| Similac Special Care 24 (Ross) | 24 | | C: Lactose and polycose glucose polymers | 86.1 | 42 | 300 | 156 | 410 |
| | | | P: Cow's milk and whey | 22 | 11 | | | |
| | | | F: MCT, corn and coconut oils | 44.1 | 47 | | | |
| Similac 24 LBW (Ross) | 24 | | C: Lactose and polycose glucose polymers | 85.3 | 42 | 290 | 160 | 360 |
| | | | P: Cow's milk | 22 | 11 | | | |
| | | | F: MCT, coconut and soy oils | 44.9 | 47 | | | |
| Enfamil Premature Formula 24 (Mead Johnson) | 24 | | C: Lactose and corn syrup solids | 89 | 44 | 300 | 220 | 320 |
| | | | P: Cow's milk and whey | 24 | 12 | | | |
| | | | F: MCT, corn and coconut oils | 41 | 44 | | | |
| SMA "preemie" 20 (Wyeth) | 20 | LBW/VLBW | C: Lactose and corn syrups solids | 74 | 43 | 268 | 128 | 320 |
| | | | P: Cow's milk and whey | 20 | 12 | | | |
| | | | S: Coconut, oleic, and soy oils, MCT | 34 | 45 | | | |
| SMA "preemie" 24 (Wyeth) | 24 | LBW/VLBW | C: Lactose and corn syrup solids | 86 | 41 | 280 | 128 | 320 |
| | | | P: Cow's milk and whey | 20 | 10 | | | |
| | | | F: Coconut, oleic, oleo and soy oils, MCT | 44 | 49 | | | |

## Special Formulas

| Product | | Description | Composition | | | | | |
|---|---|---|---|---|---|---|---|---|
| RCF (Ross) | 12 without CHO | Formula base only for CHO-intolerant infants | C: CHO free—needs to be added | | | 64 without CHO | 131 | 320 |
| | | | P: Soy protein isolate | 20 | | without CHO 20 | | |
| | | | F: Soy and coconut oils | 36 | | without CHO 80 | | |
| Nutramigen (Mead Johnson) | 20 | Hypoallergenic. Protein is hydrolyzed for infants sensitive to milk and food proteins. | C: Sucrose and modified starch—corn syrup solids | 91 | 54 | 350 | 125 | 320 |
| | | | P: Casein hydrolysate | 19 | 11 | | | |
| | | | F: Corn oil | 27 | 35 | | | |
| Pregestimil (Mead Johnson) | 20 | For malabsorption. Protein, carbohydrate, fat in readily digestible forms. | C: Corn syrup and modified tapioca starch | 91 | 54 | 350 | 125 | 320 |
| | | | P: Casein hydrolysate | 19 | 11 | | | |
| | | | F: Corn oil and MCT | 27 | 35 | | | |
| Portagen (Mead Johnson) | 20 | For fat malabsorption | C: Corn syrup solids, sucrose, lactose | 78 | 46 | 220 | 150 | 340 |
| | | | P: sodium caseinate | 24 | 14 | | | |
| | | | F: MCT, corn oil | 32 | 40 | | | |

| *Electrolyte Preparations* | *Indications* | *Contents/Liter* | |
|---|---|---|---|
| Pedialyte (Ross) (Fruit-flavored available) | To prevent dehydration in mild or moderate diarrhea | Dextrose 25 G; Na 45 mEq; K 20 mEq; Cl 35 mEq | 100 cal/liter Osmolality = 250 |
| Pedialyte RS (Rehydration Solution) (Ross) | To manage mild to moderate dehydration 2° to moderate to severe diarrhea | Dextrose 25 gm; Na 75 mEq; K 20 mEq; Cl 65 mEq | 100 cal/liter Osmolality = 305 |
| Lytren (Mead Johnson) | To supply $H_2O$ and electrolytes for maintenance; to replace mild to moderate fluid losses | CHO 22 gm; Na 50 mEq; K 25 mEq; Cl 45 mEq | 100 cal/liter Osmolality = 220 |
| Resol (Wyeth) | To control diarrhea and prevent dehydration by replacing lost fluids and minerals | Glucose 20 G; Na 50 mEq; K 20 mEq; Cl 50 mEq | 80 cal/liter Osmolality = 265 |

**Table 5.3** Comparison of Milk and Infant Formulas (continued)

| Other Special Formulas | Indications |
|---|---|
| Lofenalac (Mead Johnson) | low phenylalanine diet for patients with PKU |
| Phenyl-free (Mead Johnson) | phenylalanine-free diet for patients with PKU |
| MSUD Diet Powder (Mead Johnson) | for maple-syrup urine disease |
| Product 3200 AB (Mead Johnson) | low phenylalanine/low tyrosine for patients with hereditary tyrosemia |
| Product 3200 K (Mead Johnson) | low methionine diet for homocystinuria |
| Product 80056 (Mead Johnson) | protein-free diet formula base for several metabolic diseases requiring specific mixtures of amino acids |
| Product 3232A (Mead Johnson) | mono- and disaccharide-free formula base for mono/disaccharide intolerance |

References
1. Product literature:
   Mead Johnson
   Ross Laboratories
   Wyeth
   Loma Linda

NOTE: This table contains selected formulas that were available at press time. Readers should be aware that new formulas are being generated continuously, and this table therefore does not reflect any produced after publication.

- Use spoons
  - when suture line trauma is not a factor
  - that are rubber coated for children who bite
- Use covered, spouted cups with
  - older infants
  - children who are learning to drink from a cup
- Use flexible straws
  - when a child cannot sit upright to drink
  - just for fun

Consult physical therapy and occupational therapy professionals when special implements are needed, e.g., spoons with straps, spoons with special grips, or hand splints.

**Childhood Nutritional Requirements.** During the childhood years, nutritional needs and dietary patterns change rapidly. In general, protein and calorie requirements (per kilogram) are high at the beginning of life when most rapid growth occurs, level off during the slower growth period of school-age, and increase again during the adolescent growth spurt. The sources of nutrients change as the maturing infant gradually learns to take solid foods, develops fine motor skills, and develops likes and dislikes. Therefore, each age group has specific nutritional and feeding needs. Additional calories are necessary for premature infants, children who are very active, or whose illness requires it (AAP, 1979). Protein needs may also increase with illness.

The nurse can also assist nutritionally compromised children outside of the hospital or clinic by referring families in need to their local Women, Infants, and Children (WIC) office. Federally funded and locally administered, WIC is designed to make nutritious foods available to low income women, infants, and children. To be eligible, one must be a pregnant or a nursing woman or an infant or child under 5 years of age. Occasional medical evaluations are necessary, as well as an income standard to determine eligibility.

Foods available in the program include milk, fortified cereals, pure juices, eggs, cheese, and iron fortified formulas. These specific items must be purchased at a WIC-approved store by the eligible woman. Amounts of foods are rationed according to each individual family's needs.

The WIC phone number can be found in the federal government section of the local phone book. A simple referral can be a major nursing step toward ensuring the continuing health of the pediatric patient.

# Age-appropriate Feeding Approaches/Techniques

**Infants.** Developmentally, infancy is a period of rapid growth and rapid improvement in feeding ability:

- First 3 months: involuntary rooting, sucking, and swallowing reflexes dominate.
- After 3 months: the extrusion reflex (pushing out with the tongue) decreases and sucking becomes more voluntary.

- 5–6 months: the infant can grasp some objects and bring them to the mouth, chewing movements begin in this period, and lip coordination enables the child to drink from the rim of a cup (Howard).
- After 6 months: chewing and swallowing improve, and teeth come in, enabling the child to take more textured foods.

Feeding schedules and volume of feedings should be individualized; the infant will regulate itself if allowed. Bottle-fed infants should not be forced to "finish the bottle"if they are satiated with less. Infants will regurgitate formula if their stomach capacity cannot accommodate the volume. General guidelines for formula feeding are offered in table 5.4.

**Table 5.4** Guidelines for Formula-fed Infants

| Age (in months) | Ounces/Feeding | Number of Feedings/Day |
|---|---|---|
| 0–1 | 2–3 | 6–8 |
| 1–2 | 3–5 | 5–6 |
| 2–4 | 5–7 | 4–5 |
| 4–6 | 7–8 | 4–5 |
| 6–12 | 8 | 3–4 |

Encourage breast-feeding mothers to continue breast-feeding in the hospital if it is not contraindicated by the condition of the infant. When breast-feeding is not possible, a variety of nipples and bottles is available to bottle-feed infants (see table 5.5). A mother may want to express her breast milk and give it in a bottle or she may want to maintain her milk supply until the baby can breast-feed after the illness. Provide sterile water bottles for mothers on the unit. Frozen breast milk is safe for use for 24 hours after thawing, if kept refrigerated.

**Table 5.5** Types of Nipples for Bottle Feeding

| Nipple Type | Use | Description |
|---|---|---|
| Regular | Normal newborn | |
| NUK | Normal newborn | Wide, flat tip that fits the mouth and palate |
| Playtex | Normal newborn | Short, squared |
| Premature | Infants with weak suck | Soft, large hole or crosscut |
| Special Care (Ross) | Infants with weak suck | Short, soft, large hole |
| Lamb's nipple | Infants with cleft lip/palate | Extra long and wide, large hole, soft rubber |
| Flanged | Infants with cleft palate | Regular shape, side flaps to cover the palate |
| Cleft Palate Assembly (Ross) | Infants with cleft palate | Long nipple with a tip shaped like tubing, large hole or cross cut |

Do not use nipples intended for use with prepared formula bottles as pacifiers.

**NURSING TIPS**
- Feed infants "on demand" as much as possible, although in the hospital this may not be possible.
- Keep feeding schedules flexible.
- Use a nipple, bottle, or cup familiar to the infant to facilitate feedings.
- Hold the bottle up so the nipple is always filled with formula.
- Burp small infants frequently—after every ounce; older infants may need to burp halfway through the feeding and at the end.
- Hold infants who cannot sit alone in a semi-upright position.
- Always keep children in safe positions while feeding—sitting upright, on the side, or prone.
- Involve parents or caretakers in the feeding process, perhaps even have them share their techniques.

Switching from breast to bottle (and the reverse) is confusing to many infants since the sucking mechanisms differ. Although switching is frustrating it is sometimes done to

- allow fathers to feed infants
- allow career mothers to return to work
- supplement breast-feeding, e.g., water

Introduce the cup at 5–6 months. Delay solid feedings until the infant has the developmental ability to control mouth and tongue movements (4–6 months). Add foods one at a time and observe the child for allergic reactions for several days (see list of significant allergens, table 5.6). A recommended sequence is: rice cereal, fruits, vegetables, and meats. Avoid whole eggs and orange juice (frequent allergy-producing foods) until late in the first year. Plain, strained baby foods are best nutritionally, compared to baby food

**Table 5.6** Significant Allergens

Egg albumin
Corn syrup solids
Wheat (gluten) products
Cow's milk formulas and products (lactose intolerance or casein allergy)
Citrus fruits and juices
Tomatoes
Strawberries
Seafood (protein and iodine)
Spices
Chocolate

"dinners" and "desserts." Textured foods can be introduced at 4–6 months starting with strained foods, advancing to mashed foods (7–8 months) and finally to finely cut foods (12 months) as tongue and mouth movements become more mature.

## NURSING TIPS
- **Offer solid foods before formula.**
- **Place solids in the center of the tongue, using a small spoon, and press downward slightly to facilitate swallowing.**
- **An infant will push out solids, when first learning to eat them. This does not mean dislike, just inexperience (Howard).**
- **Allow the older infant as much independence as possible— holding its own bottle or cup, feeding self with fingers.**
- **Offer finger foods.**
- **Review table 5.7, Precautions for Feeding Infants and Toddlers**

**Table 5.7**   Precautions for Feeding Infants and Toddlers

- Avoid tiny, easily aspirated foods (e.g., nuts, hard candies, popcorn kernels) in children under age 3.
- Do not offer foods that expand upon ingestion (e.g., popcorn).
- Avoid carrot sticks since they are difficult for most toddlers to chew well; pieces are often aspirated.
- Shred, grind, or finely dice meat.
- Observe for allergic reactions to foodstuffs.

Dietary expansion is a key indicator of developmental progress, and developmental status must be considered in the dietary management of young children. The inpatient setting is not the place for the introduction of new foods to infants unless hospitalization continues for many months. An allergic reaction to unfamiliar food may be confused with hypersensitivity to a much needed drug or with a pathologic process.

Recently, two nurse-investigators (Measel & Anderson, 1979) reported on a study in which pacifiers were supplied to premature infants restricted to gavage feedings. When non-nutritive sucking opportunities were offered during and following tube feedings, statistically significant alterations in the clinical course were revealed. "Premature infants who received sucking opportunities during and following every tube feeding were given their first bottle feeding an average of 3.4 days earlier than infants in the control group ($p$ less than .05), and received 27 fewer tube feedings each ($p$ less than .05). The treated infants gained 2.5 grams more per day, but this difference was not significant. The treated infants were hospitalized four days less (*p* less than .025) from date of entry to discharge." When infants must receive tube feedings, it is helpful in most cases for the nurse to provide pacifiers. An exception would be if the rationale for tube feeding is respiratory compromise.

**Toddlers (1–3 years).**    The toddler can eat most table foods, but may have problems chewing tough meat or vegetables (see table 5.7). Iron, folate, and zinc may be lacking when meats and vegetables are refused (Howard). In many cases, milk intake decreases because of refusal to take milk from a cup during weaning, possibly resulting in vitamin A and calcium deficiencies.

Use a variety of foods to meet nutritional requirements of this age group. The Four Basic Food Groups can be used as a guide (see table 5.8). Suggested serving size for this age group is 1 tablespoon per year of age (Bonner).

Toddlers prefer plain foods (no sauces or mixtures). Independence-seeking behavior in the form of negativism, always eating the same foods, and variable appetite/food intake, though common in this period, may be frustrating to the pediatric nurse. Varying the color, shape, and texture of foods helps to maintain interest in eating. The toddler may be ritualistic and want foods special ways or in certain places on the plate.

---

**NURSING TIPS**
- **Place appropriate portions on a small plate since large trays sent from the kitchen may be overwhelming.**
- **Allow independence in eating; hands will be used more than utensils.**
- **Expect a mess and spills; don't scold child for this.**
- **Set limits with this age group.**
- **Don't offer choices when there is no choice; ask, "Which one?" rather than, "Do you want this?"**
- **Do not use force and do not use food as a bribe, punishment, or reward.**

---

**Preschoolers (4–6 years).**    This period is characterized by slow but steady growth with increased nutrient demands because of increased activity level. Continue to encourage milk intake for adequate calcium and vitamin A, and supplement the child's diet with iron as necessary (Bonner). Preschoolers will imitate adult behavior, avoiding foods they have seen adults avoid.

**School-age Children.**    More and more, the diet of school-age children is influenced by school, peers, and the outside world, and less by the family. Growth spurts and plateaus characterize this period. Appetite is generally good. Loose or missing teeth may present problems with nutrient intake.

**Table 5.8**   Age-Appropriate Diets Using the Four Basic Food Groups

| Food Group | Servings/ Day | Age Groups (Serving Size) | | | |
| --- | --- | --- | --- | --- | --- |
| | | Toddler | Preschooler | School-Age | Adolescent |
| *Milk* Whole milk, yogurt, cheese, ice cream, pudding | Child: 3 Adolescent: 4 | ½–¾ cup | ¾ cup | ¾–1 cup | 1 cup |
| *Meat* meats, poultry, fish, eggs, cheese, dried beans, peanut butter | 2 | 1 tbsp per year of age | 1 tbsp per year of age | 2 oz meat, fish, poultry 2 eggs 4 tbsp peanut butter | 2 oz meat, fish, poultry 2 eggs 4 tbsp peanut butter |
| *Fruit-Vegetable* juices, cooked, raw | 1 serving citrus fruit 3 or more others | 4 oz juice ½ whole fruit 1 tbsp per year of age cooked or raw | 4 oz juice ½ whole fruit 1 tbsp per year of age cooked or raw | 4 oz juice 1 whole fruit ½ cup cooked or raw | 4 oz juice 1 whole fruit ½ cup cooked or raw |
| *Grain* bread, cooked and ready-to-eat cereal, pasta, grits, rice | 4 | ½ slice bread ½ c cereal 1 tbsp per year of age others | ½ slice bread ½ c cereal 1 tbsp per year of age others | 1 slice bread ¾ c cereal ½ c others | 1 slice bread ¾ c cereal ½ c others |

Use the Four Basic Food Groups to guide nutrient intake with serving size as recommended for adults (Bonner) (see table 5.8). Nutritious snacks are important in this period.

## NURSING TIPS
- Involve the school-age child in own nutrition to spark interest.
- Allow the school-age child to fill out own menu, keep count of the calories, or help to prepare own snacks.
- Offer simple nutritional information and guidelines to promote understanding.
- Have children of similar ages eat together, since peers are important at this age.
- Allow children to eat in an unhurried manner

**Adolescents.**   The adolescent experiences dramatic body-image changes since growth and maturational changes are occurring rapidly. Diet and body image are closely related, and peer group frequently influences choice of food.

It is important to remember that diet is an adolescent's personal choice (Howard). Flexibility is the key to getting adolescents to eat.

Again, use a variety of foods to meet nutritional needs. The Four Basic Food Groups Guide can be used; portions will be adult-sized as recommended by the guide. Adolescent diets are frequently lacking calcium, iron, vitamin A, and vitamin C (Bonner).

---

## NURSING TIPS

- **Include favorite, popular foods in the diet if at all possible.**
- **Give guidelines for food selection and allow independence in deciding meals.**
- **Have heart-to-heart conversations about diet problems, rather than confrontations, to increase compliance. The nurse learns why the adolescent is not complying, and the adolescent learns why compliance is important.**
- **Serve foods that look pleasant.**
- **Substitute foods from home or take-out foods if the adolescent "can't stand hospital food."**
- **Allow the adolescent to eat with peers.**

---

## Special Diets

Ill infants and children may require dietary changes because of altered metabolism of nutrients. Consultation with the dietician and the diet manual should be undertaken before any diet modification. Include lists of foods permitted and not permitted on special diets in the nursing care plan and make the lists available for the child and family to consult. The information on the following special diets is adapted from Levine and Casolaro (1982):

**Sodium-Restricted Diet.**  Sodium-restricted diets are used for children with cardiac disease, though sodium may also be restricted in renal, hepatic, and oncologic diseases with complications. Sodium-restricted diets are ordered in "milligrams (or grams) allowed"; 250 mg, 500 mg ($\frac{1}{2}$ gm), and 1,000 mg (1 gm) sodium diets are very restricted, while 2,000 mg (2 gm), 3,000 mg (3 gm), and "no added salt" diets are more liberal. In general, foods are not cooked with salt, any foods preserved with salt are avoided (such as many meats and canned foods), and low sodium-unsalted substitutes are used. Refer to diet manuals or consult with the dietician for exact foods permitted and to be avoided. Low-sodium infant formulas are SMA and Similac PM 60/40.

**Protein-Restricted Diets.**  Protein-restricted diets are used for renal disease to prevent the accumulation of uremic wastes from protein breakdown, and for hepatic disease to reduce accumulation of ammonia, thus decreasing the severity of hepatic encephalopathy. Protein-restricted diets are also used in some inborn error of metabolism disorders. Electrolytes such as sodium and potassium may also be restricted with this diet. Protein-restricted diets are ordered "grams allowed" with 1–20 gm being severely restricted, and 40–60 gm moderately restricted. The allowed protein should be of high quality (eggs, meat, milk, fish, or poultry). High-calorie/low-protein supplements are sometimes used to increase calories. Low-protein substitute foods and elemental diets such as Amin-Aid (McGraw) or Hepatic Aid (McGraw) are sometimes required. Consult a dietician and diet manual for the specifics of this diet.

Nutramigen and Pregestimil are infant formulas with modified protein that may be used in protein-restricted diets. Mead Johnson makes several modified-protein formulas for specific metabolic problems (Lofenalac, MSUD Diet Powder, Product 3200 AB, Product 3200 K) and offers a protein-free formula base (Product 80056). See table 5.3.

**High-calorie/High-protein Diet.**    High-calorie/high-protein diets are used for pediatric patients with disorders such as cancer and cystic fibrosis, and for malnourishment in cases of failure-to-thrive or neurologically impaired children with decreased intake. As long as all metabolic systems are functioning, there are no restrictions on this diet. Food intake is increased as much as possible; three meals and three snacks per day are suggested. Calories and protein are added by increasing milk and cream content of foods (e.g., double-strength milk and cream soups), adding cheese to meats and eggs, using more fats (butter, gravies), and more peanut butter; giving child milkshakes made with eggs, ice cream, and milk-supplement foods. (Note: Children with cystic fibrosis may not tolerate increased fats; therefore, increase simple carbohydrates). Many infant formulas are being made with increased calories per ounce. Additives such as corn syrup, Polycose, and medium chain triglyceride (MCT) oil mixed with formula can increase the calorie value. Adding baby foods/cereals to the infant's diet will increase calories, but the infant's digestive tract must be mature enough to handle these foods.

**Diabetic Diet.**    The diabetic diet is a calorie-controlled diet necessitating specific amounts of carbohydrate, protein, and fat. Exchange lists for meats, vegetables, fruits, breads, milk, and fats are used to plan three meals and two snacks (midafternoon and evening) per day. The goal is to distribute calories throughout the day to avoid hyperglycemic peaks and hypoglycemic episodes. Juvenile diabetics should be taught to incorporate some of their favorite foods into the exchange lists to increase compliance. Sugar-free substitutes may be used. The patient and family will require thorough diet teaching, which can be carried out by the nurse and dietician in consultation.

**Lactose Intolerance Diet.**    Lactase deficiency causes intolerance of the sugar lactose that is found in milk and dairy products. These products are avoided, as well as products made or processed with milk, lactose, or glutamate. (Note: read product labels carefully.) The following infant formulas can be used: Prosobee, Isomil, Nursoy, Soyalac, Pregestimil, Portagen, and Nutramigen. Ensure, Citrotein, and Precision are supplemental feedings that may be used. LactAid, an enzyme product, may be added to milk to break down lactose. Refer to a diet manual for specifics.

**Ketogenic Diet.**    Ketogenic diets have been used in young children (less than 5 years old) in the control of seizures. The diet is low in carbohydrate and high in fat. It must be initiated in the hospital. The goal is ketosis, which affects the nervous system, thus decreasing seizure activity.

## Alternative Feeding Methods

**Tube Feedings.**    Tube, or enteral, feedings are indicated when food or adequate nutrients cannot be taken by mouth but the GI system function remains intact (see table 5.9).

**Table 5.9**    Indications for Tube Feedings

| Type of Patient | Examples |
| --- | --- |
| Physically impaired | Dental problems<br>Facial fractures<br>Head and neck surgery<br>Burns<br>Upper GI surgery |
| Neurologically impaired | Head injury<br>Paralysis<br>Loss of consciousness |
| Mentally disturbed | Depression<br>Anorexia nervosa |
| Weak | Premature<br>(Harvey, 1981) |
| Other indications | Chemotherapy<br>Radiation therapy<br>Hypermetabolic states<br>Malabsorption<br>(Konstantinides, 1983) |

Oro- and nasogastric (OG, NG) routes are used for short term feedings. The advantages of feeding directly into the stomach are that this organ has a) a large reservoir capacity and b) a high tolerance for variations in osmolality (Konstantinides, 1983). Aspiration is a risk with OG and NG feedings.

The nasal-jejunal (NJ) route (feeding beyond the pyloric sphincter), gastrostomy, and jejunostomy routes are more often used for long-term feeding. The risk of aspiration is reduced, though volume and osmolality of feedings become problems.

**Types of Tubes.**    Polyvinylchloride and newer polyurethane and silicone tubes (5–10 Fr) can be used for OG and NG feedings. The newer, softer, longer, weighted polyurethane and silicone feeding tubes are being used for NJ and jejunostomy feedings. Large bore rubber tubes are used for gastrostomy feedings. Size and type of tube depend on the child's age, as well as the route, type, volume, and purpose of the feedings. In general, use the smallest bore tube possible.

### *Procedure for NG/NJ Tube Placement*

1.  Use clean procedure.
2.  Obtain equipment: proper feeding tube (check bore size and length), tape, emesis basin, appropriate size syringe, stethoscope, pH test paper, water for older child to sip. (Benzoin should not be used unless tape has not stuck well before.)
3.  Position child at a 45 angle or on right side.
4.  Explain procedure to child if age appropriate.
5.  Tear tape and place it where it can be easily reached.
6.  Remove guide wire if it is needed to insert a soft tube, lubricate it and reinsert it into the tube.
7.  Measure length of tube
    *   NG: tip of nose to earlobe to just below the sternum at the stomach
    *   NJ: NG measurement plus 4–6 inches
8.  Mark measurement with pen or tape.
9.  Have an assistant restrain the child's hands if necessary.
10. Lubricate the tip with water-soluble jelly.
11. Insert the tip in a nostril, push gently up and back to pass the nasal ridge and continue pushing until desired length is inserted.
12. Tell the child to swallow while the tube is passing (sips of water may be given if not contraindicated).
13. Remove the tube at once if there is any respiratory difficulty. Resistance, gagging, and vomiting may occur.
14. Temporarily tape the tube in position.
15. Check the back of the throat for kinking or curling of the tube.
16. Withdraw the guide wire if present and attach syringe.
17. Inject 2 cc (small infants) to 5 cc (large infants and children) air while listening with stethoscope over
    *   right upper quadrant (stomach area) for NG placement
    *   right lower quadrant for NJ placement.
18. Aspirate contents; observe and test
    *   gastric: semi-digested food or formula
        - greenish color
        - pH: below 6
    *   jejunal: golden yellow color
        - pH: 6 or above
        If no aspirate is obtained from the NJ tube, leave it open to air and check again in ½ hour.
19. Always replace aspirate because not replacing contents consistently can lead to fluid and electrolyte imbalances similar to those occurring with persistent vomiting.
20. Tape the tube securely to patient's nose. DO NOT tape tube UP against nares. It may erode skin, causing permanent disfigurement.
21. Use x-rays to confirm placement (if necessary).

**22.** Place the child on the right side with the head of the bed elevated and allow gravity and peristalsis to assist movement of the tube if NJ tube has not passed the pylorus and is not kinked behind the throat.

**23.** Softer tubes may collapse when contents are aspirated. If this happens, inject 5 cc sterile water and aspirate it immediately to open the tube.

**24.** Allow the child time to calm down before starting feedings.

### Tube Maintenance

- Nasogastric tubes
  - Change hard plastic tubes every 3–5 days. Use alternate nostrils.
  - Soft tubes may remain in place for long periods. They may be removed, rinsed, inspected, and reinserted periodically (use the guidewire).
  - Alternate positions of tape on the skin.
  - Rinse tube with sterile water or saline after intermittent feedings and medications.
  - Tape all connections to tubing or syringes securely.
- Gastrostomy tubes
  - A cut-off nipple can be used around the tube to support it or a gauze bolster may be taped under the tube.
  - Clean the skin around the tube and the nipple daily with peroxide or Betadine (check hospital procedure).
  - Change tapes daily and as necessary; alternate position on the skin.
  - Use gauze dressings or stomahesive around the tube if the child's skin breaks down.

**Methods of Tube Feeding Administration.**    Intermittent bolus (gravity-drip) feedings deliver relatively large volumes of food over periods of a few minutes to an hour, several times a day.

### Procedure for Bolus Feedings

**1.** Use clean technique.

**2.** Obtain and measure correct formula, placing it in a sterile container. (Note: mixed formulas should be made freshly every 24 hours, labeled with date and time of reconstitution, and refrigerated.)

**3.** Warm the formula if it has been refrigerated.

**4.** Check tube placement by injecting air and listening over the appropriate site.

**5.** Aspirate and note the type and amount of residual contents. *Always* replace aspirated contents. It is a good idea to collaborate with the physician to determine a schedule of how much formula to give with residuals and when to hold feedings.

**6.** Position child upright at a 45° angle, on the side, or prone.

**7.** Explain the feeding to the child if old enough to understand.

**8.** Add room temperature formula to feeding administration set, attach to feeding tube (or, with syringe attachment, pinch tube while adding feeding to syringe), start the flow, and observe the rate.

9. Suspend the entire apparatus. Control the speed of administration by changing the drip rate of the administration set, or by adjusting the height of the syringe (no more than 12–18 inches above the stomach).
10. Never force a bolus feeding.
11. Check the tubing for kinks and clogs if the feeding does not flow.
12. Stay with the child during the entire feeding, observing for gagging and vomiting.
13. Have suction equipment nearby to clear airways if vomiting occurs.
14. Flush tubing with 10–15 cc $H_2O$ after feeding if appropriate. (Children with fluid restrictions may not tolerate this.)
15. The syringe may or may not be removed after the feeding. (Allowing excess formula to reflux back into the suspended syringe may be more desirable than allowing the infant to vomit excess feeding.)
16. Remove administration set after the feeding; clamp the feeding tube.
17. Rinse and reuse or discard the administration set.

Continuous infusion pumps are used to administer small volumes of food to children over extended periods (16–24 hours). This method *must* be used for jejunal feedings.

### Procedure for Continuous Infusion Feedings
- Connect the administration set to infusion pump tubing and attach to a pump.
- Use different types of pumps for feedings and IV fluids to avoid confusion and *clearly label* which are feeding tubes and which are IV tubes.
- Label feeding sets and tubes with the type of formula infusing and set rate (volume/hour) on the pump.
- Check the pump and reservoir hourly for progress.
- Rinse feeding set and tubing every 4 hours (adding fresh formula at this time); change set and tubing every 24 hours to prevent build-up and clogging and to discourage bacterial growth along the line.
- Always use clean technique when handling feeding equipment.

### Beginning and Advancing Feedings
- Start slowly with a low volume and strength. Never advance both at the same time.
- Start with ½ strength, advance to ¾ and to full strength as tolerated.
- Determine a schedule for advancing feeding volume and strength for the nursing care plan.

**Tube Feeding Formulas.**   Consider these factors when choosing a tube feeding formula:
- nutritional completeness
- content and type of carbohydrate, protein, and fat
- viscosity
- osmolality
- specific needs of the patient

*Categories of Tube Feeding Formulas*   (Konstantinides)
  *Blenderized*
  • nutritionally complete, commercially prepared table food
  *Milk-based*
  • nutritionally complete, containing nutrients found in milk
  *Lactose-free*
  • nutritionally complete, made with soy protein
  *Chemically-defined*
  • nutritionally incomplete, containing nutrients in simple, predigested forms
  *Specialty Formulas*
  • usually nutritionally incomplete, designed for patients with specific organ failures
  *Modules*
  • nutritionally incomplete, additives of single or several nutrients
  Table 5.10 lists commonly used tube feeding formulas and their composition.

**Total Parenteral Nutrition.**   Total parenteral nutrition (TPN) is indicated when GI function is inadequate and nutrient needs cannot be met via the enteral route. Harvey (1981) lists four groups of patients for whom TPN is indicated. Those

  • who are malnourished and need nutritional replacement before surgery
  • with prolonged postoperative complications
  • with inflammatory bowel disease when bowel rest is needed
  • with inadequate oral intake

TPN can be administered by peripheral or central routes. Because high concentrations of glucose irritate peripheral veins, dextrose concentrations greater than 12.5% should be administered via central line. Broviac or Hickman catheters are used for central lines. The catheter passes from an external site (head, neck, or chest in children) through a jugular vein into the subclavian vein or superior vena cava (Whaley & Wong, 1983). The central line is always sutured in place and covered with a sterile, occlusive dressing. TPN solutions are always administered by a pump (such as IMED) to maintain a constant rate of flow. TPN lines should not be used for anything other than TPN solutions; a second IV line or use of a multiple-bore catheter is recommended for medications, blood drawing, and blood administration.

Monitor sugar and acetone in the urine to follow tolerance of TPN. Monitor the child's temperature immediately after new bottles of solution are hung. Temperature spikes indicate possible solution contamination. If this occurs, discontinue the infusion and replace with fresh solution and IV tubing. Culture the solution and notify the MD of the fever.

To provide all nutrients, two separate solutions are used: hyperalimentation (HAL) solution and intralipid (IL).

**Table 5.10** Commonly Used Tube Feeding Formulas

| Product (Manufacturer) | Classification | Indications for Use | Osmolality | Nutrition Source | Cal/Oz | Gm/100 ml Pro/CHO/Fat | | | Normal Dilution |
|---|---|---|---|---|---|---|---|---|---|
| Portagen (Mead Johnson) | Milk-based | For patients who do not efficiently digest conventional food fats or lactose | 236 354 | CHO—corn syrup solids, sucrose PRO—sodium caseinate FAT—MCT, corn oil | 20 | 2.4 | 7.8 | 3.2 | Powder 1.6 |
| Sustacal (Mead Johnson) | Lactose-free | Lactose intolerance, anorexia, malnutrition, requiring caloric supplementation and/or high-protein diet | 625 | CHO—sucrose, corn syrup PRO—calcium caseinate, soy protein isolate, sodium caseinate FAT—partially dehydrogenated soy oil | 30 30 | 3.5 6.1 | 11.5 14 | 4.8 2.3 | 8 oz to 29 oz $H_2O$ Ready-to-feed, powder |
| Sustacal HC (Mead Johnson) | Lactose-free, high calorie | For hypermetabolic, fluid restricted, and volume-sensitive patients | 650 | CHO—corn syrup solids, sucrose PRO—calcium and sodium caseinate FAT—partially hydrogenated soy oil | 45 | 6.1 | 19 | 5.8 | Ready-to-feed |
| Ensure Plus (Ross) | Lactose-free, high calorie | For patients with increased nutrient needs, volume restricted | 600 | CHO—hydrolyzed corn starch, sucrose PRO—sodium and calcium caseinate, soy protein isolate FAT—soy oil | 45 | 5.5 | 20 | 5.3 | Ready-to-feed |

| | | | | | | | | | |
|---|---|---|---|---|---|---|---|---|---|
| Ensure (Ross) | Lactose-free | For patients requiring nutrition in liquid form | 450 | CHO—hydrolyzed corn starch, sucrose PRO—sodium and calcium caseinate, soy protein isolate FAT—corn oil | 30 | 3.7 | 14 | 3.7 | Ready-to-feed |
| Osmolite (Ross) | Chemically defined | For patients sensitive to hyperosmotic tube feedings | 300 | CHO—hydrolyzed corn starch PRO—sodium and calcium caseinate, soy protein isolate FAT—MCT, corn oil, soy oil | 30 | 3.7 | 14 | 3.8 | Ready-to-feed |
| Compleat-B (Doyle) | Blenderized | Meat-based | 390 | Contains beef puree, cereal solids, vegetable puree, nonfat dry milk, corn oil, maltodextrin, fruit puree | 30 | 4.0 | 12 | 4.0 | Ready-to-feed |
| Isocal (Mead Johnson) | Lactose-free | For patients unable to tolerate oral feedings | 300 | CHO—maltodextrin PRO—calcium and sodium caseinate, soy protein isolate FAT—soy oil, MCT | 30 | 3.4 | 13 | 4.4 | Ready-to-feed |
| Isocal HCN (Mead Johnson) | lactose-free, high calorie, nitrogen | For patients requiring increased calories and limited fluids | 740 | CHO—corn syrup PRO—calcium and sodium caseinate FAT—soybean oil, MCT | 60 | 7.5 | 23 | 9.1 | Ready-to-feed |

**Table 5.10** Commonly Used Tube Feeding Formulas (continued)

| Product (Manufacturer) | Classification | Indications for Use | Osmolality | Nutrition Source | Cal/Oz | Gm/100 ml Pro | CHO | Fat | Normal Dilution |
|---|---|---|---|---|---|---|---|---|---|
| Travasorb HN (Travenol) | | For debilitated patients | 400–450 | CHO—glucose oligosaccharides PRO—hydrolyzed lactalbumin FAT—MCT, sunflower oil | 30 | 4.5 | 18 | 1.3 | Powder: 1 packet (2.94 oz) to 285 ml $H_2O$ |
| Travasorb MCT (Travenol) | | For patients with limited digestion and absorption, low fat tolerance | 250 at 1 cal/ml 475 at 2 cal/ml | CHO—corn syrup solids PRO—lactalbumin, potassium caseinate FAT—MCT, sunflower oil | 30 60 | 4.9 9.8 | 12 24 | 3.3 6.6 | Powder |
| Criticare HN (Mead Johnson) | Chemically-defined | For patients with impaired digestion and absorption | 650 | CHO—Maltodextrin, modified corn starch PRO—hydrolyzed casein, amino acids FAT—safflower oil | 30 | 3.8 | 22 | 0.3 | Ready-to-feed |
| Vivonex (Eaton) | Chemically-defined | For patients with impaired digestion and absorption | 500 | CHO—glucose oligosaccharides PRO—amino acids FAT—safflower oil | 30 | 2.2 | 23 | 0.1 | Powder: 1 packet (80 gm) to 300 ml $H_2O$ |
| Precision Isotonic (Doyle) | Lactose-free | For patients with intolerance to normal foods, lactose intolerance | 300 | CHO—glucose oligosaccharides, sucrose PRO—egg albumin FAT—vegetable oil | 30 | 2.9 | 15 | 3.0 | 5,814 gm powder to 1,440 ml $H_2O$ |

*HAL*

- Provides glucose and amino acids.
- Glucose and amino acid content are determined from child's needs—vitamins, minerals, and trace elements are added.
- Must be filtered to remove particulate matter and microorganisms.
- Run at a constant rate because of high glucose concentration; do not try to "catch up" by increasing the rate or suddenly stop the infusion.
- Glucose concentration and rate of administration should be gradually increased when HAL is first started, and gradually decreased when HAL is no longer needed.

*IL*

- Provides fats.
- Contains soybean oil, egg yolk phosphatide, and glycerol (Levine & Casolaro, 1982).
- Not filtered since it provides fat particles the size normally found in circulation.
- Hypersensitivity reactions to IL can occur; give a test dose of 1 ml over 15–30 minutes before starting the infusion.
- The IL solution is piggybacked into the HAL line at the Y-connection closest to the child.

## GENERIC CARE PLAN FOR THE NURSING DIAGNOSIS
# ALTERATION IN NUTRITION: LESS THAN BODY REQUIREMENTS

## 1. General Information

### a. Etiology
- Metabolic deficiencies: JDM, hypoglycemia, PKU, CHO metabolic disorders, cystic fibrosis
- Congenital defects of GI tract: cleft lip/cleft palate, GE reflux, TE fistulas/atresia, biliary atresia
- Inadequate intake: child neglect, failure to thrive, lack of parental knowledge of appropriate diet, dyspnea, respiratory insufficiency
- Increased metabolic needs: prematurity, burns, infections
- Anorexia: loss of appetite, anorexia nervosa
- Congenital anomalies: muscle wasting syndrome, mental retardation, heart disease, renal disease
- Diarrhea, chronic or infectious

### b. Clinical Manifestations
- Body weight 20% (or more) less than height percentage on standard growth grids

  - Loss of weight with appropriate food intake
  - Poor muscle tone
  - Lack of energy
  - Hyperactive bowel sounds
  - Lack of interest in food

c. **Multidisciplinary Approaches**
  - Replacement of deficient hormone or enzyme
  - Surgical repair of GI defect
  - High-calorie, high-protein diet
  - Administration of vitamins and/or minerals
  - Psychologic counseling, behavior modification

## 2. Nursing Process

a. **Assessment**
  - Weight (at the 5th percentile or lower on the appropriate pediatric growth grid, maintenance or loss of weight as height increases)
  - Food intake (inadequate)
  - Muscle weakness
  - Energy (apathy)
  - Mood (irritability, crying)
  - Sucking reflex (poor)
  - Bowel elimination (diarrhea, hyperactive bowel sounds)
  - Colic
  - Skin (breakdown)
  - Serum albumin (decreased)
  - Lymphocyte count (decreased)
  - Heart rate (tachycardia)
  - Respiration (dyspnea/tachypnea)
  - Causative factors for nutritional deficit
  - Sucking reflex and number of teeth of infants
  - Food intolerances

b. **Goal**
Child will ingest needed nutrients for maintenance and growth while conforming to the necessary dietary restrictions.

c. **Interventions**
  • Estimate the child's daily caloric requirement for maintenance and growth.
  • Give small frequent feedings.
  • Offer solid foods (if appropriate) before formula or milk.
  • Record and describe food intake and bowel movements.
  • Weigh child daily.
  • Encourage adequate rest.
  • Promote relaxing nonstressful mealtimes.

- Evaluate caretaker's financial status and ability to prepare prescribed formula or diet.
- Teach the caretakers (and child as appropriate) the principles of good nutrition within the framework of the child's health problem.

**d. Evaluation**
- Child's
  - daily intake of food/formula contains essential calories and nutrients.
  - skin turgor is adequate.
- Toddlers and older children eat adequate amounts of milk, meat, fruits, vegetables, breads, and cereals.

**e. Possible Related Nursing Diagnoses**
Activity intolerance
Alteration in bowel elimination
Fluid volume deficit
Impairment of skin integrity
Knowledge deficit

# Selected Health Problems Frequently Associated with the Nursing Diagnosis ALTERATION IN NUTRITION: LESS THAN BODY REQUIREMENTS

## 1. Cystic Fibrosis

**a. Definition:** An autosomal disorder of the exocrine glands affecting multiple organ systems, particularly the GI and respiratory systems.

**b. Multidisciplinary Approaches**
- Diagnostic studies
  - pilocarpine iontophoresis (sweat test): the cholinergic drug pilocarpine is introduced into the skin by electrodes to stimulate the production of sweat. The sweat is collected and measured for chloride content. If sweat chloride values are more than 60 mEq/liter, the test is positive. If values are 40–60 mEq/liter, results are questionable and the test is repeated. Values below 40 mEq/liter are normal.
  - measurement of duodenal enzyme activity: trypsin and chymotrypsin content of the stools is analyzed
  - fat absorption: measured by calculating the fat content of a 5-day stool collection and comparing it with the child's fat intake

- Diet therapy
  - high-calorie, high-protein diet
  - twice the RDA of fat-soluble vitamins A, D, and E
  - administration of vitamin K if hypoprothrombinemia is present
  - supplementary iron
  - pancreatic enzyme replacement with all meals and snacks

## Additional Nursing Care That Can Be Incorporated into the Generic Care Plan

a. **Assessment**
   - I&O (dehydration)
   - 24-hour dietary recall; does patient have poor tolerance of fat?
   - stools (steatorrhea—excessively fatty, foul-smelling bulky stool; may appear frothy)
   - GI system (rectal prolapse, rectal polyps, abdominal obstruction, distention, vomiting, meconium ileus in newborns)

b. **Goals**
   Parents will verbalize symptoms of dehydration and sodium depletion, emphasizing special instances such as fever, increased exertion, hot weather.
   Parents/child will
   - titrate enzymes appropriately prior to discharge.
   - list foods in which enzymes may be mixed with minimal immediate chemical reactions.
   - select a sample menu that contains foods high in protein and calories, low in fat.
   - develop a reasonable schedule for administration of vitamins and minerals.

c. **Interventions**
   - Teach parents to titrate pancreatic enzymes according to appearance of stool and child's status.
   - Give more enzymes if stools are frothy, loose, or steatorrheic; give fewer enzymes if child becomes constipated.
   - Place enzymes in food that won't be easily digested (e.g., applesauce), not in foods high in starch, such as tapioca or mashed potatoes, since they are easily digested by the enzymes.
   - Administer enzymes during the middle of the meal. Provide small, frequent meals high in carbohydrates and protein, and having the desired amount of added salt.
   - Monitor laboratory values; report significant deviations to MD.
   - Maintain I&O.
   - Administer enzymes during the middle of the meal.

**d.  Evaluation**
  - Parents/child
    - identify variations in the character of stools based on enzyme administration.
    - select appropriate foods, such as applesauce or strained fruits as a medium for administration of enzymes.
    - select foods for minimal fat content (yet allowing enough dietary fat to provide essential fatty acids for myelination in young children).
  - Child takes vitamins and minerals with food (if appropriate).
  - Parents describe salt supplementation strategies.

## Other Possible Nursing Diagnoses

Alteration in bowel elimination
Alteration in family process
Ineffective airway clearance

## 2.  Gastroesophageal Reflux (GER)

**a.  Definition/Discussion**
  - Persistent and debilitating GER is the frequent return of stomach contents into the distal esophagus.
  - All infants, to some extent, have regurgitation and reflux. It is often accompanied by apnea, and in severe, sometimes insidious cases, aspiration. Etiologies can be chronic pulmonary disease, esophagitis, peptic ulceration, esophageal stricture, rumination, organic failure to thrive, and sudden infant death syndrome.

**b.  Multidisciplinary Approaches**
  - Surgical intervention such as a Nissen fundoplication is indicated occasionally

## Additional Nursing Care That Can Be Incorporated into the Generic Care Plan

**a.  Assessment**
  - Return of large amounts of formula; frequency
  - Weight gain

**b.  Goal**
Infant will retain feedings and maintain weight.

**c.  Interventions**
  - Observe chalasia (reflux) precautions (will often be effective)

- feed infant in a prone position with 30° head elevation (use pillow for significant GER); normal feeding positions are satisfactory for less problematic infants
- place infant on abdomen with head of crib elevated to 30°; do not place infants in pyloric chairs (infant seats) after feedings, since they tend to slide down, bend at the waist, and thereby force gastric contents upward
- give small, frequent feedings thickened with commercial thickening agents (Nestargel or Carobel) or 2 tablespoons rice cereal per 120 cc liquid (amount recommendations may vary per MD)
- bubble and burp over shoulder (upright position)
- Use cardiorespiratory monitoring when indicated.
- Teach parents strict chalasia precautions.
- Teach parents first aid (airway clearance) measures.
- Teach parents to place crib mattress at home on an inclined plane (plywood or pegboard generally work nicely).

  d. **Evaluation**
  - Child
    - ingests formula with regurgitation of less than 10 cc
    - gains weight at an appropriate level for age.

## Other Possible Nursing Diagnoses

Fluid volume deficit
Impairment of skin integrity
Parental anxiety
Parental knowledge deficit

# 3. Juvenile Diabetes Mellitus (JDM), Type I

  a. **Definition:** A metabolic disease in which carbohydrate utilization is reduced and that of lipid and protein enhanced. Nutritional deficit is caused by a deficiency of insulin.

  b. **Multidisciplinary Approaches**
  - Medical therapy: administration of insulin; see table 5.11

**Table 5.11**   Insulin Chart

| Product Name (Manufacturer) | Concentrations Available | Species Source | Action (In Hours) | | |
|---|---|---|---|---|---|
| | | | Onset | Peak | Duration |
| Actrapid Regular (Squibb-Novo)* | U-100 | Pork | .5 | 2.5–5 | 6–8 |
| Regular (Squibb-Novo)* | U-40 or U-100 | Pork | .5 | 2.5–5 | 6–8 |
| Regular-Iletin I (Lilly)* | U-40 or U-100 | Beef/pork mixture | .5 | 2–4 | 6–8 |

**Table 5.11**    Insulin Chart (continued)

| Product Name (Manufacturer) | Concentrations Available | Species Source | Action (In Hours) | | |
|---|---|---|---|---|---|
| | | | Onset | Peak | Duration |
| Regular-Iletin II | U-100 | Beef or pork | .5 | 2–4 | 6–8 |
| Velosulin Regular (Nordisk)* | U-100 | Pork | .5 | 2–4 | 6–8 |
| Humulin R (Lilly)* | U-100 | Human Recombinant DNA | .5 | 2–4 | 6–8 |
| Novolin R (Squibb-Novo)* | U-100 | Human Semi-synthetic | .5 | 2.5–5 | 6–8 |
| Semilente Iletin I (Lilly) | U-40 or U-100 | Beef/pork mixture | 1–2 | 3–8 | 10–16 |
| Semilente (Squibb-Novo) | U-100 | Beef | .5–2 | 5–10 | 12–16 |
| Semitarde (Squibb-Novo) | U-100 | Pork | .5–2 | 5–10 | 12–16 |
| Insultard NPH (Nordisk) | U-100 | Pork | 1–4 | 6–12 | 16–28 |
| Lentard (Squibb-Novo) | U-100 | Beef/pork mixture | 1–7 | 7–15 | 15–24 |
| Lente Iletin I (Lilly) | U-40 or U-100 | Beef/pork mixture | 1–3 | 6–12 | 18–26 |
| Lente Iletin II (Lilly) | U-100 | Beef or pork | 1–3 | 6–12 | 18–26 |
| Lente (Squibb-Novo) | U-40 or U-100 | Beef | 1–4 | 7–15 | 18–24 |
| Monotard (Squibb-Novo) | U-100 | Pork | 1–5 | 7–15 | 15–22 |
| NPH Iletin I (Lilly) | U-40 or U-100 | Beef/pork mixture | 1–2 | 6–12 | 18–26 |
| NPH Iletin II (Lilly) | U-100 | Beef or pork | 1–2 | 6–12 | 18–26 |
| NPH Isophane (Squibb-Novo) | U-40 or U-100 | Beef | 1–2 | 4–12 | 16–23 |
| Protophane NPH (Squibb-Novo) | U-100 | Pork | 1–3 | 4–12 | 14–23 |
| Mixtard (Nordisk) | U-100 | Pork | .5–4 | Variable | 16–28 |
| Humulin N (Lilly) | U-100 | Human Recombinant DNA | 1–2 | 6–12 | 18–24 |
| Novolin N (Squibb-Novo) | U-100 | Human Semi-synthetic | 1–5 | 7–15 | 16–22 |
| Protamine Zinc Iletin I (Lilly) | U-40 or U–100 | Beef/pork mixture | 4–6 | 14–24 | 26–36 |
| Protamine Zinc Iletin II (Lilly) | U-100 | Beef or pork | 4–6 | 14–24 | 26–36 |
| Ultralente (Squibb-Novo) | U-100 | Beef | 3–7 | 10–30 | 30–36 |
| Ultralente Iletine I (Lilly) | U-40 or U-100 | Beef/pork mixture | 4–6 | 14–24 | 28–36 |
| Ultratard (Squibb-Novo) | U-100 | Beef | 3–9 | 10–30 | 30–36 |

- Dietary therapy: American Dietetic Association (ADA) calorie, carbohydrate, protein, and fat-controlled diet; see diabetic diet, page 138
- Diabetes clinical nurse specialist

## Additional Nursing Care That Can Be Incorporated into the Generic Nursing Care Plan

a. **Assessment**
   - Polydipsia, polyphagia, polyuria, and/or eneuresis
     • weight loss
     • signs of impending diabetic ketoacidosis (see page 158.)
     • monitor for signs of hypoglycemia (e.g., irritability, tremors, headache, and blurred vision)
   - Time since diagnosis of JDM
   - Experience with and/or knowledge of diabetes
   - Manual skills

b. **Goal**
   Child will ingest prescribed diet.
   Family and affected member will
   - achieve an acceptable level of glycemic control.
   - maintain the child's growth and development within normal limits.
   - integrate the treatment regimen into life-style.
   - develop a plan for reviewing and updating information regularly.

c. **Interventions**
   • Use exchange lists for meats, vegetables, fruits, breads, milk, and fats to plan three meals and two snacks (mid-afternoon and evening) per day.
   • Distribute calories throughout the day to avoid hyperglycemic peaks and hypoglycemic episodes.
   • Teach juvenile diabetics to incorporate some of their favorite foods into the exchange lists to increase compliance.
   • Use sugar-free substitutes.
   • Teach parents/child as soon as feasible after diagnosis is made. Include
     - general information about diabetes mellitus
       * simplified explanation of pathophysiology
       * three-pronged approach to management: insulin, diet, exercise
       * concept of chronicity: controllable, not curable
     - glucose testing
       * blood glucose monitoring—why? how? when?
       * recording and reporting results
       * urine testing for ketones—how? when?
       * reporting results

- insulin (see table 5.11)
  * what kind(s)
  * how to administer
  * when to give
  * what it does
  * action—onset, peak and duration
  * site rotation plan (see medication chapter for chart on various insulins)
- hypoglycemia
  * signs and symptoms
  * treatment
  * prevention
- hyperglycemia and ketonuria
  * signs and symptoms
  * appropriate management
  * etiologies
- 3–4 weeks after initial diagnosis and teaching, instruct on
  - nature of diabetes
    * pathophysiology
    * etiology
    * effects of growth spurts, illness, and stress
    * need for identification, i.e., Medic Alert tag
  - insulin
    * review injection techniques, site rotation, etc.
    * needs and actions
    * adjustment schedules or "sliding scales" (if used)
  - diet
    * normal nutrition and review of exchange lists
    * incorporation of cultural preferences and life-style effects
    * adjustments for growth changes
    * adjustments for exercise
    * guidelines for illness
    * eating away from home
  - monitoring and record keeping
    * review monitoring techniques
    * when to do tests
    * when to get assistance from health care providers
    * what other information to record
      † exercise and activity
      † feelings
      † responses to problems
  - review hypo- and hyperglycemia
  - exercise
    * effect on blood sugar
    * importance of regular exercise
    * how to adjust diet and insulin when exercise changes
  - hygiene
    * treatment of cuts and scratches

  * importance of regular eye and dental examinations
  * correct nail trimming
  * avoidance of injury to extremities
 — complications
  * research regarding prevention of long-term complications
  * discussion of effects of diabetes on future plans
   † sexuality and dating
   † marriage and childbearing
   † career
 — self-management and problem solving
 — continuing education
  * review of previously learned skills and knowledge
  * update on new information, techniques, and research (American Diabetes Association, 1983; Etzwiler, 1983; Whaley & Wong)

**d.   Evaluation**
 • Child has no hyperglycemic peaks or hypoglycemic episodes.
 • Child's
  — urine sugar and acetone readings are within normal limits.
  — blood glucose levels are within normal limits.
 • Child/parents
  — consistently perform basic survival skills (e.g., insulin injection, glucose monitoring, diet selection).
  — describe in their own words what diabetes is and the management approach used.
  — state type, amount, and peak action times of insulin being used.
  — state signs, treatment and prevention of hypoglycemia.
  — state signs and appropriate responses to hyperglycemia.
  — accurately explain what diabetes is and applicable components of its management.
  — apply the knowledge to hypothetical situations that may arise in the child's experiences.
  — seek appropriate assistance from health care team.
  — recognize the need for continuing education and follow-up.

# Other Possible Nursing Diagnoses

Activity intolerance
Alteration in family process
Fluid volume deficit
Impairment of skin integrity
Knowledge deficit
Noncompliance
Sensory-perceptual alteration
Social isolation

## 4.  Hypoglycemia

a.  **Definition:** The presence of a lower than normal concentration or level of glucose in the blood; most cases are preventable. Occurs relatively quickly in known diabetics, generally as a result of decreased caloric intake, increased exercise, overdosage of insulin, or gastroenteritis.

b.  **Multidisciplinary Approaches**
   – Administration of IV dextrose is necessary to prevent permanent brain damage
   – IM or SQ glucagon

## Additional Nursing Care That Can Be Incorporated into the Generic Nursing Care Plan

a.  **Assessment**
   – *Mild reaction*: hunger, tachycardia, increased respiratory rate, and weakness, followed by lethargy, irritability, and confusion
   – *Moderate reaction*: diaphoresis, tremors, nervousness, headache, abdominal pain, vomiting, dizziness, and blurred vision
   – *Severe reaction*: seizures and coma

b.  **Goal**
   Child's blood sugar will remain within normal limits.

c.  **Interventions**
   • For mild reactions give food that increases the glucose level (e.g., sugar, honey, orange juice, milk).
   • For moderate reactions give a simple concentrated sugar.
   • Teach patients and their parents the early signs and symptoms.

d.  **Evaluation**
   • Child has
      – no adverse reactions, e.g., periods of being hungry, tachycardic, weak, lethargic, irritable, confused, nervous.
      – no episodes of tremors, headache, abdominal pain, vomiting, and dizziness.
   • Child and/or parents recognize early signs and symptoms of hypoglycemia.

## Other Possible Nursing Diagnoses

Activity intolerance
Alteration in comfort: pain
Potential for injury
Sensory-perceptual alterations

## 5.  Diabetic Ketoacidosis

**a.  Definition:** A possible complication of diabetes mellitus in which there is a low pH and reduced bicarbonate concentration in the blood due to a build-up of ketone bodies; a presenting condition in children not previously diagnosed as diabetic. Infection, trauma, or noncompliance with diabetic regimen can trigger an episode.

**b.  Multidisciplinary Approaches**
- IV fluids (fluid losses may reach 10% of body weight)
- Insulin either bolus (half IV, half SC) or continuous infusion; adjusted according to blood sugar
- Potassium (when urine output established); adjusted according to blood levels and EKG changes
- Bicarbonate (if necessary) to correct acidosis
- NG tube, Foley catheter (if necessary)
- 5% dextrose infusion when blood sugar is about 300 mg%, if acidosis has not been corrected

## Additional Nursing Care That Can Be Incorporated into the Generic Nursing Care Plan

**a.  Assessment**
- Polydipsia, polyuria, dehydration
- Abdominal pain, nausea, vomiting, and drowsiness
- Kussmaul respirations, fruity odor on breath, stupor, and eventually coma (develop if no treatment given)

**b.  Goal**
Child's blood glucose will remain within normal limits.

**c.  Interventions**
- Record changing lab values and report significant deviations.
- Monitor IV infusion rates and adjust rates as ordered to maintain blood suguar within normal limits.
- Monitor cardiac rhythm, serum potassium levels; regulate IV potassium as ordered.

**d.  Evaluation**
- Child's
    - blood sugar is within normal limits.
    - serum potassium level and EKG tracing are within normal limits.
- Child
    - has no nausea, vomiting, or abdominal pain.
    - is alert and oriented.

## Other Possible Nursing Diagnoses

Alteration in cardiac output
Fluid volume deficit
Ineffective breathing pattern
Potential for injury
Sensory-perceptual alteration

## 6.  Phenylketonuria (PKU)

a.  **Definition:** A nutritional deficit caused by an inborn error of phenylalanine metabolism. Lack of the enzyme that converts phenylalanine to tyrosine leads to high levels of phenylalanine in blood, urine, and spinal fluid. The untreated disease causes mental retardation.

b.  **Multidisciplinary Approaches**
   – Serum phenylalanine level (Guthrie test) done after infant has been on breast milk/formula for at least 3 days
   – Dietary therapy
      • low phenylalanine diet
      • low-protein diet; restrict meat, fish, poultry, dairy products, nuts, some breads and cereals
      • may have fruit, vegetables, some breads and cereals
      • Lofenalac, a synthetic milk product

## Additional Nursing Care That Can Be Incorporated into the Generic Care Plan

a.  **Assessment**
   – Signs of decreased melanin production (e.g., fair hair, blue eyes, eczema)
   – Signs of decreased epinephrine and thyroxine (e.g., hyperactivity, irritability, seizure activity)

b.  **Goal**
   Child will ingest needed nutrients in a low-phenylalanine diet.
   Child's phenylalanine blood level will remain within normal limits.

c.  **Interventions**
      • Individualize the diet to maintain serum phenylalanine level between 4–10 mg/100 ml.
      • Use Lofenalac infant formula with small amounts of milk formula added to it to provide some phenylalanine.
      • Use equivalency lists for older children.
      • Teach family regarding diet; consult a dietician and diet manual for diet specifics.

    d.  **Evaluation**
        •   Child's serum phenylalanine level remains between 4–10 mg/100 ml.
        •   Child is properly nourished.

## Other Possible Nursing Diagnoses

Parental anxiety
Sensory-perceptual alteration

7.  **Celiac Disease** (gluten-induced enteropathy, nontropical sprue, or idiopathic steatorrhea)

    a.  **Definition:** A nutritional deficit, either an inborn error of gluten metabolism or an immunologic response.

    b.  **Multidisciplinary Approaches**
        –   Gluten-restricted diet
        –   Encourage breast-feeding
        –   Delay introduction of solid foods

## Additional Nursing Care That Can Be Incorporated into the Generic Nursing Care Plan

    a.  **Assessment**
        –   Fatty stools, steatorrhea or constipation, nausea, and vomiting
        –   Protuberant abdomen and thin extremities
        –   Failure to regain weight or appetite after an episode of diarrhea

    b.  **Goal**
        Child will ingest prescribed diet in sufficient quantity to meet body needs.

    c.  **Interventions**
        •   Give diet free of wheat, rye, oats and barley.
        •   Use Prosobee formula for infants.
        •   Give nutritional supplements without glutens: Hycal, Citrotene, Precision LR, Meritene, Sustacal, and Vivonex.
        •   Teach parents to plan adequate menus free of gluten.
        •   Consult a dietician and diet manual for more information.

    d.  **Evaluation**
        •   Child
            –   is free from steatorrhea.
            –   maintains age-appropriate height and weight.

## 8.  Breast-feeding Difficulties

a.  **General Information**
- Initial instruction regarding breast-feeding almost always is the responsibility of the nurse; the new mother and the infant both have to learn correct techniques to ensure that the infant gets adequate nutrition and that problems are prevented or solved quickly.
- Potential breast-feeding problems
  - *infant*: crying, sleepiness, too-vigorous or too-weak suck, colic, illness
  - *mother*: delayed let-down reflex, inadequate milk supply, engorgement, sore nipples, mastitis, stress, poor nutrition, lack of knowledge, lack of support from significant others
  - any reason that necessitates separation of mother and child, e.g., hospitalization, working mother
- Successful breast-feeding can be initiated following a cesarean birth.

b.  **Multidisciplinary Approaches**
- Lactation aids, counselors
- Support groups

# Additional Nursing Care That Can Be Incorporated into the Generic Care Plan

a.  **Assessment**
- Previous instruction
- Maternal-child behaviors (bonding; how the mother holds [*en face*] and talks to the newborn)
- Support system (other family members' views on breast-feeding (husband, boyfriend, child's grandparents, mother's peer group)
- Breasts: fullness, sore, cracked, or inflamed nipples
- Mother's weights during breast-feeding
- Infant's sucking ability (slow rhythmic movement of infant's jaw followed by "click" sound means infant is nursing correctly [and swallowing liquid])
- Infant's sleep pattern, hydration status, weight gain and activity level
- Infant's blood glucose levels

b.  **Goals**
Mother will
- breast-feed confidently and without discomfort to the mutual satisfaction of both her and her baby.
- maintain her weight during breast-feeding.
Baby will regain birth weight within 2 weeks of delivery.

c.  **Interventions**
  - Provide opportunity for early breast-feeding, during the first hour of life, if possible.
  - Discuss with the mother the advantages of breast-feeding
    - breast milk contains exact nutritional requirements of baby
    - needs no mixing or warming
    - is economical
    - is free of contamination
    - contains antibodies
    - fosters a close mother-child relationship
  - Discuss principles of "on demand" feeding.
  - Explain how breasts will begin to become full
    - first milk expressed will be clear (colostrum)
    - regular milk comes in 3rd–4th day
  - Discuss let-down reflex.
  - Explain rooting reflex
    - can be aroused by contact with the areola causing the infant's mouth to open to a wide "ah" position
    - the tongue will extend out along the lower lip and feel for the nipple
    - when contacted, the lips encompass the areola, sealing it and compressing the collecting ductules against the palate, expressing colostrum from areola to the nipple, resulting in the swallowing reflex
  - Teach that the tongue's expressing action must be on the areola and not on the nipple (nipples act only as a pipeline for the milk).
  - Suggest prefeeding massage if breasts are engorged and difficult to grasp.
  - Stress need to wash hands and to assume comfortable position, sitting or lying down.
  - Discuss need to change positions and to rotate around the nipple.
  - Suggest feeding 5 minutes on one breast and switching to other one for rest of feeding. Alternate first breast each feeding; use both breasts each feeding.
  - Provide frequent encouragement.
  - Describe technique of inserting finger between baby's lips and areola before pulling baby away from breast to break suction.
  - Explain need to keep nipples clean using clear water, that soaps can irritate and lead to cracking; allow breasts to air dry after feeding and remove any plastic lining from brassieres.
  - Discuss measures to be taken to assure mother gets adequate rest, and how breast-feeding will fit into her schedule.
  - Instruct need for diet with increased calories (1,000 more per day), increased protein (from usual of 46 gm/day to 66 gm/day) and high fluid intake (2,500–3,000 ml/day).
  - Instruct to notify MD if mastitis or abscess develops.
  - Discuss possibility that all drugs can be transferred to infant in breast milk, and mother should consult with MD before taking any medication.

- Discuss possibility of manual expression or breast pump for busy or working mothers.

**d. Evaluation**
- Mother and father identify benefits of breast-feeding and express their concerns.
- Mother describes physical changes in breasts, rooting and let down reflex.
  - explains initiation of breast-feeding, correct sucking action of infant on nipple/areola.
  - describes breast care, feeding schedule, principles of infant demand, necessary changes in her fluid and nutritional intake.
  - maintains stable weight.
- Baby
  - is adequately hydrated, nourished.
  - regains birth weight after 2 weeks.
- Breast-feeding is successful, with no discomfort.

# Fluid and Electrolyte Balance

Hydration status must be meticulously monitored, particularly in young children. The nurse must be aware of not only intake and output but also insensible fluid loss.

Electrolytes are regulated jointly by the brain, kidneys, skin, lungs, GI tract, and various hormones (e.g., cortisone, aldosterone, antidiuretic hormone, parathormone, and thyrocalcitonin). When neurons in the thirst center become dehydrated and shrink, there is decreased cardiac output and drying of the mucous membranes.

**Total Body Water (TBW).**    The percentage of total body water varies among individuals and is related to body fat. Females have less water in relation to weight, as do the obese because of their higher percentage of fatty tissue. TBW ratios in the neonate are approximately 20% greater than those of the adult, but decrease rapidly in the neonatal period until the approximate adult percentage (58%) is reached at the age of about 2 years. A full-term neonate is approximately 73% water.

**Antidiuretic Hormone (ADH).**    Changes in the blood volume stimulate baroreceptors (volume receptors) in veins of the thorax. Standing or sitting for prolonged periods, or use of a positive pressure ventilator decreases thoracic blood volume, increasing production of ADH and stimulating fluid retention. A reclining position increases intrathoracic blood volume, decreasing ADH and increasing diuresis.

ADH is produced in the posterior pituitary; however, the hypothalamus may assume this role in neurohypophysis disease. When the osmolarity of body fluids increases, cells shrink and osmoreceptors in the hypothalamus are stimulated. A natural trigger stimulates ADH production at this point. Water is reabsorbed when ADH increases the permeability of the distal and collecting tubules. Conversely, when the osmolarity of body fluids decreases, cells swell and ADH secretion is inhibited.

**Aldosterone.** Aldosterone is an adrenocortical hormone crucial in sodium and potassium regulation. Renal vasoconstriction, stimulation of the juxtaglomerular apparatus, and fluid retention all occur related to increased aldosterone levels. In such cases, sodium is retained (edema) and potassium excreted by the kidneys (see figure 5.1 for an illustration of fluid retention mechanisms). The clinical symptoms of this mechanism, notably puffiness in the eyes and extremities and irritability, occur in healthy people under stress as well as in compromised individuals.

**Table 5.12** Electrolyte Imbalances

| Condition | Associated Factors | Signs and Symptoms | Nursing Management |
|-----------|--------------------|--------------------|--------------------|
| *Hyperkalemia* | | | |
| Serum-potassium level greater than 5 mEq/1 iter | Increased dietary potassium intake Excess or too rapidly administered IV fluid Administration of old blood (cells break down and release potassium) Decreased urinary excretion (oliguric renal failure) Potassium-sparing diuretics (spirono-lactone) Decreased aldos-terone effect (hypocorticism) Movement of potas-sium into extracellular fluid (cellular damage or death) Acidosis (hydrogen ions migrate into the cell, liberating potassium) Insulin deficiency (insulin drives potas-sium into the cell) | Early stages; skeletal muscle excitability Cramps, twitching Intestinal colic and diarrhea Muscle weakness (beginning in the lower extremities) and flaccid paralysis (exacerbated by hyperkalemia) Peaked T waves, widened QRS complexes (ECG) | Monitor IVs carefully. Give fluids to encourage urinary output (if no renal failure). Avoid high-potassium salt substitutes. Provide adequate carbohydrates to prevent tissue breakdown. Monitor effects of Kayexalate if ordered. |
| *Hypokalemia* | | | |
| Serum potassium level less than 3.5 mEq/liter | Decreased potassium intake GI loss (e.g., diarrhea, vomiting, laxative abuse) High licorice ingestion Diaphoresis | Muscle cells unrecep-tive to stimuli (firing potential decreased) Distention of the abdomen Anorexia, nausea and vomiting | Encourage patients taking digoxin and diuretics to eat high-potassium foods (e.g., bananas, dried figs, peaches, oranges). Teach patients about |

**Table 5.12**   Electrolyte Imbalances (continued)

| Condition | Associated Factors | Signs and Symptoms | Nursing Management |
|---|---|---|---|
| | Hyperaldosteronism Large steroid doses Hypomagnesemia Diuretics and alkalosis | Paralytic ileus Muscle weakness Flaccid paralysis and paresthesias Polyuria Flattened T waves, prominent U waves, peaked P waves, prolonged PR intervals (ECG) Potentiation of digitalis derivative leading to paroxysmal atrial tachycardia | diuretics and to report side effects. Request physician prescription for salt substitute containing potassium. Never give IV potassium push since it can lead to cardiac dysrhythmias and death. Administer oral doses in a well diluted solution (e.g., orange juice) so that it does not precipitate necrosis of the small bowel. |
| *Hypercalcemia* | | | |
| Serum calcium level greater than 5 mEq/liter | Increased GI absorption of calcium (hypervitaminosis D or milk-alkali syndrome) Increased release of calcium from bone (hyperparathyroidism, malignancy, bone tumors, or prolonged immobilization) Increase in physiologically available calcium (acidosis) | Decreased cell membrane permeability (lowers neuromuscular excitability) Anorexia, nausea and vomiting Abdominal pain, constipation Confusion, lethargy Fatigue, CNS depression Polyuria, calculi Pathologic fractures Shortened QT interval Development of U waves (ECG) | Teach patient to avoid excess vitamin D intake. Encourage mobility. Administer prescribed normal saline to encourage diuresis, decrease blood osmolality, and prevent kidney stones. Give supplemental phosphorus and diuretics as ordered. Maintain acid urine to increase calcium solubility. Prevent urinary tract infections because they make urine alkaline, permitting calcium to precipitate into stones. Handle child gently to prevent pathologic fractures. Warn patient on digitalis derivatives that calcium potentiates effect of digitalis. |

**Table 5.12**    Electrolyte Imbalances (continued)

| Condition | Associated Factors | Signs and Symptoms | Nursing Management |
|---|---|---|---|
| *Hypocalcemia* | | | |
| Serum calcium level less than 3.5 mEq/liter | Decreased calcium intake or poor absorption<br>Steatorrhea, sprue<br>Diarrhea<br>Antacid overuse<br>Lack of milk, poor vitamin D intake<br>Decreased calcium storage from alkalosis<br>Massive transfusion of citrated blood<br>Rapid plasmanate infusion<br>Hypoparathyroidism<br>Hypomagnesemia<br>Overdose of phosphate-containing laxative/enemas<br>Increased renal calcium excretion<br>Calcium loss through exudation | Tetany (severe depletion)<br>Muscle twitching/cramping<br>Positive Chvostek's and Trousseau's signs<br>Grimacing<br>Perioral and digital paresthesias<br>Carpopedal spasms<br>Laryngospasm (may lead to asphyxia if not corrected)<br>Seizure and cardiac dysrhythmias<br>Infants appear jittery | Teach patients careful administration of antacids.<br>Explore tolerable dietary supplements of calcium and vitamin D for children with milk allergies or lactose intolerance.<br>Have calcium gluconate available for rapid IV adminstration after thyroid or cardiac surgery.<br>Do not administer calcium in electrolyte solution since it precipitates and forms an insoluble salt.<br>Give calcium-containing oral medications before meals for best absorption.<br>Eliminate all dietary sources of phosphorus. |

# GENERIC CARE PLAN FOR THE NURSING DIAGNOSIS FLUID VOLUME DEFICIT

## 1. General Information

- There are three classes of dehydration
  - *isotonic*: fluids are lost in physiologic proportion to one another (70% of dehydration cases)
  - *hypertonic*: fluid losses are proportionately greater than solute losses; serum sodium greater than 145 mEq/liter, a high plasma volume, alkalosis and high renal solute loads (20% of dehydration cases)
  - *hypotonic* (also known as water intoxication): sodium is lost in increased proportion to fluid losses; serum sodium is less than 137 mEq/liter, and hemoglobin values are low; brain cells swell with

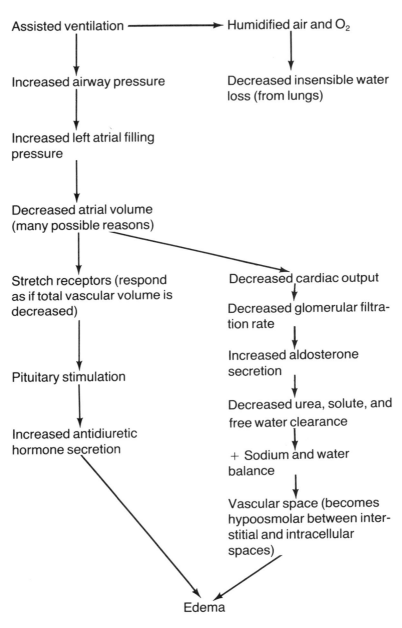

This mechanism is the same for chronic and episodic stress of other kinds as well.

**Figure 5.1**    Fluid Retention Mechanisms Related to Stress of Continuous Mechanical Ventilation

fluid, and cerebral edema may produce permanent secondary brain injury if untreated (10% of dehydration cases)

— *Third spacing* may be defined as an insidious form of dehydration in which fluid is shifted to a "third space" and becomes physiologically unavailable (e.g., burn wound exudates, ascites, a traumatized operative site with a localized inflammatory response, thrombophlebitis with resultant venous obstruction, or intestinal obstructions in which fluid accumulates due to decreased peristalsis).

Fluid maintenance requirements are generally based on individual metric weight, although some institutions use body surface area to determine replacement needs. Replacement is based on serum electrolyte values that indicate specific deficits. Whether the child is drinking enough is a frequent problem in toddlers who are undergoing severe separation and stranger anxiety and who may choose to exercise control by refusing oral fluids. The pediatric nurse must be well versed in use of the metric system, which is much more precise and easier to use than common household measures (see table 5.13 for recommended maintenance fluids based on body weight). Metric-to-avoirdupois conversion tables appear in Chapter 2. Table 5.14 will be useful in identification of possible problems.

**Table 5.13**    Recommended Maintenance Fluids and Electrolytes Based on Body Weight

| Substance | Dose |
|---|---|
| Water | 100/ml/kg/24 hours for each kg below 10 kg (first 10 kg) |
| | Add 50 ml/kg/24 hours for each kg from 11–20 kg |
| | Add 20 ml/kg/24 hours for each kg over 20 kg |
| Glucose | 100–200 mg/kg/hour |
| Electrolytes | |
| Sodium ($Na^+$) | 4 mEq/kg/24 hours |
| Potassium ($K^+$) | 2 mEq/kg/24 hours |
| Chloride ($Cl^-$) | 4 mEq/kg/24 hours |
| Calcium ($Ca^{++}$) | 50–200 mg/kg/24 hours |
| Magnesium ($Mg^{++}$) | 1 mEq/kg/24 hours |

(Levin, 1979)

Some therapies induce dehydration, e.g., radiant warmer, phototherapy for hyperbilirubinemia, mechanical ventilation. Maintenance requirements in these children must be increased by 10%–20%.

Several studies have demonstrated that rehydration occurs as rapidly with oral as with parenteral rehydration therapy, even when there is a related increase in stools (Behrman & Vaughn, 1983). Traditionally, oral feedings have been omitted in the initial treatment of

**Table 5.14**  Levels of Severity of Dehydration

| Dehydration | Level | Signs and Symptoms |
| --- | --- | --- |
| 1%–5% | Mild | Thirst (if child is able to indicate) |
| 5%–8% | Moderate | Increased pulse rate, weariness |
| 11%–15% | Severe | Significant circulatory impairment, deafness, renal failure, shock, delirium |
| 20% | Irreversible | Cracked, bloody skin, bloody tears, lost sensorium |

The percentage of dehydration is calculated in reference to total body weight (TBW). An infant weighing 3.5 kg who is 10% dehydrated has lost approximately 350 gm (11½ oz). This loss of fluid significantly impairs circulation.

small children and infants with moderately severe diarrhea. However, during an acute episode, the small bowel may absorb up to 60% of ingested nutrients; therefore, there is no physiologic basis for "resting" the bowel.

a.  **Etiology**
  — Excess fluid loss
    • shock, hemorrhage
    • overuse of diuretics
    • nasogastric suctioning
    • heat prostration
    • diarrhea, vomiting, diaphoresis
    • burns, draining wounds/fistulas
  — Medical conditions
    • diabetes mellitus or insipidus
    • TE fistula/atresia
    • Cushing's syndrome
    • hyperaldosteronism
    • cystic fibrosis
    • inappropriate secretion of ADH
    • renal disease, adrenal insufficiency
  — Physiologic conditions
    • fever
    • fluid shifts, third spacing
    • electrolyte imbalance
    • starvation
    • hyperventilation.
    • osmotic diuresis (excess blood glucose or urea)
  — Therapy related
    • mechanical ventilation without humidification
    • high solute intake without accompanying proportionate water ingestion (tube feedings)
    • excess administration of greater than 0.9% saline or sodium bicarbonate

- prolonged sodium-restricted diet
- excess administration of 5% dextrose without electrolyte replacement
- frequent tap water enemas
- frequent irrigations with hypotonic solutions

**b. Clinical Manifestations**
- Isotonic
  - dry mucous membranes
  - "tenting" of skin
  - lack of tears
  - sunken fontanels
  - oliguria
- Hypertonic
  - intense thirst
  - sticky mucous membranes
  - confusion
  - lethargy (brain cells shrink, interstitial edema occurs)
  - convulsions, coma
  - muscle weakness/twitching
  - flushing, dry skin, fever
  - oliguria
  - firm tissue turgor (sodium retention)
- Hypotonic
  - headache, malaise
  - confusion, coma
  - leg cramping
  - decreased urine output
  - decreased urine specific gravity

**c. Multidisciplinary Approaches**
- Intravenous fluids (see table 5.15)
- Oral hydration
- Hypodermoclysis (rare)

**Table 5.15**  Purposes and Tonicity of Commonly Used IV Solutions

| IV Solutions | Purpose | Tonicity |
|---|---|---|
| 5% dextrose/0.45% saline | Hydration | Hypertonic |
| 5% dextrose/0.9% saline | Replacement | Hypertonic |
| 5% dextrose/water | Fluid, calories | Isotonic |
| 2.5% dextrose/0.45% salies | Hydration | Isotonic |
| 5% dextrose/0.25% saline | Hydration | Hypertonic |
| Lactated Ringer's | Replacement | Isotonic |
| 0.45% saline | Hydration | Hypotonic |
| 0.9% saline | Replacement | Isotonic |
| 10% dextrose/water | Fluid, calories | Hypertonic |

## 2.  Nursing Process

a.  **Assessment**
  - Thirst
  - Generalized weakness
  - Daily fluid intake (less than daily requirement for child's weight [see table 5.13])
  - Skin and mucous membranes
  - Weight
  - Perspiration (salty)
  - Urine output (decreased)
  - Urine specific gravity (increased)
  - Hematocrit and RBC (increased)
  - Serum electrolytes
  - Heart rate (increased)
  - Temperature (elevated)
  - Prior to the initiation of parenteral fluid therapy
    • the kind, amount, and quantity of administered fluids
    • how they have been given (po, NG, clysis)
    • additional electrolytes, glucose, proteins, medications given
    • child's output during the period of the illness
    • amount, color, contents, and consistency of urine
    • diarrhea, perspiration, vomitus, sump drainage, chest tube or other drainage
    • estimated blood loss, etc.
  - Child's age and significant medical history (renal, cardiovascular, respiratory, metabolic, or CNS disease)

b.  **Goal**
Child will be adequately and safely hydrated.

c.  **Interventions**
  • Know normal fluid and electrolyte values in order to provide safe care and adequate replacement in pathologic states.
  • Maintain appropriate fluid intake for child's weight (see table 5.13) by offering a selection of fluids, and giving small, frequent drinks.
  • Substitute bouillon or fruit juices for water when clear liquids are indicated.
  • Rehydrate the child orally with Pedialyte, Lytren, or similar solution.
  • Irrigate tubes with normal saline instead of water.
  • Increase dietary sodium intake to protect the child at risk.
  • Avoid tap water enemas.
  • Use infusion pumps to administer IV therapy to any infant or to children requiring fluid restrictions.
  • Use infusion pumps that monitor fluid lines for occlusions, air bubbles, and infusion completion when they are available.

- Put only hourly amount of fluid in drip chamber and on pump dial so that "infusion complete" alarm will "remind" nurse to check site hourly.
- Check pediatric IV therapy every half hour.
  - inspect the site with each IV check for signs of infiltration, puffiness, or leaking
  - document hourly the amounts infused, site condition, location, changes, and reasons for observed alteration
- If infiltrations occur, stop the infusion and apply warm soaks. (If a caustic medication was being infused, notify the MD or follow standard treatment protocol.)
- Change infusion tubing and solutions within product guidelines recommended by specific pharmaceutical companies or hospital policy.
- Restrain armboards to crib sheets at the end of the armboard closest to the patient.
- Maintain strict intake and output for all children on continuous IV therapy.
- Do not give potassium unless renal function is established.
- Encourage parents to hold and comfort their child despite an IV.
- Record termination of an IV site and attempts to start new sites.

**d. Evaluation**
- Child regains adequate hydration as evidenced by
  - no thirst
  - daily fluid intake equal to daily requirement
  - moist skin and mucous membranes
  - adequate skin turgor
  - weight within normal limits
  - adequate urinary output
  - urine specific gravity between 1.0015–1.025
  - hematocrit and RBC within normal limits
  - normal temperature and pulse
  - flat fontanels
  - tears when crying

# Selected Health Problems Frequently Associated with the Nursing Diagnosis FLUID VOLUME DEFICIT

## Shock

**a. Definition:** An inadequate perfusion of the vital organs—brain, heart, lungs, kidneys, and liver.
- Hypovolemic shock may be related to hemorrhage (e.g., cardiac tamponade, GI bleeding), burn wound exudation (or other forms

of third spacing), peritonitis, or severe dehydration from fluid shifts, diarrhea, or similar losses.
- Infants and young children are especially prone to and endangered by hypovolemia. A 2.5 kg infant has an approximate total blood volume of only 200 cc. A 10cc (5%) blood loss is the equivalent of 250 cc loss to an adult.
- Septic shock is the inadequate perfusion of the vital organs secondary to a specific infection. In overwhelming infection, capillary permeability is increased, permitting fluid loss from the intravascular compartment. Organisms commonly responsible for septic shock in children are rickettsials (e.g., Rocky Mountain Spotted Fever), gram positive organisms (e.g., meningococci), and viruses (e.g., hepatitis B).

**b.  Clinical Manifestations**
- Weak cry, poor responsiveness
- Irritability, anxiousness
- Confusion, lethargy
- Apprehension or restlessness
- Lost skin elasticity (poor turgor)
- "Tented" position of pinched skin
- Poor capillary filling
- Warm and dry mucous membranes
- Pallor
- Elevated or decreased temperature and pulse
- Tachycardia
- Tachypnea
- Shallow respirations in infants
- Thirst
- Decreased urinary output, concentrated urine (high specific gravity)
- Renal shutdown
- Septic shock: delirium, petechiae, and disseminated intravascular coagulation (DIC)

**c.  Multidisciplinary Approaches**
- Treatment is based on symptoms and underlying pathologies and usually consists of resuscitation with IV fluids (physiologic saline, lactated Ringer's, etc.). Whole blood and plasma are rarely used (unless there is an actively bleeding artery) because of the increased risk of emboli in this severely compromised state (Behrman & Vaughn).
- Airway and ventilation maintenance, oxygen administration
- Fluid replacement
- Drug therapy (dopamine or isuprel may be used to maintain blood pressure and urine output)
- Treatment of underlying cause (e.g., infection, blood loss)

## Additional Nursing Care That Can Be Incorporated into the Generic Care Plan

a. **Assessment**
   - Appearance
   - Activity
   - Skin
   - Mucous membranes
   - Temperature, pulse, respiration
   - Intake and output

b. **Goal**
   Child's vital organs will function adequately.

c. **Interventions**
   - Place child in supine position with legs elevated (except in cases of head injury).
   - Monitor
     - effects of replacement fluid and electrolytes, blood products, and plasma expanders
     - effects of medications administered (e.g., insulin, pitressin, ADH)
     - effects of oxygen therapy
     - vital signs and lab values
     - compromised or post-op patients carefully for such subtle early changes as pallor, tachycardia, or anxiety

d. **Evaluation**
   - Child's
     - vital signs and laboratory values are returning to normal.
     - intake and output are balanced.
   - Child is active and alert.

## Other Possible Nursing Diagnoses

Alteration in cardiac output
Impaired gas exchange
Impairment of skin integrity
Potential for injury
Sensory-perceptual alteration

## GENERIC CARE PLAN FOR THE NURSING DIAGNOSIS
## FLUID VOLUME EXCESS

1. **General Information:** Major fluid shifts from the plasma to the interstitium or vice versa can severely compromise the injured or ill child.

-   *Edema* is an accumulation of an excessive amount of watery fluid in cells, tissues, or serous cavities; it may be a generalized accumulation of fluid or localized to small areas.
-   *Interstitial-fluid-to-plasma shifts* are essentially a remobilization of edema fluid. This may occur when volume is restored after a hypovolemic episode or after recovery from other injuries. When a large amount of fluid is remobilized over a short period of time, the following symptoms may develop: bounding pulse, peripheral vein engorgement, rales, weakness, pallor, and rapid breathing. Hemodilution occurs and there is a fluid overload. This is particularly significant in a child with compromised cardiac function, because it may precipitate or enhance congestive heart failure.
-   *Plasma-to-interstitial-fluid shifts* occur under the following conditions: portal hypertension, decreased oncotic pressure with increased capillary permeability, renal compromise, vasodilation, and decreased venous return. Patients admitted with certain high-risk medical diagnoses, e.g., chronic liver disease, malnutrition, starvation edema, burns, massive crushing injuries, nephrotic syndrome, shock, should be watched carefully for this problem.

a.  **Etiologies**
    -   Renal and liver disease
    -   Decreased cardiac output
    -   Inflammation
    -   Hormonal disturbances
    -   Steroid therapy
    -   Nephrotic syndrome
    -   Starvation
    -   Increased venous pressure
    -   Capillary permeability
    -   Diminished plasma proteins
    -   Lymphatic obstruction
    -   Excessive fluid intake
    -   Excessive sodium intake

b.  **Clinical Manifestations**
    -   Edema (orbital edema usually appears first in younger children), taut shiny skin
    -   Weight gain
    -   Bounding pulse
    -   Increased blood pressure
    -   Increased venous filling
    -   Intake larger than output
    -   Hepato-, splenomegaly

c.  **Multidisciplinary Approaches**
    -   Diuretics
    -   Fluid restriction
    -   Sodium restriction

## 2. Nursing Process

### a. Assessment
- Skin
- Weight
- Pulse, blood pressure, respirations
- Hydration
- Size of liver, spleen

### b. Goal
Child will be adequately hydrated free from fluid overload.

### c. Interventions
- Distribute fluid allowances over 24 hours.
- Give small frequent drinks.
- Provide fluid selection.
- Provide cold water for rinsing mouth between drinks if child will not swallow the water.
- Use mouthwash and hard candy.
- Monitor IV rate closely.
- Place child on bedrest if necessary.
- Elevate the head of the bed if child has difficulty breathing.
- Monitor BP, CVP, and pulse every 1–2 hours.

### d. Evaluation
- Child's
  - fluid intake is equal to urinary output over a 24-hour period.
  - BP, CVP, and pulse are returning to normal parameters.
- Child has no respiratory difficulty.

### e. Possible Related Nursing Diagnoses
Alteration in cardiac output
Impairment of skin integrity
Ineffective breathing pattern

## GENERIC CARE PLAN FOR THE NURSING DIAGNOSIS
# IMPAIRMENT OF SKIN INTEGRITY

## 1. General Information

### a. Etiology
- Burns
- Chronic illness
- Diarrhea
- Dehydration

b.  **Clinical Manifestations**
  – Itching
  – Pain
  – Numbness
  – Disruption of skin surface

c.  **Multidisciplinary Approaches**
  – Debridement for burns
  – Dietary consultation

## 2.  Nursing Process

a.  **Assessment**
  – Sensory deficits
  – Inability to change position or to move self
  – Incontinence of urine or feces
  – Current appearance of skin: redness, tenderness, warmth, coolness, dryness, poor turgor, discoloration, edema, blistering or blanching
  – Evidence of scratching, bleeding, or discharge
  – Current medications; exposure to any new medications, soaps, lotions
  – Presence of lesions: locations, configuration, color
  – Need for bedrest, traction, casts or splints
  – Obesity
  – Nutritional deficits

b.  **Goal**
  Child will maintain/regain an intact skin surface.
  Child/parents will participate in strategies to sustain skin integrity.

c.  **Interventions**
  • Assess skin condition at least every 2 hours.
  • Provide child and family simple, accurate explanations about factors that contribute to skin irritation.
  • Explain why an intact skin surface is important.
  • Engage child and family in active participation in maintaining skin integrity.
  • Develop an individualized bowel and bladder emptying schedule to prevent incontinence.
  • Assure adequate diet and fluid intake.
  • Implement range-of-motion exercises at least every 8 hours.
  • Turn or reposition every 2 hours.
  • Provide skin care using mild soap, clear water rinse, and massage.
  • Use sheepskin, egg-crate mattresses, heel and elbow pads.
  • Teach family skin care techniques, importance of daily skin assessment, and turning schedules.

**d.  Evaluation**
- Child's skin is intact.
- Child/family
  - state contributing factors to skin irritation and why intact skin is important.
  - assist in maintaining skin integrity.

**e.  Possible Related Nursing Diagnoses**
Alteration in comfort: pain
Alteration in nutrition: less than body requirements
Disturbance in self-concept: body image
Fluid volume deficit
Knowledge deficit
Potential for infection

# Selected Health Problems Frequently Associated with the Nursing Diagnosis IMPAIRMENT OF SKIN INTEGRITY

## 1.  Burns

**a.  Discussion:** Children under 5 years suffer especially severe effects, while those under 2 have the highest associated mortality rate. The most critical burn injuries are those to the face, hands, feet, and genitalia. The most common childhood burns are

- *Thermal* (caused by hot liquids or open flames)
- *Chemical* (caustic ingestion)
- *Electrical* (objects in electrical outlets, contact with electrified railroad tracks)
- *Radiation* (x- or ultraviolet ray overexposure)

As many as 25%–30% of all burns reported in children may result from parental abuse and neglect (Helberg, 1983).

Calculating the affected body surface area (BSA) to determine the percentage of the body that has been burned can be especially difficult in children. Because of the proportional differences between adults and children, standard "rule of nines" charts do not apply. Special charts have been developed to account for the child's relatively large head and small legs (see table 5.16). Burns may be classified according to the depth or degree of the burned tissue.

**Table 5.16**   Percentage of Body Surface Area According to Age (Burn Estimate)

| Area (%) | Birth–1 year | 1–4 years | 5–9 years | 10–14 years | 15 years | Adult |
|---|---|---|---|---|---|---|
| Head | 19 | 17 | 13 | 11 | 9 | 7 |
| Neck | 2 | 2 | 2 | 2 | 2 | 2 |
| Anterior trunk | 13 | 13 | 13 | 13 | 13 | 13 |
| Posterior trunk | 13 | 13 | 13 | 13 | 13 | 13 |
| Each buttock | 2$^1/_2$ | 2$^1/_2$ | 2$^1/_2$ | 2$^1/_2$ | 2$^1/_2$ | 2$^1/_2$ |
| Genitalia | 1 | 1 | 1 | 1 | 1 | 1 |
| Each upper arm | 4 | 4 | 4 | 4 | 4 | 4 |
| Each lower arm | 3 | 3 | 3 | 3 | 3 | 3 |
| Each hand | 2$^1/_2$ | 2$^1/_2$ | 2$^1/_2$ | 2$^1/_2$ | 2$^1/_2$ | 2$^1/_2$ |
| Each thigh | 5$^1/_2$ | 6$^1/_2$ | 8 | 8$^1/_2$ | 9 | 9$^1/_2$ |
| Each leg | 5 | 5 | 5$^1/_2$ | 6 | 6$^1/_2$ | 7 |
| Each foot | 3$^1/_2$ | 3$^1/_2$ | 3$^1/_2$ | 3$^1/_2$ | 3$^1/_2$ | 3$^1/_2$ |

Note: From *Manual of Emergency Pediatrics* (pp. 52–53) by R. Reece and J. Chamberlain, 1974. Philadelphia: Saunders, 52–53. Copyright 1974 by Saunders. Reprinted by permission.

- Depth of injury
  - *first degree* (epidermal): minor burn; systemic effects are extremely rare
  - *second degree* (partial thickness): superficial or extends deeper into the dermal layer
  - *third degree* (full thickness); severe burn, extends through all layers of skin
- Severity
  - minor injury: less than 15% of BSA (20% in children under 2) is covered with partial thickness burns or full-thickness burns covering less than 2% BSA
  - moderate injury: partial-thickness burns over 15%–30% of BSA (10%–20% in children under 2) or full-thickness burns over 2%–10% of noncritical BSA (2%–5% in children under 2)
  - major injury
    * partial-thickness injury to more than 30% of BSA (20% in children under 2) *or* full-thickness burns to more than 10% BSA (less than 5% in children under 2), especially in critical areas (e.g., face, hands, toes)

* often involves associated trauma (crushing or head injuries, fractures), respiratory injury (generally from prolonged exposure to heat and smoke; common with fires in enclosed areas)
* electrical burns
* concurrent chronic illness (e.g., diabetes, cardiac, pulmonary, or renal disease)
* concurrent malnutrition

b. **Multidisciplinary Approaches**
   - Intubation if necessary
   - High concentration of oxygen
   - ABGs (arterial blood gases)
   - Hydration to prevent shock
     • two large bore IV lines (may be started through burned skin)
     • administration of Ringer's Lactate without glucose (2–4 ml/kg/ % BSA burned) over the first 24 hours: half during the first 8 hours, half over the next 16 hours
   - NPO status (for burns over 20%–25% of BSA, NG tube to avoid ileus, distention, vomiting)
   - Pain relief (usually with IV morphine)
     • no IM injections because of poor absorption
     • dosage titrated to child's response
   - Tetanus prophylaxis if necessary
   - Medication (Silvadene or similar agent; antibiotics are not normally used in initial burn treatment)
   - Dressing changes
   - Plastic surgery consultation (especially for facial burns)
   - Dietary, social service consultation

# Additional Nursing Care That Can Be Incorporated into the Generic Care Plan

a. **Assessment**
   - Nature and extent of burn injuries
     • percentage of body surface area (BSA) burned
     • burn type
     • depth and location
     • age of child
   - Associated injuries
     • respiratory: check for cough, soot in mouth or nose, facial or neck burns; assess continuously for tachypnea, dyspnea, stridor, cyanosis, nasal flaring, restlessness
     • trauma (head and cervical fractures); see "Assessment" in *Potential for Injury: Trauma,* page 103
     • shock (requires continuous assessment); see "Assessment" in *Fluid Volume Deficit,* page 171

- Pertinent history (circumstances surrounding injury, preexisting conditions, date of last tetanus shot)

---

**NURSING TIP: Children with increased carbon monoxide levels from smoke inhalation are especially susceptible to cerebral edema and respiratory arrest.**

---

b. **Goal**
Child will be free from burn complications (e.g., shock, infection, respiratory distress).

c. **Interventions**
- For minor burns, cool burned area (if not already done) and clean with soap if necessary. Apply medications and dressings as ordered.
- Maintain airway, control bleeding, perform CPR as required.
- Contact burn center immediately if the patient is to be transferred to make arrangements and receive instructions; if that transfer will be completed promptly, no treatment of the burn itself is necessary.
- Preserve circulation
  - remove jewelry from burned extremities
  - observe for circumferential burns that may obstruct vascular flow as they heal and scar tissue forms
- Avoid hypothermia (use warm blankets); monitor temperature.
- Cover burned areas with dry sterile sheets or dressings.
- Wrap burned extremities in bulky gauze dressings.
- Instruct parents about dressing changes and signs of infection.
- Refer for professional follow-up if necessary (e.g., dietician, social service).

d. **Evaluation**
- Child is afebrile, vital signs are stable.
- Wounds are free of purulent drainage, heal with minimal scarring.

## Other Possible Nursing Diagnoses

Alteration in comfort: pain
Alteration in family process
Alteration in nutrition: less than body requirements
Anxiety
Disturbance in self-concept
Diversional activity deficit

Fear
Fluid volume deficit
Impaired physical mobility
Potential for injury (infection)
Self-care deficit
Social isolation

## 2. Cleft Lip/Palate

a. **Definition**
   - *Cleft lip*: a unilateral or bilateral lack of fusion of the facial process that may produce a small opening or ridge in the upper lip extending even to the nasal septum and dental ridge
   - *Cleft palate*: lack of closure of the hard palate and dental ridge; can be unilateral, bilateral, or midline

b. **Multidisciplinary Approaches**
   - Cleft lip: surgically repaired around 3 months of age
   - Cleft palate: surgically repaired around 18 months of age

## Additional Nursing Care That Can Be Incorporated into the Generic Care Plan

a. **Assessment**
   - Airway (for patency and child's ability to expectorate secretions)
   - Incision site (for approximation and signs of infection, discharge amount and character)
   - Feeding methods (question parents)
   - Parents' attitude toward facial defect
   - Pain
   - Crying, activity level, and ability of parents to calm child
   - Parents' understanding of reasons for treatment measures
   - Comfort measures that calm/quiet child
   - Hydration level

b. **Goals**
   Child will
   - be free from compromised skin integrity postoperatively.
   - maintain adequate hydration and nutrition postoperatively.
   Parents will be able to properly care for child pre- and postoperatively.

c. **Interventions**
   - Teach parents to place child in arm restraints periodically before admission.
   - Train child to lie on his back a great deal of time to reduce post-op irritability and resistance; allow child with cleft palate repair to lie on abdomen.

- Position child on back or in infant seat when reactive from anesthesia; place child in side-lying position if there is difficulty in handling secretions; reposition every 2 hours.
- Place in mist tent with cool air to keep secretions loose.
- Aspirate mouth and nasopharyngeal secretions gently as necessary.
- Maintain protective appliance or butterfly closure to the cheeks to prevent tension on suture line.
- Use arm restraints and pin cuff to bed or clothing; use jacket restraints in older infant.
- Remove restraints periodically to exercise arms, one at a time (demonstrate to parents).
- Teach parents how to use restraints and why they are important; ask for return demonstration.
- Hold and cuddle infant frequently.
- Encourage parents to participate in child's care.
- Administer pain medication (e.g., acetaminophen) as ordered and note effectiveness.
- Discuss with parents importance of not allowing child to cry (tension on suture line).
- Avoid placing objects in child's mouth (e.g., pacifier, fingers).
- Avoid trauma to suture line when feeding by
  - using rubber-tipped syringe
  - feeding child with a cleft palate repair only with soup spoon or from the side of spoon, being careful not to insert spoon into child's mouth
  - placing child on right side after feedings
  - rinsing mouth with clear water before and after each feeding
  - cleaning suture line after each feeding with cotton or gauze-tipped swab and a half and half solution of normal saline and hydrogen peroxide if ordered
- Remove crusts on suture line gradually and gently every 4 hours to prevent buildup.
- Keep suture line dry.
- Demonstrate proper restraining, position, feeding, and cleaning of suture line to parents.
- Encourage other family members to learn to feed infant to enable mother to rest.
- Before discharge
  - discuss with parents the need to avoid hard items in diet (e.g., hard cookies, pizza, carrots, celery, tough meat)
  - caution parents to continue elbow restraints until suture line is healed
  - explain to parents the reason for continuing side lying position when child returns home
  - demonstrate temperature taking to parents
  - describe signs of infection and necessary actions
- Refer parents to genetic counseling, local cleft lip/palate group if desired.

   **d.  Evaluation**
   - Child's suture line remains well approximated, facial edema decreases.
   - Operative site is trauma-free.
   - Child has good skin turgor and urinary output; vital signs are stable.
   - Parents
     - remove and apply elbow restraints correctly.
     - feed child without disrupting suture line.
     - gently cleanse suture line as directed and maintain good oral hygiene after feedings.

## Other Possible Nursing Diagnoses

Alteration in comfort: pain
Alteration in nutrition: less than body requirements
Fear
Fluid volume deficit
Ineffective airway clearance
Parental anxiety
Potential for injury, infection

## References

American Academy of Pediatrics. (1979). *Pediatric nutrition handbook.* Evanston, IL: Academy.

American Diabetes Association. (1983). *Curriculum for youth education.* New York: Author.

Behrman, R., & Vaughn, V. (1983). *Nelson's textbook of pediatrics.* (12th ed.). Philadelphia: Saunders.

Bonner, J. (1981). Nutrition during the growing years. In M. Green & J. Harry (Eds.), *Nutrition in contemporary nursing practice.* New York: Wiley.

Children's Hospital of Philadelphia. *Nutrition support service comprehensive nutritional assessment sheet.* Philadelphia: Author.

Etzwiler, D. (1983). Patient education and management: A team approach. In M. Ellenberg & H. Rifkin (Eds.), *Diabetes mellitus: Theory and practice.* New Hyde Park, NY: Medical Examination.

Harvey, P. (1981). Tube feedings and nutritional supplements. In M. Green & J. Harry (Eds.), *Nutrition in contemporary nursing practice.* New York: Wiley.

Howard, R. (1982). Nutrition through the growing years. In R. Howard & N. Herbold (Eds.), *Nutrition in clinical care.* New York: McGraw-Hill.

Konstantinides, N., & Shronts, E. (1983). Tube feeding: Managing the basics. *American Journal of Nursing, 83,* 1312-1320.

Levin, D. (1979). Abnormalities in fluids, minerals, and glucose. In D. Levin, F. Morris, & G. Moore (Eds.). *A practical guide to pediatric intensive care.* St. Louis: Mosby.

Malasanos, L., Barkauska, V., Moss, M., & Stoltenberg-Allen, K. (1981). *Health assessment.* (2nd ed.). St. Louis: Mosby.

McFarland, M., & Grant, M. (1982). *Nursing implications of laboratory tests.* New York: Wiley.

Moore, W. (1981). *Recognition and prevention of cow-milk-induced enteric blood loss in infancy.* Columbus, OH: Ross Laboratories.

Salmond, S. (1980). How to assess the nutritional status of acutely ill patients. *American Journal of Nursing, 5,* 922–924.

Walker, W. (1977). Development of intestinal host defense mechanisms and the passive protective role of human milk. *Mead Johnson symposium on perinatal and developmental medicine No. 11: Selected aspects of perinatal gastroenterology,* (p. 43).

Whaley, L., & Wong, D. (1983). *Nursing care of infants and children.* (2nd ed). St. Louis: Mosby.

# CHAPTER 6

# ELIMINATION
## FUNCTIONAL HEALTH PATTERN

The elimination functional health pattern includes excretory function (bowel and bladder) in childhood. This pattern includes the development of bowel and bladder control, patterns of elimination, and elimination problems.

## Childhood Urinary Tract Problems

The most common urinary tract problem seen in childhood is urinary tract infection (UTI). Most UTIs are of the lower urinary tract, i.e., bladder and urethra. In infants, UTIs are usually blood borne; in older children they are urethral. Girls have more frequent UTIs because of their short urethras. The antibacterial properties of prostatic secretions also help prevent UTIs in boys.

Most UTIs are caused by *E. coli*. The symptoms of pain and bleeding in UTIs result from irritation and inflammation of the urinary mucosa by bacteria. If the infection is not treated with antibiotics early and thoroughly enough, urine can flow back through the ureters to the kidneys (vesicoureteral reflux), causing urine to enter the ascending tubule of the kidney and bacteria to damage the renal parenchyma. If obstruction (from pus or inflammation) is also present at the vesicoureteral junction, hydronephrosis (dilation of the pelvis and calices) can also occur, leading to further renal impairment.

There are several congenital urinary tract disorders that are repaired in childhood. Phimosis (narrowing of the prepuce of the penis, preventing retraction of the foreskin) and cryptorchidism (failure of one or both of the testes to descend into the scrotum) can be corrected surgically in early childhood with minimal sequelae. However, epispadias (abnormal placement of the urinary meatus on the dorsum of the penis) and extrophy of the bladder (congenital malformation in which the lower portion of the abdominal wall and anterior wall of the bladder fail to fuse during fetal development) require more extensive surgical repair, including the formation of a urinary diversion such as an ileal loop conduit.

## Urinary Elimination Management

**Bladder Regulation.**   The child with a neurologic, neuromuscular, or physical disability will often be maintained on an individualized pattern of bladder training. When such a child is admitted to an acute care setting, the child's usual elimination regimen must be observed by nurses in order to prevent discomfort or more serious complications (e.g., hydronephrosis, renal failure).

The child will generally have appliances from home. Often, acute care institutions do not purchase the same brands or sizes to which the child has become accustomed. In any case, it is important for the nurse to carefully observe the processes that families or long-term care institutions have developed, and to continue to use effective strategies and to modify other patterns.

**Long-Term Urinary Elimination Management.**   Occasionally, the child with a physical impairment to normal voiding will have an indwelling Foley catheter. This is rare, however, because of the device's attendant risks. Generally, some type of diversion such as a urostomy or cystostomy or other methods to empty the bladder are employed. If bladder emptying is transurethral, the Credé procedure is often used, and is discussed in detail below. Another method frequently employed to empty a child's bladder is the use of intermittent straight catheterizations.

When a child is following an intermittent urinary catheterization program, it is imperative that the nurse continue the program. Generally, the intermittent catheterization schedule will be every 3–4 hours. Probably (if the child is old enough to sleep all night) there will be a period between procedures lasting 6–8 hours. Often, the child will undergo the Credé process first, followed by straight catheterization for residual urine.

Catheters come in a variety of materials, including surgical steel (for more thorough disinfecting), red rubber, and plastic. Use the type of catheter the child is used to if possible. While clean procedure is often used at home, use sterile technique in an inpatient setting to decrease the possibility of nosocomial infection and protect the patient. Fidelity to the child's individual regimen will maintain bladder tonus and prevent complications such as hydroureter.

The child with a urinary tract-to-surface stoma presents several challenges. If there is no collecting appliance, the problems of ammoniacal dermatitis or candida albicantia infections may occur. When a collecting bag is used, breakdown around the stoma site may be a problem. If no skin disorders are present around a functioning stoma when the child is admitted, the care regimen has been successful and should continue to be followed. Intervention may be necessary in other cases to regain and maintain skin integrity.

Some children with neurogenic bladders, for example, as a complication of myelomeningocele are unable to control their urinary elimination with the use of intermittent straight catheterization. They may find the use of a urinary appliance difficult. In some circumstances, they have the option of having a continent urinary diversion.

The Kock pouch is a collection reservoir for urine created from a portion of the small intestine. Two nipple valves are formed from intussuscepted portions of the ileum. The ureters are implanted near the inlet nipple valve. The urine leaves the pouch through the outlet nipple valve and a stoma. The child or family empties the pouch by inserting a catheter through the stoma into the pouch. This is done 4–6 times a day. At other times the stoma is covered with a Band-Aid or small dressing (Brogna & Lakaszowski, 1986).

**Dialysis.**    When renal function has been severely impaired (usually after a loss of more than 50%–75% of the nephrons) signs of renal failure become apparent and the child must be treated with dialysis to survive.

Dialysis is the movement of a fluid across a semipermeable membrane resulting in the separation of molecules by

- *osmosis:* passive movement of fluid from an area of lower concentration to one of higher concentration
- *diffusion:* random movement from areas of greater concentration of a substance to areas of lesser concentration
- *ultrafiltration:* the movement of fluid under pressure through a filtering medium with very small pores

With dialysis, the child's blood is cleansed of metabolic wastes. Two types of dialysis are commonly used for children in renal failure

- *peritoneal dialysis:* filtration of blood by the use of a dialysate administered through the abdominal cavity. The peritoneal membrane serves as the semipermeable membrane across which the water and solutes move. This type of dialysis is used frequently for acute renal failure or other acute conditions such as severe metabolic acidosis, accidental poisoning, intractible heart failure, and hepatic coma.

    *Continuous ambulatory peritoneal dialysis (CAPD)* can be used for some children with chronic renal failure in their homes. Dialysate is introduced into the peritoneal cavity through a catheter that has been permanently sutured in place. The dialysate remains in the peritoneum for 4–6 hours. This allows children to remain relatively active at home.

- *hemodialysis:* filtration of blood across a dialyzer through an artificially constructed arteriovenous fistula or shunt, or through a graft.

## GENERIC CARE PLAN FOR THE NURSING DIAGNOSIS
# ALTERATION IN PATTERNS OF URINARY ELIMINATION: RETENTION

## 1.  General Information

### a.  Etiology
  - Neurogenic bladder
  - Myelomeningocele
  - Mechanical trauma
  - Surgical intervention
  - Infection
  - Obstruction

### b.  Clinical Manifestations
  - Bladder distention
  - Lower abdominal pain or discomfort
  - Low urine output
  - Restlessness

### c.  Multidisciplinary Approaches
  - Medications
    - antibiotics
    - antispasmodics
    - urinary antiseptics
    - urecholine
    - Foley catheter
  - Urinary diversion

## 2.  Nursing Process

### a.  Assessment
  - Usual urinary elimination pattern
  - Urine output
  - Bladder distention
  - Discomfort

### b.  Goals
Child will
  - have an adequate urinary output.

     – be free from complications of urinary retention (e.g., hydronephrosis, renal damage).

**c. Interventions**
- Encourage voiding by use of warm washcloth over perineum, running water, allowing child to get up to bathroom, etc.
- Use intermittent straight catheterization every 4 hours for residual urine as ordered.
- Perform bladder Credé if appropriate: general procedure
  - position child on back in bed or on toilet (if developmentally appropriate)
  - check for bladder level; if unable to palpate, begin Credé below umbilicus
  - place hand in semi-fist (fingers flexed to second knuckle but not to palm of hand)
  - place hand on abdomen, pressing toward spine and downward toward feet; continue to hold pressure while urine is being evacuated
  - remove hand and wait for 1 minute
  - reposition hand slightly below initial starting point and repeat cycle
  - reposition hand just above symphysis pubis and repeat this cycle; if a moderate amount of urine is expressed, repeat entire cycle
  - record output
  - do not do the Credé procedure on males if they have erections, as they are unable to void at this time
  - delay Credé procedure if a child is crying and the abdomen is tense
- For child with unrepaired myelomeningocele
  - relax for one minute after each cycle and repeat cycle, beginning at the symphysis pubis
  - repeat cycle if a large amount of urine is expressed at level of symphysis pubis

**d. Evaluation**
- Child is free from renal damage as evidenced by
  - clear, yellow, odorless urine output of at least 1 ml/kg/hour
  - normal BUN and creatinine

**e. Possible Related Nursing Diagnoses**
Alteration in comfort: pain
Fluid volume deficit
Ineffective breathing patterns
Knowledge deficit
Potential for infection
Sleep pattern disturbance

# Selected Health Problems Frequently Associated with the Nursing Diagnosis ALTERATION IN PATTERNS OF URINARY ELIMINATION

## 1. Renal or Bladder Trauma

### a. Discussion
- *Renal trauma* includes contusions, lacerations, rupture, and fragmentations. Renal damage is frequently associated with twelfth rib fracture and can lead to hemorrhage, extravasation of urine, and permanent damage to renal function.
- *Bladder trauma* is less common than renal trauma; frequently associated with fracture of the pelvis.

### b. Multidisciplinary Approaches
- Cystogram; may be done for definitive diagnosis
- IV fluids/blood
- Surgical treatment generally indicated for renal lacerations, rupture and fragmentation; may be indicated for bladder trauma
- Urinary catheterization

# Additional Nursing Care That Can Be Incorporated into the Generic Care Plan

### a. Assessment
- Flank or abdominal pain
- Hematuria
- Palpable flank mass
- Inability to void with severe bladder trauma

### b. Goal
Child's urine output will return to normal.

### c. Interventions
- Inspect child for bruises, contusions, masses, etc.
- Monitor every 1–4 hours
  - urine output
  - BUN and creatinine levels for signs of renal failure
  - vital signs
  - Hct and Hgb
- Measure abdominal girth daily.
- Provide catheter care per hospital protocol.

    **d.**  **Evaluation**
- —  Child's urine is free from blood, WBCs; Hct and Hgb are within normal limits; abdominal girth is stable.

## Other Possible Nursing Diagnoses

Activity intolerance
Alteration in comfort: pain
Alteration in tissue perfusion

## 2.  Nephrotic Syndrome

    **a.**  **Definition:**   Increased glomerular permeability resulting in massive plasma protein loss via urine.

    **b.**  **Etiology**
- —  Congenital nephrotic syndrome is caused by a recessive gene.
- —  Secondary nephrotic syndrome occurs after glomerular damage of known etiology (e.g., acute or chronic glomerulonephritis, systemic lupus erythematosus, drug toxicity).
- —  Minimal change nephrotic syndrome is ideopathic but often follows a nonspecific viral illness.

    **c.**  **Multidisciplinary Approaches**
- —  Corticosteroid therapy
- —  Cytoxan for children who are steroid resistant
- —  Diuretics (usually thiazides, but Spironolactone may be used with thiazides)
- —  Intravenous albumin
- —  Paracentesis

## Additional Nursing Care That Can Be Incorporated into the Generic Care Plan

    **a.**  **Assessment**
- —  Nutritional status
- —  Weight
- —  Skin (edema, breakdown)
- —  Respiratory function
- —  Hydration
- —  Abdominal girth
- —  Urinalysis (specific gravity, protein)

    **b.**  **Goal**
Child's urine will be free from protein.

c. **Interventions**
   - Provide small frequent meals with increased protein.
   - Monitor effects of prescribed fluid and sodium limits.
   - Examine urine for amount and protein every four hours
   - Measure abdominal girth daily.
   - Weigh child daily.

d. **Evaluation**
   - Child is free from edema around eyes, abdomen, extremities, and/ or scrotum; weight was lost during diuresis.
   - Child's urine tests negative for protein on dipstick.

## Other Possible Nursing Diagnoses

Alteration in nutrition: less than body requirements
Disturbance in self-concept: body image
Fluid volume excess
Impairment of skin integrity
Ineffective breathing patterns

## 3. Acute Renal Failure (ARF)

a. **Definition:** Sudden and potentially reversible loss of kidney function

b. **Etiology**
   - Prerenal (outside kidney)
     - loss of blood or body fluid
     - circulatory inadequacy (e.g., CHF)
     - peripheral vasodilation
   - Renal (damage to kidney)
     - renal disease
     - tubular dysfunction
     - vascular occlusion
     - hypoxia
   - Postrenal (urinary tract obstruction)
     - stones or crystals
     - strictures
     - tumors

c. **Multidisciplinary Approaches**
   - Prevention by adequate hydration of children at risk and/or cautious use of nephrotoxic drugs
   - Fluid replacement
   - Foley catheter
   - Diuretics (e.g., Mannitol, Lasix)
   - TPN as necessary
   - EKG monitoring

- Reduction of serum potassium
  - calcium gluconate
  - sodium bicarbonate
  - Kayexalate
- Phosphate binders (e.g., Amphojel, Basaljel)
- Dialysis

# Additional Nursing Care That Can Be Incorporated into the Generic Care Plan

a. **Assessment**
   - Serum electrolytes (especially $K^+$) and BUN
   - Weight
   - Urine (volume, specific gravity)
   - Vital signs (especially blood pressure)
   - PMI

b. **Goal**
   Child will regain normal renal function.

c. **Interventions**
   - Monitor
     - I&O hourly
     - heart rate hourly
     - for indications of electrolyte imbalances
     - for peripheral edema
   - Weigh child daily.
   - Teach child and family the importance of eating a limited amount of high quality protein (i.e., foods containing essential amino acids such as meat, milk).
   - Decrease child's tissue catabolism by decreasing stresses (thermal, emotional).
   - Provide low-potassium foods and fluids (e.g., canned fruits, apple or cranberry juice, refined cereals).

d. **Evaluation**
   - Child gradually regains normal renal function as evidenced by stable weight, lack of edema, normal BUN and creatinine.
   - Child and/or family can list foods permitted in child's diet, i.e., those with essential amino acids and low in potassium.

# Other Possible Nursing Diagnoses

Activity intolerance
Alteration in cardiac output
Alteration in family process
Alteration in nutrition, less than body requirements

Impairment of skin integrity
Sensory-perceptual alteration

# 4. Chronic Renal Failure

### a. Definition
- A progressive, irreversible deterioration of kidney function over a prolonged time in which more than 50% of nephrons have been destroyed by disease or injury.
- Results in fatal uremia without dialysis or kidney transplant.

### b. Etiology
- Urinary obstruction
- Congenital renal and urinary tract malformations (e.g., renal hypoplasia and dysplasia)
- Glomerular diseases (e.g., acute glomerulonephritis, systemic lupus erythematosus)
- Hereditary disorders (e.g., Alport's syndrome, polycystic kidney, congenital nephrotic syndrome)
- Renal vascular disorders (e.g., hemolytic uremic syndrome)
- Metabolic disease (e.g., diabetes)
- Nephrotoxic chemicals and drugs

### c. Multidisciplinary Approaches
- Low-protein diet (high quality proteins)
- Restriction of dietary phosphates
- Phosphorus binding agents (e.g., Amphojel)
- Medications
  - calcium
  - vitamin D
  - sodium bicarbonate
  - folic acid and iron
  - antihypertensives
  - antibiotics
- EKG
- Dialysis
- Renal transplant: an increasingly common therapeutic measure for treatment of chronic renal failure in children. Selection criteria for transplant in children is fairly liberal. Most institutional transplant programs exclude children who
  - would require extensive continual custodial care for mental retardation
  - have metastatic cancer
  - have active systemic fungal infection
  - have a multisystem disease.

    Young children usually have the graft placed in their abdomen. Older children have it placed in the extraperitoneal space. The child's own kidneys are usually left in place. Rejection of the transplanted kidney is the major complication. There are 3 types of rejection

- *hyperacute:* occurs immediately due to an antibody antigen reaction; irreversible
- *acute:* occurs in the first few days through the first 6 months; usually responds to the administration of Solu Medrol
- *chronic:* occurs 6 or more months after transplant by a slow, but irreversible process

One of the major nursing implications for the care of children who have received a renal transplant is to protect them from infection. These children require careful monitoring for possible infections since they receive continuous immunosupressive therapy (usually Imuran and Prednisone) to counteract rejection.

## Additional Nursing Care That Can Be Incorporated into the Generic Care Plan

a. **Assessment**
   - Blood gases
   - Cardiac function
   - Edema
   - Level of consciousness
   - Nutritional status
   - Renal function (I&O, BUN, creatinine)
   - Skin
   - Vital signs
   - Weight

b. **Goal**
   Child will maintain fluid balance.

c. **Interventions**
   - Monitor diet: restrict foods high in
     - phosphorus (e.g., milk products)
     - proteins
     - sodium (crackers, commercially prepared soups, sodas, instant cereals, smoked meats)
     - potassium (nuts, bananas, oranges)
   - Monitor child for indications of impending seizures
     - blood pressure
     - electrolyte imbalance
     - level of consciousness
   - Regulate fluids per amount prescribed.
   - Monitor for signs of cardiac decompensation (e.g., tachycardia, PMI).

d. **Evaluation**
   - Child maintains a normal fluid balance as evidenced by

- BUN and creatinine within normal limits
- stable weight
- lack of edema
- vital signs within normal limits
- appropriate level of consciousness
- serum potassium within normal limits.

## Other Possible Nursing Diagnoses

Activity intolerance
Alteration in cardiac output
Alteration in family process
Alteration in nutrition: less than body requirements
Diversional activity deficit
Impairment in skin integrity
Knowledge deficit
Sensory-perceptual alteration
Social isolation
Powerlessness

## Bowel Elimination Management

Bowel elimination programs for the chronically disabled are very individualized. They vary greatly, and may involve the use of cathartics, enemas, laxatives, digital disimpaction, and dietary bulk. A careful history to determine what works best for the child is imperative. Failure to promote elimination may not be immediately damaging to health, but will result in discomfort, loss of regular pattern, and constipation or impaction. An uncomfortable autonomic response may be triggered. Symptoms of this include discomfort, diaphoresis, and lack of a sense of well-being.

## GENERIC CARE PLAN FOR THE NURSING DIAGNOSIS
## ALTERATION IN BOWEL ELIMINATION: CONSTIPATION

### 1. General Information

a. **Etiology**
- Immobility
- Intestinal obstruction
- Painful elimination
- Dietary intake
- Behavioral disorders

   **b. Clinical Manifestations**
- Colicky abdominal pain
- Distention
- Hypomotile bowel sounds
- Nausea
- Anorexia
- Failure to pass stools for prolonged periods of time (it is normal for some children to have as few as one or less stools per day)

   **c. Multidisciplinary Approaches**
- Enemas
- Stool softeners
- Therapeutic bowel regimen

## 2. Nursing Process

   **a. Assessment**
- Amount, color, consistency and characteristics of stool (e.g., hard, pellet-shaped, dry)
- Presence of fecal mucus, blood streaks, character of blood if present (e.g., bright red, occult)
- Passage of liquid stool accompanied by palpable fecal mass in abdomen (impaction)

   **b. Goal**
Child will eliminate soft stools on a regular basis.
Parents will verbalize safe methods of eliciting normal pattern.

   **c. Interventions**
- Perform digital examination of older children or insert a lubricated rectal thermometer in infants.
- Use gloves to manually remove stool (disimpaction).
- Continue usual long-term bowel regimens for children with chronic illness, physical, or neurologic disabilities.
- Encourage defecation at same time each day.
- Praise children in process of toilet training.
- Promote increased fluid (water and fruit juice) intake when not contraindicated.
- Provide dietary management with high-fiber foods (e.g., bran, whole wheat).
- Monitor effects of stool softeners, bulk agents, or mineral oil (older children), cathartics if ordered by MD, or enemas (lubricated and pediatric approved, e.g., Fleet, normal saline) if indicated for severe constipation.
- Caution parents regarding dangers of fluid and electrolyte imbalance if enemas are used excessively.

   **d. Evaluation**
- Child passes softer stools without undue anxiety or discomfort.

      – Child develops regular defecation pattern.
      – Parents state dangers of overuse of cathartics, mineral oil, or enemas.

**e.  Possible Related Nursing Diagnoses**
Anxiety
Disturbance in self-concept: body image
Self-care deficit: toileting
Impaired physical mobility
Fluid volume deficit
Alteration in nutrition, less than body requirements (for high-fiber foods)

# Selected Health Problem Frequently Associated with the Nursing Diagnosis ALTERATION IN BOWEL ELIMINATION: CONSTIPATION

## Intussusception

**a.  Discussion**
      – Obstruction can occur in any area of the GI tract but is most common in the intestines.
      – One kind of obstruction seen almost exclusively before age 2 is intussusception, the folding back or telescoping of one portion of intestine onto another.

**b.  Multidisciplinary Approaches**
      – Therapeutic barium enema; usually resolves the obstruction completely
      – NG tube is sometimes necessary
      – Surgical treatment when barium enema fails, child goes into shock, or bowel perforates

## Additional Nursing Care That Can Be Incorporated into the Generic Care Plan

**a.  Assessment**
      – Colicky abdominal pain
      – Nausea and vomiting
      – Constipation
      – Abdominal distention
      – Symptom progression depends on the location of the obstruction
      – Listlessness

- Dehydration
- "Currant jelly" stools
- Palpable mass in the RUQ

b. **Goal**
Child's pattern of bowel elimination returns to normal.

c. **Interventions**
- Prepare child for barium enema and possible surgical intervention.
- Monitor effects of replacement fluids and blood products if necessary.
- Monitor NG output.
- Measure abdominal girth daily.

d. **Evaluation**
- Child
    • passes a normal brown formed stool.
    • is free from abdominal distention or cramping.

## Other Possible Nursing Diagnoses

Alteration in comfort: pain
Alteration in nutrition: less than body requirements
Fluid volume deficit
Parental anxiety
Potential for injury: infection

## GENERIC CARE PLAN FOR THE NURSING DIAGNOSIS
# ALTERATION IN BOWEL ELIMINATION: DIARRHEA

1. **General Information:** Diarrhea is particularly significant in the pediatric population because of children's susceptibility to dehydration following the loss of fluids and electrolytes through the GI tract.

a. **Etiology**
- Gastroenteritis
- Antibiotic therapy
- Ingestion of toxins
- Food/formula allergy

b. **Clinical Manifestations**
- Abdominal pain and cramping
- Urgency

- Increased frequency of bowel sounds and stools
- Loose, liquid, green or yellow-green stools
- Ring of water around stool in diaper

c. **Multidisciplinary Approaches**
- NPO status
- In cases of severe diarrhea, bowel rest is indicated.
- IV therapy; hydration takes precedence over nutrition initially. IV fluids do not, however, provide all nutrients and cannot therefore be used for more than a few days.
- Fluid orders may be written "IV/PO on sliding scale," which means the IV rate will decrease as more is taken by mouth.
- Dietary therapy

## 2. Nursing Process

a. **Assessment**
- General symptoms of dehydration (see page 169)
- Frequency, amount, color, characteristics of stool

b. **Goal**
Child will have formed stool at expected frequency for usual pattern and dietary intake.

c. **Interventions**
- When diarrhea has decreased, advance (as ordered and as tolerated) to a clear liquid diet.
  - infants may take 5% glucose water or special electrolyte preparations such as Pedialyte or Lytren; plain, sterilized water will not provide calories or electrolytes and should not be used
  - give older children weak tea, flat soda, gelatin or gelatin water, broths, flavored ices, and ice popsicles. NOTE: avoid red dye products if hematesting the stool; red dyes cause false positive readings
  - offer 15–30 cc clear liquid at first, advancing to "ad lib" as tolerance is noted
  - offer breast-feeding to breast-fed infants since breast milk is easily digested
- As the infant/child tolerates clear liquids
  - for the infant on formula, advance only to half-strength formula (mix 1 part formula to 1 part sterile water, glucose water, or clear electrolyte preparation as ordered)
  - for the infant who has been on foods and older children, advance to a BRAT diet (bananas, rice, applesauce, and toast with no butter); these foods are very easy to digest; continue clear liquids with the BRAT diet
- As the BRAT diet is tolerated
  - advance the child gradually to a regular diet, avoiding known irritating foods (e.g., high-bulk foods, spicy foods, caffeine, and milk)

         – advance the formula-fed infant to full-strength formula but give a soy-based formula for a few days before resuming the regular formula since lactose intolerance is sometimes a postdiarrhea problem in infants

**d. Evaluation**
- Child eliminates stools that are normal in number and consistency for 24 hours.

**e. Possible Related Nursing Diagnoses**
Alteration in nutrition: less than body requirements
Fluid volume deficit
Impaired skin integrity

# Selected Health Problem Frequently Associated with the Nursing Diagnosis ALTERATION IN BOWEL ELIMINATION: DIARRHEA

## Ileostomy/Colostomy

**a. Etiology**
- Congenital anomalies (e.g., gastroschisis, intestinal atresias)
- Bowel ischemia (e.g., volvulus, necrotizing enterocolitis)
- Trauma
- Chronic inflammatory bowel disease

**b. Multidisciplinary Approaches**
- Bowel antiseptics (e.g., Neomycin)
- NG tube
- Enterostomal therapist or CNS
- Dietary consultation

# Additional Nursing Care That Can Be Incorporated into the Generic Care Plan

**a. Assessment**
- Preoperatively
  - nutritional status
  - acceptance of need for ostomy
  - financial status
  - parent/child knowledge of procedure
  - health (presence of sepsis, shock)
  - hydration
- Postoperatively
  - stoma

- parent/child knowledge of stoma care, diet, and activity
- acceptance of change in body image

**b. Goal**
Child is able to eliminate solid wastes effectively.

**c. Interventions**
- Preoperatively
  - cleanse bowel by oral, IV, or rectal administration of antibiotics as ordered
  - record I&O
  - monitor vital signs
  - explain preoperative procedures to child and family
  - allow child to tour recovery room and ICU if possible and if indicated
  - show child and family ostomy appliances
  - allow child to manipulate equipment
  - allow young child to use dolls or puppets with "ostomies"
- Postoperatively
  - observe site for bleeding, drainage, and color
  - change dressings as needed to prevent skin breakdown
  - apply occlusive ointment (e.g., Karaya, Stomahesive) around stoma site if it is draining
  - apply ostomy bag to site to collect drainage when appropriate
  - empty bag frequently
  - encourage child and family to observe, then assist with, and finally to perform stoma care
  - arrange a visit from another child with a stoma

**d. Evaluation**
- Preoperatively
  - bowel is clean.
  - child is hydrated (skin turgor good, I&O balanced).
  - child and family state reason for surgery and describe appliances.
- Postoperatively
  - no bleeding or maceration at stoma site
  - parent and/or child demonstrate appropriate stoma care.

# Other Possible Nursing Diagnoses

Disturbance in self-concept: body image
Impairment of skin integrity

# Reference

Brogna, L., & Lakaszowski, M. (1986). The continent urostomy. *American Journal of Nursing, 86*(2), 160–163.

# CHAPTER 7

# ACTIVITY-EXERCISE
## FUNCTIONAL HEALTH PATTERN

T he activity-exercise functional health pattern covers exercise, activity, and diversional activity or play. In childhood these activities are vital as the child grows and develops increasing ability or skill. Cardiopulmonary function assumes major importance in childhood since a deficit in cardiac or respiratory functions influences all areas of a child's growth and development. Immobility can be a major influence on children's adjustment to hospitalization. Play or diversional activity is not only important in the formation of the child as a complete person, but is often the best way to prepare a child for unpleasant hospital experiences.

## Cardiopulmonary Arrest—Basic and Advanced Life Support

Most situations requiring cardiopulmonary resuscitation (CPR) in children are preventable. Frequent causes include airway obstruction secondary to a foreign body, smoke inhalation, drowning, trauma—with chest injuries and/or hypovolemia—secondary to motor vehicle accidents. Children are anatomically and physiologically different from adults and some adaptation of CPR technique is necessary. Every apneic child requires airway management and ventilatory assistance. If bag and mask resuscitation with 100% oxygen does not initiate respiration, intubation is needed. Use an uncuffed endotracheal tube in children under eight. Use a straight laryngoscope blade size 0 for newborns, size 1 or 2 for infants or young children.

The primary aims of emergency drug therapy are 1) correction of hypoxemia, acidosis, and hypotension and 2) cardiac acceleration. Many of the same drugs are used for both children and adults. Some however, are more effective

205

for one age group or the other (see table 7.1 for the drugs most commonly used in pediatric code situations). Every ER and treatment room should have dosage charts by weight prominently displayed in the pediatric area.

**Table 7.1**    Drugs Most Commonly Used in Pediatric Codes

| Drug | Indication | Dose | Frequency | Maximum Dose | How Supplied |
|------|-----------|------|-----------|--------------|--------------|
| Atropine | Bradycardia | .01–.03 mg/kg | Once | — | 0.1 mg/ml |
| Sodium bicarbonate | Metabolic acidosis | 102 mEq/kg *Titrate according to ABGs* | Every 5 minutes | 50 mEq | 1 mEq/ml (pediatric dilute preparation available) |
| Calcium chloride* ** | Low cardiac output | 2.5 mg/kg 0.2–0.3 ml/kg | Every 10 minutes | 300 mg | 100 mg/ml |
| Calcium gluconate** | Low cardiac output | 30–100 mg/kg | Every 10 minutes | 100 mg/ml | |
| Dextrose 25% | Low glucose | 2 ml/kg | Every 15 minutes | — | As 50% solution; must be diluted. |
| Epinephrine | Bradycardia | 0.1 ml/kg | Every 4–5 minutes | 5–10 ml | Use 1:10,000 solution. |

*Calcium chloride is very caustic to veins and given only via central lines in children.
**Efficacy of calcium is not proven; check current protocols.

(Chameides, Melker, Raye, Todres, & Viles, 1983)

Defibrillation is useful only in the presence of ventricular fibrillation, which is uncommon in children.

- Paddle diameter
  - 4.5 cm (infants/toddlers)
  - 8.0 cm (older children)
- Position: same as that for adults; take care that there is no "bridge" of conducting gel between paddles.
- Joules: 2 joules/kg initial defibrillation; double the dose if that is ineffective (Chameides, Melker, Raye, Todres, & Viles, 1983)
  OR
  - first attempt: 2 watt/seconds/kg
  - second attempt: 4 watt/seconds/kg
  - third attempt: 8 watt/seconds/kg

## Cardiopulmonary Resuscitation

1. **Establish airway**
   - Do not hyperextend the neck since it will occlude an infant's airway.
   - Suspect foreign body obstruction in unmonitored pediatric arrests (see *Foreign Body Aspiration,* page 243).

- Use "sniffing position" in children under age five to open the airway. Pull the child's chin up and slightly forward. Slightly extend the neck by placing the head back. A small roll can be placed under the child's shoulders to keep the neck from flexing.
- Use head tilt/chin lift for older children.

2.  **Ventilate**
    - Without ET tube
      - give small puff of air into infant's nose *and* mouth
      - cover only the mouth of an older child, pinch nostrils shut
      - observe for chest rising
    - With ET tube
      - use appropriate bag-valve devices
      - humidify air to prevent obstruction by dried secretions

3.  **Assist circulation (cardiac compression)**
    - After airway is established and ventilation is initiated, assess for presence of effective circulation. Because the infant's carotid pulse is difficult to palpate, use the brachial pulse. If no pulse is present, continue ventilation and initiate cardiac compression.
    - Cardiac compression technique in infants and children differs from that of adults due to the position of the heart within the chest, smaller chest size, and faster normal pulse rates (American Heart Association, 1980):
      - *infants:* area of compression is midpoint of line drawn from nipple to nipple. Use two or three fingers to compress the chest ½–1 inch, at the rate of 100 compressions/minute. For extra support, the hand not being used in compression may be placed under the child's back. Ventilate after every fifth compression.
      - *children*: area of compression is one to two fingers above sternal notch. Use the heel of one hand (keeping the fingers off the chest) to compress the chest 1–1½ inches, at the rate of 80/minute. Ventilate after every five compressions.

4.  **Evaluate effectiveness of interventions**
    - Following intubation, equal breath sounds should be heard bilaterally.
    - Presence of peripheral pulses, pupils of normal size, and return of normal skin color signal return of adequate cardiac functioning.

# Cardiorespiratory Monitoring

Cardiorespiratory monitors may be exceptionally helpful for early detection of problems, but should not replace clinical assessment. Routinely auscultate heart and breath sounds and make sure that the auscultated rates are synchronous with monitor readouts. Cardiac monitors are especially useful for observing children receiving vasoactive drugs, such as an aminophylline bolus or an isuprel nebulization.

**Monitors.**    Most health care facilities use the traditional three-wire ECG lead. For apnea monitoring, a two-lead approach is used sometimes. Lead wires may be attached to pregelled electrodes or strapped around the chest (in infants) with a foam and Velcro band.

**Three-Electrode Monitors.**    In traditional three-electrode placement, location of the leads depends on the weight of the child and the type of breathing.

Chest breather

- Right leg electrode near 6th or 7th intercostal space on right midclavicular line
- Left arm electrode near 6th or 7th intercostal space on left midclavicular line
- Right arm electrode wire near atrium or below right clavicle

Abdominal breather

- Right arm electrode directly under right clavicle
- Place left arm and right leg electrodes opposite each other at level of maximum respiration

Infants weighing less than 2.5 kg

- Right arm electrode directly under right clavicle
- Right leg electrode wire beneath right arm electrode
- Left arm electrode wire near 6th or 7th intercostal space on left midclavicular line
- Any spot that will give a reasonable trace on the oscilloscope

---

**NURSING TIPS**
- **If the monitor does not pick up a clear ECG tracing or strong, regular indication of a QRS complex, change the electrodes. If problem persists, change the lead wires and/or cable.**
- **Determine alarm limits, based on the child's age and underlying pathology. For example, a child with a pacemaker set at a rate of 100 should have the lower cardiac alarm limit at about 99 or 100 as that is considered a safe rate by that child's physician. The lower limit should not be set at the lower end of the range of normal for the age group.**
- **Alarm limits should be checked and tested for function at the beginning of each shift.**

## GENERIC CARE PLAN FOR THE NURSING DIAGNOSIS
## ALTERATION IN CARDIAC OUTPUT: DECREASED

### 1. General Information

  a. **Etiology**
   - Cardiac dysfunction (e.g., congestive heart failure, congenital heart disease, acquired heart disease)
   - Respiratory disorders
     - cor pulmonale
     - asthma
   - Other disorders
     - endocrine (e.g., adrenocortical deficiency, diabetes mellitus)
     - hematologic (e.g., polycythemia, anemia)
     - fluid and electrolyte disorders

  b. **Clinical Manifestations**
   - Low blood pressure
   - Tachycardia
   - Irritability
   - Cyanosis
   - Dyspnea
   - Dysrhythmias
   - Edema
   - Cough

  c. **Multidisciplinary Approaches**
   - Medications
     - diuretics
     - digoxin
     - sedation (usually morphine sulfate 0.1 mg/kg) as needed
   - Oxygen
   - Surgery
     - palliative, e.g., pulmonary artery banding, shunt procedures
     - corrective (one or more surgeries)

### 2. Nursing Process

  a. **Assessment**
   - General appearance: color, position of comfort, facial expression, respiratory effort, level of activity, responsiveness to environment
   - Tachycardia, tachypnea, moist grunting respirations, orthopnea, paroxysmal nocturnal dyspnea (PND)
   - Location and depth of retractions
   - Signs of venous engorgement
     - periorbital edema
     - hepatomegaly

- Decreased urine output, diaphoresis
- Abnormal heart sounds, rhythm; pulsus alternans
- Prolonged feeding times followed by vomiting, irritability
- Cool and clammy skin that is mottled, with poor capillary refill
- Serum electrolytes
- Dose of digoxin for weight, serum digoxin levels

**b.  Goals**

Child's
- cardiac function will be improved as demonstrated by an increase in the force of contraction, decrease in heart rate, and increased renal perfusion.
- respiratory rate will be within normal range, and free from retractions, grunting, orthopnea, or PND.

Child will
- achieve adequate rest with age-appropriate sleep pattern.
- have adequate nutritional intake without excessive fatigue.

Child/parents will be able to describe the disease, reasons for treatments used, and how they will care for child after discharge.

**c.  Interventions**
- Maintain bedrest in semi-Fowler's position; preserve body temperature by use of blankets, warmer, Isolette, or hyperthermia blanket as necessary.
- Avoid restrictive clothing or restraints around abdomen and chest.
- Organize nursing activities to allow for uninterrupted periods of sleep.
- Provide humid atmosphere (vaporizer, mist tent, or hood).
- Perform percussion, vibration, postural drainage, and suction as needed and as tolerated.
- Administer digoxin loading and maintenance doses as ordered; hold if apical rate less than 100/minute in infant, less than 80/minute in older child; compare dose calculation with another staff member before giving medication.
- Assess for signs of digoxin toxicity, such as bradycardia, loss of appetite, nausea, vomiting, and diarrhea.
- Record I&O; note all sources of fluid loss (e.g., diaphoresis, fever, elevated respiratory rate).
- Note time and response to diuretics.
- Have child urinate prior to bedtime, if possible.
- Maintain fluid restriction if imposed (carefully calculated to avoid dehydration).
- Feed small amounts when hungry according to wake and sleep patterns, if possible, to avoid stress (every 2–3 hours); consider gavage feeding if respiratory rate of infant is greater than 60/minute, or oral intake is less than 2 oz over an hour.
- Provide formulas with higher calorie count per ounce.

- Encourage parents to stay with child and to participate in care as much as possible to decrease child's anxiety and therefore decrease cardiac workload.
- Counsel parents regarding child's activity and possible activity restrictions; teach child and parent the knee-chest or squatting position to facilitate breathing.

**d. Evaluation**
- Child's heart rate decreases, peripheral pulses become stronger.
- Child
  - eliminates excess fluid.
  - has clear, unlabored respirations without use of accessory muscles.
  - has adequate rest, is as comfortable as possible, neither lethargic nor irritable.
  - ingests sufficient fluids and calories to meet metabolic needs (Whaley & Wong, 1983; Hazinski, 1984).

---

**NURSING TIP: Parent Teaching: Discuss disease process, therapies used, and how child will be cared for at home. To evaluate, have parents describe home care, medications, how they are taken, their side effects, and when to call the doctor.**

---

**e. Possible Related Nursing Diagnoses**
Activity intolerance
Anxiety
Fluid volume deficit
Fluid volume excess
Impaired gas exchange
Ineffective breathing pattern
Knowledge deficit

# Selected Health Problems Frequently Associated with the Nursing Diagnosis ALTERATION IN CARDIAC OUTPUT: DECREASED

## 1. Congenital Cardiac Anomalies, Preoperative

**a. Discussion**
The incidence of congenital cardiac anomalies is approximately 8–10 of every 1,000 live births (Whaley & Wong). Although there is much in

the recent literature linking certain forms of congenital cardiac anomalies with specific teratogens or genetic factors, most congenital cardiac anomalies are the result of a complex interaction of genetic and environmental factors.

Years ago the anatomic complexity of many cardiac defects were prohibitive of long survival, and generally only supportive therapy was recommended. Recently, pioneers in surgery have sought to palliate and, in many centers, now attempt physiologic repair of complex congenital heart anomalies. Cardiac surgery pertains to both open- and closed-heart procedures for the palliation and correction of congenital heart defects. Closed-heart procedures may be accomplished through a thoracotomy or modified thoracotomy. Open-heart procedures include the use of cardiopulmonary bypass (i.e., the use of the "heart-lung" machine to divert the blood from the operative site and oxygenate the body while the heart is being repaired and deep hypothermia to reduce the body's oxygen needs).

Common complications of cardiac surgery include
- Respiratory insufficiency following pulmonary artery banding
- Hemorrhage (more likely with pre-op cyanosis and compensatory polycythemia)
- Cardiac tamponade
- Postpericardiotomy syndrome: fever, leukocytosis, pericardial friction rub, pericardial or pleural effusion
- Conduction disturbances: heart block, dysrhythmias
- Thoracotomy-associated problems: chylothorax, phrenic nerve paralysis
- Leaks of baffle, conduit, anastamosis sites; valve malfunction
- Low cardiac output
- Congestive heart failure (CHF)
- Thromboembolus, cerebrovascular accidents

## Acyanotic Defects

1.  **Atrial Septal Defect (ASD):** an opening between the right and left atrium

    *Classification*
    - Ostium primum
      • the most common
      • occurs low in the atrial septum just above the tricuspid valve
      • incomplete form of the endocardial cushion defect
    - Ostium secundum
      • located in the center of the atrial septum
    - Sinus venosus
      • located high in the septum
      • involves anomalous drainage of right pulmonary veins into the right atrium

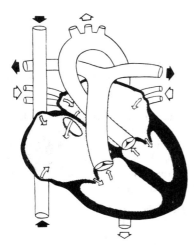

**Figure 7.1**    Atrial Septal Defect

*Hemodynamics*
– Pressure in the left atrium is higher than in the right atrium therefore blood is shunted from the left atrium, through the septal defect, to the right side of the heart
– Congestive heart failure is not common because the pressure increase on the pulmonary circulation is small

*Management*
– Treatment of congestive heart failure
– Primary or patch closure of the defect using cardiopulmonary bypass
– Atrial umbrella
    • eliminates the need for corrective surgery for ostium secundum
    • during cardiac catheterization a catheter is advanced from the right atrium into the left atrium through the septal defect
    • a patch graft with claws that adheres to the atrial wall is carefully placed over the defect
    • graft held in place by high left atrial pressure

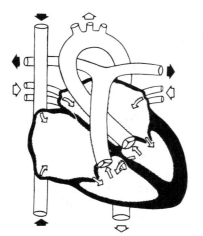

**Figure 7.2**    Ventricular Septal Defect

2.  **Ventricular Septal Defect (VSD):** an opening between the right and left ventricles

    *Hemodynamics*
    – Small defect
        • may be asymptomatic
        • may close spontaneously
    – Large defect
        • increased pulmonary blood flow under high pressure resulting in pulmonary hypertension
        • CHF after 4–6 weeks of age

    *Management*
    – Asymptomatic children
        • treated conservatively
        • high incidence of spontaneous closure in the first two years of life

- Large defect
  - treatment of CHF
  - pulmonary artery banding: palliative procedure to reduce volume and pressure of pulmonary blood flow
  - repair is accomplished through patch or suture closure using cardiopulmonary bypass

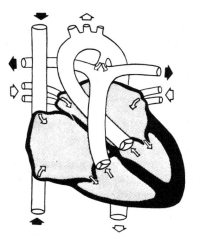

**Figure 7.3**    Patent Ductus Arteriosus

3. **Patent Ductus Arteriosus (PDA):** a persistence of the fetal ductus arteriosus beyond the perinatal period; occurs with increased frequency in premature and hypoxic infants

   *Hemodynamics*
   - Large PDA
     - permits a large aorta-to-pulmonary-artery shunt under high pressure
     - CHF may occur
   - Small PDA
     - less clinically significant
   - May be life saving in infants with cyanotic heart disease and compromised pulmonary blood flow

*Management*
- Medical: indomethacin (prostaglandin inhibitor); promotes ductus closure in neonates
- Surgical ligation and/or division through a left thoracotomy

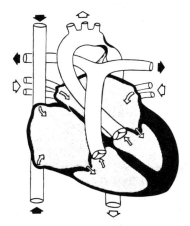

**Figure 7.4**    Coarctation of the Aorta

4. **Coarctation of the Aorta:** congenital constriction of the aorta

   *Classification*
   - Preductal, infantile type: narrowing of the aorta occurs proximal to the ductus arteriosus
   - Postductal, adult type: narrowing occurs distal to the ductus

   *Hemodynamics*
   - Constriction of the aorta reduces the amount of oxygenated blood to the descending aorta (lower extremities may be cyanotic)

- Preductal
  - severe CHF within hours or days of birth if the aortic arch is small
  - if the narrowing is in the arch of the aorta, there may be a difference of blood pressure between right and left arms
- Postductal
  - provides large resistance to flow
  - collateral vessels develop during fetal life
  - blood pressure in the upper extremities is increased
  - left ventricular hypertrophy
  - CHF may occur if coarctation is severe

### Management
- Excision of the narrowed aortic area
  - reanastomosed directly
  - closed using a patch
- Cardiopulmonary bypass may be used

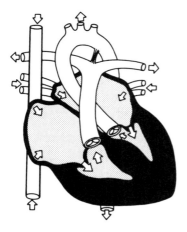

**Figure 7.5**   Aortic Stenosis

5. **Aortic Stenosis:** an obstruction of the aorta interfering with left ventricular outflow

### Classification
- Valvular stenosis (usually bicuspid)
  - the most common form
  - thickening and increased rigidity of the valve tissue
  - varying degrees of commisural fusion
  - obstruction to flow
- Supravalvular
- Subvalvular (subaortic) obstruction (due to fibrous ring or muscular obstruction)

### Hemodynamics
- Vary with the degree of obstruction
- Increased left ventricular pressure causes left ventricular hypertrophy
- Outflow into the aorta becomes extremely turbulent, producing loud murmurs and palpable thrills

### Management
- Valvular stenosis: aortic valvotomy
- Aortic valve replacement
  - subvalvular stenosis
    * excising the membrane or fibromuscular ring
    * possible enlargement of the entire left ventricular outflow tract and annulus

- supravalvular stenosis
  - \* excision of a discrete membrane if present
  - \* enlargement of the aorta with a prosthetic patch if the area is extensive

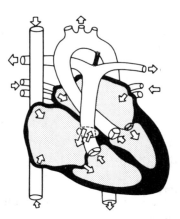

**Figure 7.6**    Endocardial Cushion
Defect

6. **Endocardial Cushion Defect:** improper fusion of the endocardial cushions during fetal development so that the right and left atrioventricular orifices are not correctly formed

   *Classification*
   - Ostium primum
     - defect low in atrial septum
   - Complete atrioventricular (AV) canal
     - common AV septal defect
     - severe mitral insufficiency

   *Hemodynamics*
   - Ostium primum: similar to an atrial septal defect
   - Complete AV canal
     - left-to-right shunt of blood
     - increased pulmonary blood flow
   - If ventricular defect is large
     - CHF
     - right and left ventricular hypertrophy

   *Management*
   - Pulmonary artery banding if CHF occurs
   - Definitive repair
     - patch closure of ASD and VSD on cardiopulmonary bypass
     - possible mitral valve replacement
     - possible division of common AV valves

# Cyanotic Defects

1. **Tetralogy of Fallot:** a lack of development of the subpulmonary conus during fetal life producing pulmonary infundibular stenosis and malalignment of the conal septum (Castaneda & Norwood, 1981). Includes four associated defects:
   - Pulmonary infundibular stenosis
   - Ventricular septal defect
   - Overriding aorta
   - Right ventricular hypertrophy

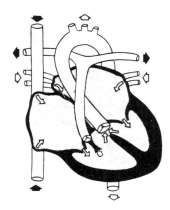

**Figure 7.7**   Tetralogy of Fallot

*Hemodynamics*
– Mild stenosis (vary depending on severity of obstruction of pulmonary flow)
  • minimal right-to-left shunting of blood
  • cyanosis
– Severe stenosis
  • decreased pulmonary blood flow
  • right-to-left shunting of blood
  • cyanosis
  • hypoxemia

*Management*
– Palliative: aortopulmonary shunt
– Corrective
  • closure of the ventricular septal defect
  • resection of the pulmonary stenosis
  • possible patch enlargement of the pulmonary outflow tract

2. **Hypoplastic Left Heart Syndrome:** a constellation of defects including
   – Aortic valve atresia associated with mitral atresia or stenosis
   – Diminutive or absent left ventricle
   – Severe hypoplasia of the ascending aorta and aortic arch (Norwood, Lang, & Hansen, 1983)

*Hemodynamics*
– Resistance to flow into the aorta
– Inadequate perfusion of the systemic circulation
– Flow of blood from the pulmonary artery through the ductus arteriosus supports life

*Management*
– Prostaglandin $E_1$ to keep the ductus arteriosus open
– Surgical repair
  • stage I (infancy)
    * reconstruction of the diminutive ascending aorta and aortic arch
    * systemic artery-to-pulmonary artery shunt
    * creation of large ASD
  • stage II (early toddler period)
    * removal of systemic artery-to-pulmonary artery shunt
    * anastamosis of the right atrium to the pulmonary arteries
    * insertion of an interatrial baffle to connect the left atrium to the right ventricle via the atrial septal defect

- Other options
  - heart transplantation; limited due to small number of donor hearts

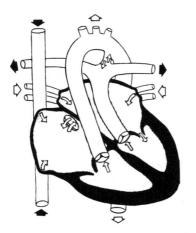

**Figure 7.8**   Transposition of the Great Arteries

3. **Transposition of the Great Arteries:** the aorta arises from the right ventricle and the pulmonary trunk arises from the left ventricle

*Hemodynamics*
- Unoxygenated systemic venous blood enters the right heart and aorta and returns to the systemic circulation and oxygenated pulmonary venous blood enters the left heart and pulmonary artery and is returned to the lungs resulting in severe systemic arterial hypoxemia
- A communication such as a VSD, ASD, and/or PDA must exist between the two circulations to allow survival

*Management*
- Palliative
  - Rashkind balloon atrioseptostomy via a cardiac catheterization
  - pulmonary artery banding
  - Blalock-Hanlon septectomy
- Corrective
  - Mustard procedure
    * excision of the atrial septum
    * use of a pericardial baffle to redirect venous return
  - Senning repair
    * similar to Mustard procedure
    * the atrial septum is preserved and utilized
  - the atrial switch procedure (performed during the first few weeks of life)
    * pulmonary artery and aorta are transected several millimeters above the semilunar valves
    * pulmonary artery is sutured to the stump of the aorta; the aorta is sutured to the stump of the pulmonary artery
    * the coronary arteries are detached from the aorta and reimplanted after the switch.
  - Rastelli procedure (if VSD or pulmonary atresia)
    * VSD closed with a baffle
    * pulmonary valve is sewn closed

* a conduit connects the right ventricle to the main pulmonary artery (Ng, 1983)

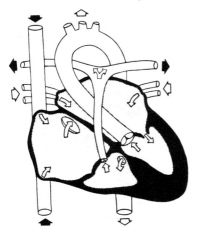

**Figure 7.9**    Tricuspid Atresia

4. **Tricuspid Atresia:** lack of formation of the tricuspid valve during fetal cardiac development preventing blood flow between the right atrium and right ventricle

    *Hemodynamics*
    − All systemic venous blood must enter the left heart through a patent foramen ovale or an atrial septal defect
    − Pulmonary blood flow depends on left-to-right shunt through a ventricular septal defect, patent ductus arteriosus, or surgical shunt
    − CHF may be present
    − Cyanosis is usually severe

    *Management*
    − If the foramen ovale is too small to allow adequate right-to-left atrial shunting
    • Rashkind balloon septostomy
    • Blalock-Hanlon septectomy
− Pulmonary artery banding (when CHF is unresponsive to medical management)
− If severe hypoxemia is present
    • systemic-to-pulmonary artery shunt
    • Fontan procedure
        * connection of the right atrium to the main pulmonary artery
        * closure of other existing shunts
        * ideally performed when the child is school age to allow insertion of a large conduit

5. **Truncus Arteriosus:** inadequate division of the truncus arteriosus during fetal life resulting in a single, large great vessel arising from the ventricles and giving rise to the pulmonary systemic and coronary circulations; a ventricular septal defect is present since the truncal septum contributes to closure of the ventricular septum (Ng)

    *Classification*
    − Truncus arteriosus types I, II, III
        • direct branching of pulmonary arteries and aorta from common trunk
    − Truncus arteriosus type IV, or pseudotruncus

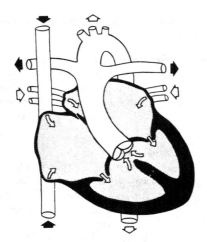

**Figure 7.10**   Truncus Arteriosus

- a single great vessel, the aorta, comes from the ventricles; blood enters this vessel through the ventricular septal defect from both right and left ventricles
- enlarged bronchial arteries and collateral vessels arising from the descending aorta carry unoxygenated and oxygenated blood to the lungs

*Hemodynamics*
- Types I, II, and III
  - both ventricles pump into a common trunk
    - increased pulmonary blood flow unless pulmonary stenosis is present
    - right and left ventricular hypertrophy
- Type IV
  - blood flow to the lungs is reduced and accomplished only through a patent ductus arteriosus or collaterial circulation

*Management*
- Types I, II, and III
  - pulmonary artery banding
  - closure of the VSD, insertion of a valved conduit using cardiopulmonary bypass
- Type IV
  - initial shunt procedures to increase pulmonary flow
  - closure of any associated septal defects and/or a PDA
  - establishment of blood flow from right ventricle to pulmonary artery via a valved conduit

6.  **Total Anomalous Pulmonary Venous Return:**   drainage of the pulmonary veins into the right atrium instead of into the left atrium; pulmonary veins may be attached directly to the right atrium or they may attach to a systemic vein above or below the diaphragm

*Hemodynamics*
- Oxygen saturation of blood in both right and left sides of the heart and the systemic circulation is the same
- Increased pulmonary blood flow because of the low resistance
- Right heart failure, systemic venous engorgement, pulmonary hypertension

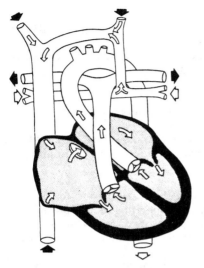

**Figure 7.11**   Total Anomalous Pulmonary Venous Return

*Management*
- Rashkind balloon septostomy to allow greater intra-atrial mixing and more flow to the systemic circulation
- Corrective surgery
  - anastomosis of the pulmonary veins to the left atrium
  - elimination of the anomalous pulmonary venous connection
  - closure of ASD

b.   **Multidisciplinary Approaches**
- Palliative or corrective surgery
- Medications
  - digoxin
  - diuretics
  - antidysrhythmics
- Child life therapist
- Social service
- Dietary management

# Additional Nursing Care That Can Be Incorporated into the Generic Care Plan

a.   **Assessment**
- General growth and development, motor and/or psychosocial skills, signs of developmental delay
- Exercise tolerance, required rest periods
- Baseline skin color, cyanosis
- Clubbing (especially thumbnails)
- Chest deformities (asymmetry)
- Baseline respiratory pattern, unusual rate, nasal flaring, grunting, retractions, or other irregularities
- Heart rate and rhythm and/or presence of murmurs
- Baseline vital signs including blood pressures and pulses in all four extremities
- Pattern and method of medication administration
- Nutritional status, tolerance of diet, growth pattern
- Parental concerns and level of understanding of child's condition, planned surgery
- Child's/parents' anxiety: observe child for anorexia, insomnia, crying and child/parent's subjective verbalization of fears and concerns

b. **Goals**

Child will be in optimal health for surgery (no sign of URI, viral syndrome or other infections, or CHF).

Child/parents will be able to describe what to expect preoperatively and postoperatively, if surgery is planned.

c. **Interventions**
   - Take vital signs every 4 hours and measure weight daily.
   - Allow child usual activity as tolerated.
   - Administer usual cardiac medications (when applicable) as ordered (some, such as digoxin, may be discontinued preoperatively); monitor effects.
   - Maintain diet as usual.
   - Provide pre-op teaching to child and/or parents including
     • tour of intensive care unit and operating room if possible
     • anesthesia npo orders and pre-op medications (oral or IM)
     • post-op pain control measures (medications, repositioning)
     • type of incision
     • pacer wires and pacemakers if planned
     • intubation, mechanical ventilation, and process of weaning to room air
     • use of cardiac/respiratory monitor
     • Foley catheter and its purpose
     • chest tubes (when necessary)
     • chest physical therapy measures such as percussion, vibration, postural drainage, endotracheal saline, and suctioning
     • arterial line/intravenous/central venous lines (including Swan-Ganz catheter, if planned)
     • level of consciousness immediately following surgery
     • slow diet progression as child recovers
   - Allow for and provide therapeutic play opportunities appropriate to child's age; see page 260.
   - Provide for a messenger ("go-between") for parents during intraoperative phase to report progress.

d. **Evaluation**
   - Child goes to surgery in best possible health status.
   - Family's anxiety is at level that promotes positive coping.
   - Parents and child (if developmentally appropriate) are able to verbalize expectations of the post-op course.
   - Family is able to cope with the child's decreased level of consciousness, multiple tubes and wires, and high technology environment post-op.

# Other Possible Nursing Diagnoses

Alteration in family process
Anxiety
Knowledge deficit

## Pediatric Respiratory Care

**Segmented Bronchial Drainage.**    Pediatric respiratory therapy involves many technologically advanced diagnostic and healing measures. Segmental bronchial drainage is a procedure utilizing gravity and physical maneuvers to stimulate movement of secretions in order to remove accumulated mucus and relieve airway obstruction. Children with respiratory problems caused by increased production of secretions, thick or sticky secretions, impaired removal of secretions, ineffective cough, or combinations of any of these factors can benefit from bronchial drainage.

As a preventive measure, it benefits those children with a predisposition for increased production or thickness of secretions and/or weakness of the muscles of respiration.

The positions to be used, as well as the frequency and duration of treatment, are individually prescribed. The lung segment to be drained is placed uppermost and the segmental bronchus leading to that segment is placed in as near a straight up-and-down position as possible to allow secretions to flow by gravity into larger airways. Maneuvers that help remove secretions from the walls of the airways and stimulate coughing include

- clapping with the cupped hand
- vibration
- deep breathing
- assisted coughing.

*Clapping* is done with the cupped hand on the chest wall over the segment to be drained. It stimulates vibrations that cause movement of secretions and may help loosen secretions sticking to the bronchial walls. Cup the hand by holding the fingers together so that the shape of the cupped hand conforms with the chest wall and traps a cushion of air, which softens the blow.

- Clapping should be vigorous, but not painful.
- Do not clap on bare skin.
- Do not administer clapping over seams or buttons.
- Remove rings before clapping.

Clapping is usually performed on the child by a therapist or a person trained in the technique. Older children, however, may be taught to self-administer the procedure.

*Vibration* is also a maneuver that helps to stimulate the flow of secretions. Press your hand firmly over the segment on the chest wall and tense the muscles of your upper arm and shoulder. Vibrate with a flattened, not cupped, hand. Perform vibration during exhalation, with the child saying "FFF" or "SSS." Exhalation should be as slow and as complete as possible. Various mechanical vibrators are available commercially, but not all physicians and respiratory therapists recommend their use.

*Deep breathing* assists in the movement of secretions and may stimulate coughing. An effective cough is an essential part of clearing the airways. A forced but not strained exhalation, following a deep inhalation, may move secretions and may stimulate a productive cough.

*Coughing* may be assisted by supporting the sides of the lower chest with the hands. This may decrease the strain of coughing and may increase its effectiveness.

**Suggestions for Bronchial Drainage.**   It is very important that the child receiving therapy and the therapist be comfortable during bronchial drainage. A substantial, firm, padded board or table can be inclined to the specific angle or height that is needed for drainage of the right middle lobe, lingular, and the basal segments of the lower lobes. Tables can be constructed to adjust to various angles or heights or can be obtained commercially. Tilt boards can be elevated at one end by placing blocks on the floor. Infants can be positioned in the therapist's lap with or without pillows.

Before beginning bronchial drainage, remove child's tight clothing. Have the child wear light, soft clothing, such as a T-shirt. Have an ample supply of tissues or a receptacle for disposal of expectorated secretions available.

Do bronchial drainage before meals or 1½–2 hours after eating to minimize the chance of vomiting. Early morning and bedtime sessions are usually best. Bronchial drainage before bedtime may reduce nighttime coughing by helping clear the airways of accumulated secretions. Work closely with respiratory therapists when they are providing bronchial drainage to schedule the most appropriate time for therapy.

Bronchial drainage is usually most effective as a treatment when done at least twice daily. Provide additional bronchial drainage during acute respiratory infections and in instances where the extent of disease requires it. For prevention, provide drainage once or twice daily.

**Oxygen Therapy.**   Prolonged oxygen administration may have toxic effects, particularly in infants. Oxygen should not be administered to any child unless a hypoxic situation exists, which is documented by serial blood gas determinations or less invasive techniques, such as transcutaneous capillary $O_2$ measurements. A physician's written order is required to administer oxygen to children in all but emergency situations.

- Do not administer oxygen over a prolonged period of time without humidification, as it may dry up secretions and parch respiratory mucous membranes.
- Sequelae of prolonged oxygen therapy include
  - reduced cerebral blood flow with neurologic damage
  - retrolental fibroplasia (RLF), which results in retinal detachment and varying degrees of blindness
  - progressive hypoxemia and decreased lung compliance
- Monitor concentrations of greater than 40% $FIO_2$ with an oximeter (including alarm), and in a setting where blood gases and other oxygenation parameters may be followed closely.
- When a child with or without an artificial airway has intermittent hyperinflation with suctioning, maintain the $FIO_2$ at the same percentage normally ordered for the child.

- For children receiving less than 40% $FIO_2$, such as in a tent or face mask, check the $O_2$ concentration with an oxygen analyzer every 2–4 hours.

When a child has an endotracheal tube, maintaining an airway is the number one nursing priority.

**Table 7.2**  Conditions Requiring Intubation

$PO_2$  less than 50 mm Hg on an $FIO_2$ of 80
$PCO_2$  greater than 50 mm Hg acutely
Decreased or absent cough and gag reflexes
Airway obstruction
Neuromuscular respiratory impairment/failure

**Table 7.3**  Neonatal/Pediatric Endotracheal Tube Guide

| Age | Size (Fr) | Internal Diameter (mm) | Length (mm) |
|---|---|---|---|
| Newborn (<1 Kg) | 11–12 | 2.5 | 10 |
| Newborn (>1 Kg) | 13–14 | 2.5–3.0 | 11 |
| 1–6 months | 15–16 | 3.0–4.0 | 11 |
| 6–12 months | 17–18 | 3.5–4.5 | 12 |
| 12–18 months | 19–20 | 4.0–5.0 | 13 |
| 18–26 months | 21–22 | 4.5–5.5 | 14 |
| 3–4 years | 23–24 | 5.0–6.0 | 16 |
| 5–6 years | 25–26 | 5.5–6.5 | 18 |
| 6–7 years | 26–27 | 6.0–7.0 | 18 |
| 8–9 years | 27–28 | 6.5–7.5 | 20 |
| 12–14 years | 32–34 | 7.5–8.5 | 24 |

Guideline for children over 2 years of age:

$$\text{Tube size} = \frac{\text{Age (years)}}{4} + 4.5$$

(Anton, 1984; Lough & Doershuk, 1980)

**Table 7.4**  Examples of Critical Airway Situations

Traumatic Tonsillectomies and Adenoidectomies
Pierre-Robin Syndrome
Tracheomalacea
Tracheostenosis
Congenital Tracheal Vascular Rings
Viral Croup
Epiglottitis

---

**NURSING TIP: Keep tracheotomy setups at the bedsides of children with critical airways in case obstruction occurs suddenly.**

---

**Inadvertent Extubation.**    Attempt repositioning or replacement of the endotracheal or tracheostomy tube but if it cannot be accomplished immediately and easily, completely remove the tube. Then establish ventilation by any means available. This may mean simple mouth-to-mouth or bag and mask with intermittent positive pressure ventilation.

## Indications for Extubation
1. Reversal of pathologic process
   - Pulmonary edema
   - Acute Respiratory Distress Syndrome (ARDS)
   - Infection
   - Shock
2. Clinical evidence of adequate cerebral function: awake, appropriate responses and reflexes
3. Evidence of effective pulmonary function and adequate gas exchange

Premature and unsuccessful attempts at weaning can have adverse psychologic effects on a child. Fear, anxiety, discouragement, low level frustration, and muscle deconditioning are major obstacles that interfere with a successful weaning process.

Respiratory care does not end when the child is extubated or successfully weaned from the ventilator. Continue close observation and therapeutic measures to prevent regression or acute exacerbation. Since many children have an ineffective epiglottic reflex after extubation, withhold oral fluids for 24 hours.

Factors increasing the chance of development of a postintubation croup include

- Age (increased chance in 1- to 4-year-olds)
- Traumatic intubation
- ETT that is too large
- Coughing with the ETT in place
- Changing the child's position or head movement in a way that causes pressure on the glottic area and/or trachea
- Lengthy duration of intubation

**Respiratory Suctioning.**    The need for tracheal suctioning is greatly dependent upon the ability to cough adequately. This can be evaluated by measuring the vital capacity (VC), the negative inspiratory force, and by judging the level of consciousness. Bronchial hygiene can be maintained without an artificial airway if there is an acceptable VC and the child is cooperative.

Suction children only when absolutely necessary, and not because orders for routine suctioning have been written. Such instances include
- Audible secretions
- Palpable rales
- Symptoms of obstruction
- Signs of hypoxia

Equipment needed
- Vacuum cannister setup or wall unit suction
- Soft plastic eye-droppers (for instillation of saline nose drops)
- Clean or sterile, unpowdered disposable gloves
- Sterile, normal saline (for artificial airways)
- Normal saline irrigation solution and paper cups
- Catheters with side holes approximately ½ diameter of artificial airways
  - infants: 6–8 French
  - children: 8–14 French

Pressure
- Nasal and oropharyngeal suctioning
  - neonates: 100 mm Hg
  - children: 150 mm Hg
- Artificial airway: no more than 150 mm Hg unless obstruction such as vomitus is present

Procedure
- Attach catheter to suction hose, leaving wrapper in place (keep sterile).
- Auscultate breath sounds.
- If artificial airway is present, instill sterile saline, and hyperinflate (10 breaths) if ordered
  - acutely ill children: use 1.0 $FIO_2$
  - chronically ill: child's normal $FIO_2$
- Put gloves on both hands, keeping one sterile (reduces cross contamination between patients and may prevent care giver infections such as herpetic Whitlow).
- Hold catheter so that natural curve follows airway or anatomic structures.
- Insert until child coughs or resistance is met.
- Draw catheter back 1 cm, then apply suction for no longer than 5–7 seconds.
- Change child's head position and repeat.
- Suction artificial airway first; then without changing catheters, suction oronasopharynx.
- Apply suction only as catheter is being withdrawn. Avoid "stabbing" or "jamming" catheter in and out repeatedly.
- Monitor child's clinical condition (e.g., heart rate, color) throughout procedure.
- Permit rest periods or hyperinflate between passes with the catheter.
- Flush connecting tubing with saline until clear.

- Remove gloves inside out with catheter tucked inside and discard.
- Wash hands.
- Record amount, color, consistency, odor of secretions, and frequency of the need for suctioning.

**Arterial blood gas sampling.**    Arterial blood gas sampling is one method of assessing oxygenation. The site of choice in a child is a superficial artery with good collateral circulation such as

- Radial artery
- Dorsalis pedis
- Brachial artery
- Superficial temporal artery
- Femoral artery

Know that prolonged crying may change the values; see table 7.5 for normal ranges and table 7.6 for primary blood gas classifications.

**Procedure**
- Lubricate barrel of syringe with heparin.
- Palpate chosen site with index and middle fingers.
- Clean the skin with povidone iodine and alcohol swab.

---

**NURSING TIP: Children do not respond well to infiltration of local anesthetics.**

---

- Enter artery in as parallel a fashion as possible to enhance arterial wall healing and avoid going completely through the artery.
- Put pressure on puncture site for at least five full minutes after obtaining sample, longer if patient has any coagulopathies.

**Table 7.5**    Normal Pediatric Arterial Blood Gas Values

|  | Infant | Older Infant | Child over 2 |
| --- | --- | --- | --- |
| pH | 7.30–7.40 | 7.30–7.40 | 7.35–7.45 |
| $PCO_2$ (mm Hg) | 30–35 | 30–35 | 35–45 |
| $PO_2$ (mm Hg) | 40–60 | 60–80 | 80–95 |
| Bicarbonate (mEq/liter) | 20–22 | 20–22 | 22–24 |

(Anton, 1984; Shapiro, 1975)

**Table 7.6**    Primary Blood Gas Classifications

| | pH | PACO$_2$ | HCO$_3$ or Base Excess | PAO$_2$ |
|---|---|---|---|---|
| *Primary Ventilatory Classifications* | | | | |
| Acute ventilatory failure | Decreased | Increased | Normal | Decreased |
| Chronic ventilatory failure | Normal | Increased | Increased | Decreased |
| Acute ventilatory insufficiency | Increased | Decreased | Normal | Decreased |
| Chronic ventilatory insufficiency | Normal | Decreased | Decreased | Decreased |
| *Primary Acid-Base Classifications* | | | | |
| Uncompensated acidosis | Decreased | Normal | Decreased | Normal |
| Uncompensated alkalosis | Increased | Normal | Increased | Normal |
| Partly compensated acidosis | Decreased | Decreased | Decreased | Normal |
| Partly compensated alkalosis | Increased | Increased | Increased | Normal |
| Compensated acidosis or alkalosis | Normal | Increased or decreased | Increased or decreased | Normal |
| Acidosis correction: mEq of bicarbonate to be infused = 0.3 x body weight (kg) x base deficit | | | | |

(Shapiro, 1975)

# GENERIC CARE PLAN FOR THE NURSING DIAGNOSIS
# INEFFECTIVE AIRWAY CLEARANCE

## 1.  General Information

### a.  Etiology
   — Foreign body aspiration
   — Bronchiolitis
   — Tracheobronchial infection or secretion (e.g., pneumonia, asthma, croup, CF)
   — Trauma

### b.  Clinical Manifestation
   — Abnormal breath sounds
   — Alterations in respiratory rate and/or rhythm
   — Fever
   — Cough
   — Cyanosis
   — Dyspnea
   — Retractions

- Lower airway (i.e., alveoli, bronchioles) pathology has a different symptom manifestation than upper airway (i.e., larynx, epiglottis) pathology (see table 7.7)

**Table 7.7**  Differences Between Upper and Lower Airway Obstruction by Observation

| Physical Sign | Upper Airway | Lower Airway |
|---|---|---|
| Voice | Hoarse* | Normal |
| Cough | Barking (croupy)* | Deep (hacking) |
| Sounds made during breathing | Stridor (high-pitched, crowing sound) more pronounced during inspiration than expiration | Wheezing (whistling sound) more pronounced during expiration than inspiration |
| Inspiratory/Expiratory ratio | Prolonged inspiratory phase | Prolonged expiratory phase |
| Chest retractions | Supraclavicular, suprasternal, and sternal retractions relatively pronounced | Intercostal and subcostal retractions relatively pronounced |
| Chest configuration | Normal | Increased anterior-posterior diameter |
| Respiratory rate | Less rapid (usually <60/minute) | Often very rapid (frequently >60/minute) |

*Hoarseness and barking cough are present only when vocal cords are involved. Children with epiglottitis are usually not hoarse.
(Waechter & Blake, 1976)

    c.  **Multidisciplinary Approaches**
- Diagnostic studies
  - chest x-ray
  - arterial blood gases
- Administration of bronchodilators, steroids, expectorants, $O_2$ therapy
- Insertion of a tracheostomy or endotracheal tube
- Chest physical therapy

## 2.  Nursing Process

    a.  **Assessment**
- Respiratory status, rate and pattern, abnormal breath sounds, and depth of respiration
- Frequency and effectiveness of cough and ability to handle secretions
- Signs of oxygen deficit (e.g., mottling, cyanosis)
- Signs of respiratory infection (e.g., increased TPR, presence of purulent sputum)

b.  **Goal**
Child will maintain a patent airway, clear of secretions.

c.  **Interventions**
    – Suction airway (trachea, mouth, nares) to remove secretions.
    – Keep head of bed elevated to facilitate breathing.
    – Change child's position at least every 2 hours to promote drainage of secretions.
    – Insert oral airway if necessary.
    – Encourage deep breathing and coughing every hour.
    – Monitor effect of croup tent if ordered to liquify secretions
        • ensure that tent is closed and tucked under bed
        • change wet clothes and linen promptly
        • ensure adequate misting in tent
    – Provide diversional activity and parental support to decrease child's anxiety.
    – Encourage fluids within prescribed restrictions.

d.  **Evaluation**
    – Child
        • has no signs of respiratory infection.
        • breathes easily without distress.
        • is free from mottling or cyanosis.
        • expectorates thin secretions.
        • has clear breath sounds.

e.  **Possible Related Nursing Diagnoses**
    Anxiety
    Fluid volume deficit
    Impaired gas exchange
    Ineffective breathing pattern

# Selected Health Problems Frequently Associated with the Nursing Diagnosis INEFFECTIVE AIRWAY CLEARANCE

## 1.  Cystic Fibrosis (respiratory complications)

a.  **Discussion:**  Respiratory obstruction occurs because of the thick, sticky, mucus plugs; atelectasis; and alveolar hyperinflation.

b.  **Multidisciplinary Approaches**
    – Diagnostic tests
        • pilocarpine iontophoresis (sweat test): a sweat chloride greater than 60 mEq/liter is considered diagnostic
        • chest x-ray

**Table 7.8** Some Common Childhood Respiratory Disorders

| Disorder | Onset | Fever | Tachypnea | Inspiratory Stridor | Prolonged Expiration | Wheezing | Specific Diagnostic Findings | Common Infectious Agents |
|---|---|---|---|---|---|---|---|---|
| Viral croup | Sudden | ± to + + | + + + | + + + | − | ± | "Barking sound" | Parainfluenza virus (66%), influenza adenovirus |
| Epiglottitis | Sudden | + + | + + + | + + + | − | ± | Child assumes sitting position; cherry-red epiglottis | H. influenza |
| Bronchiolitis | Progressive | ± to + + | + + + | − | + + + | + + + | − | Respiratory synctial virus, influenza |
| Pneumonia | Variable | ± to + + + | ± | − | ± | ± | − | Various viral and bacterial agents |
| Bronchial asthma | Sudden | ± | + + + | − | + + + | + + + | Rapid response to bronchodilators | − |
| Cystic fibrosis | Progressive | ± | + | − | + | + + | Sweat chloride = 60 mEq/liter | S. aureus and pseudomonas (2° invaders) |
| Tuberculosis | Progressive | ± | ± | − | ± | ± | + PPD test | M. tuberculosis |
| Foreign body | Sudden | ± | + | ± | ± | ± | Opaque foreign body on chest x-ray | |

(Kent, 1975)

Key (presence of symptoms):

- −    absent
- ±    absent or mild
- +    mild
- + +    moderate
- + + +    severe

- Medications
  - antibiotics
  - mucolytics, expectorants, or bronchodilators via aerosol
- Annual tuberculin testing

# Additional Nursing Care That Can Be Incorporated into the Generic Care Plan

a. **Assessment**
   - Chronic cough
   - Frequent throat clearing
   - Repeated bouts of bronchitis and bronchopneumonia or other respiratory infections
   - Dyspnea, grunting, flaring, retractions, pallor, cyanosis of lips and nails
   - Use of accessory muscles (which appear overdeveloped)
   - Presence of nasal polyps
   - Excessive, very thick sputum (observe for color, consistency, and send for culture and sensitivity)
   - Decreased breath sounds related to lung consolidation
   - Clubbing of fingertips
   - Barrel-shaped chest
   - Jugular venous distention (in older children)
   - Activity intolerance
   - Failure to thrive related to energy expenditure in breathing

b. **Goals**
   Child will
   - be assisted in clearing secretions and sputum.
   - actively participate in breathing exercises if developmentally capable.
   Parents will
   - perform percussion and postural drainage with vibration and suctioning according to the Cystic Fibrosis Foundation Guidelines.
   - accurately administer mucolytics and expectorants.
   - verbalize symptoms of deteriorating respiratory status and knowledge of when to notify physician.

c. **Interventions**
   - Assist with expectoration of sputum
     - administer mucolytics, expectorants, or bronchodilators as ordered via aerosol
     - perform chest physical therapy every 4 hours or more frequently during acute pulmonary exacerbation
     - encourage breathing exercises for developmentally capable children: diaphragmatic breathing, side bending, pursed lips breathing, playing a wind instrument, "blowing" games with feathers or ping pong balls

- Monitor blood levels of antibiotics (if on therapy).
- Provide protective isolation or at least guard child from contact with persons with symptoms of infectious diseases, particularly respiratory.
- Encourage ambulation and exercise as tolerated to discourage stasis pneumonia.
- Teach and involve all capable family members in above regimen.
- Involve school-age children in as much of self-care as stamina permits, including self-administered chest physical therapy.
- Encourage normal group and individual, age-appropriate activity.
- Discuss need for close pulmonary monitoring on an outpatient basis.
- Discuss with family the need to avoid cough suppressants and antihistamines.

**d. Evaluation**
- Child
  - breathes easily; skin color is pink, no cyanosis.
  - participates in "blowing" games; uses incentive spirometer, or other strategies.
- Parents use accurate and effective techniques in executing chest physical therapy.

# Other Possible Nursing Diagnoses

Alteration in family process
Alteration in nutrition: less than body requirements
Fluid volume deficit

## 2. Pneumonia

**a. Definition/Discussion**
- Acute inflammatory response in lower respiratory tract
- Alveoli fill with exudate (blood, serum, neutrophils, infectious organisms)
- Caused by chemicals, viruses, and bacteria (pneumococci, staphylococci, streptococci)
- Obstruction causes $O_2/CO_2$ diffusion difficulties

**b. Multidisciplinary Approaches**
- Diagnostic tests
  - CBC
  - sputum culture
  - chest x-ray
  - ABGs
- Antibiotics, expectorants
- Respiratory therapy

- Thoracentesis
- Chest tube insertion and closed chest drainage

# Additional Nursing Care That Can Be Incorporated into the Generic Care Plan

a. **Assessment**
   - Continuous cardiorespiratory monitoring
   - Presence of rales, rhonchi, wheezing, areas of consolidation, presence of retractions, nasal flaring
   - Chest pain, abdominal pain, pallor, or cyanosis
   - Position of comfort
   - Signs of dehydration
   - Sputum

b. **Goals**
   Child will be
   - adequately hydrated.
   - adequately rested with minimal anxiety and avoidance of excessive coughing.

c. **Interventions**
   - See CDC guidelines for isolation of respiratory infections, page 108.
   - Suction to maintain patent airway (especially in infant).
   - Provide chest physical therapy every 4 hours and prn; elevate head of bed; position for greatest comfort.
   - Provide cool, moist environment with oxygen, if indicated.
   - Provide bedrest; plan nursing activities to disturb as little as possible.
   - Minimize sources of anxiety.
   - Administer sedatives as ordered and encourage parents to stay with child when possible.
   - Maintain IV fluids as ordered.
   - Monitor I&O, daily weight, and urine specific gravity.
   - If oral feedings permitted, provide cautiously; if respirations are rapid during early acute phase, hold feedings to prevent possible aspiration.

d. **Evaluation**
   - Oral fluids are taken when respiratory rate permits; aspiration is avoided.
   - Child is adequately hydrated and urine output is at least 1 ml/kg/hour.
   - Child receives adequate rest.
   - Parents stay to help comfort child (Whaley & Wong).

## Other Possible Nursing Diagnoses

Anxiety
Fluid volume deficit
Potential for injury

## 3. Asthma/Bronchiolitis

a. **Definition/Discussion**
   - A fairly common condition characterized by paroxysmal smooth muscle spasms in the nonconducting small airways, increased mucus production and edema.
   - Bronchiolitis in the infant and younger child has pathophysiology similar to asthma. However, it is thought that bronchiolar smooth muscle is not well developed before 18 months. The diagnosis of asthma is generally not made in this age group.
   - Many people have the misconception that asthma is entirely a "psychologic" problem and are unaware of the pathophysiologic basis of the disease.
   - Children and families need to be able to recognize early signs of an asthmatic attach in order to prevent or minimize the attack.

b. **Multidisciplinary Approaches**
   - Bronchodilators, expectorants, corticosteroids, antibiotics for asthma
   - Pharmacologic treatment of bronchiolitis is minimal
   - Dietary therapy
   - Respiratory therapy
   - Occupational therapy

## Additional Nursing Care That Can Be Incorporated into the Generic Care Plan

a. **Assessment**    (use "asthma scoring" system, see table 7.9)
   - Rate and character of respirations, rales, rhonchi, retractions, inspiratory and expiratory effort, use of accessory muscles, grunting, flaring
   - Cyanosis, diaphoresis, hydration, speech patterns, poor capillary refill
   - $CO_2$ narcosis (anxiety or CNS depression)
   - Possible factors precipitating onset of condition
     • contact with allergens
     • history of allergic reactions
     • emotional factors
     • infection (viral or bacterial)
   - Diet, home, school, play environment for allergenic agents

- Medications taken at home, their benefits and side effects, and how often they are taken
- Use of aerosol medications
- Parent-child interactions

**Table 7.9**   Clinical Asthma Score

|  | 0 | 1 | 2 | Score |
|---|---|---|---|---|
| $PO_2$ | 70–100 in room air | 70 in air | 70 in 40% $O_2$ | |
| Cyanosis | None | In air | In 40% $O_2$ | |
| Inspiratory breath sounds | Normal | Unequal | Decreased to absent | |
| Use of accessory muscles | None | Moderate | Maximal | |
| Expiratory wheezing | None | Moderate | Marked | |
| Cerebral function | Normal | Depressed or agitated | Coma | Total Score |

A score of 5–6 indicates impending respiratory failure; notify MD; may require transfer to the ICU
A score of 7 with a $PCO_2$ of 65 mm Hg (except in chronic state) indicates respiratory failure requiring ventilatory support.
(Johns Hopkins Hospital)

   **b.  Goals**
Child will
- maintain patent airway with decrease in rate, free from rales, rhonchi, wheezes, inspiratory and expiratory effort.
- maintain adequate oxygenation as demonstrated by absence of pallor or cyanosis.
- remain calm and participate in activities of daily living.

Parents and child (if possible) will be able to
- describe signs and symptoms of an impending attack (increasing shortness of breath, orthopnea, diaphoresis, air gulping), measures to be taken to avoid an attack, and when to see an MD.
- describe proper administration of prophylactic medications, their side effects, and signs of toxicity.
- openly express their feelings about the disease, and realistically describe limitations on child's activity.

   **c.  Interventions**
- Position in high-Fowler's or sitting leaning forward.
- Use calm, reassuring approach, explaining procedures to child and parents.
- Administer IV fluid as ordered.
- Administer bronchodilators, corticosteroids, antibiotics and expectorants as prescribed.

- Monitor vital signs every 1–2 hours noting pulsus paradoxus.
- Obtain sputum specimen for gram stain, culture and sensitivity, and eosinophil stain (presence of eosinophils indicates allergic response).
- Maintain I&O; note urine specify gravity.
- Monitor serum electolytes, theophylline levels, and blood gas values.
- Observe for signs of theophylline toxicity noting fever, nausea, coffee-ground emesis, restlessness, hypotension, abdominal discomfort—progressing to convulsions and coma.
- Observe for signs and symptoms of "rapid metabolism" of theophylline derivatives: failure to improve despite bolus doses or continuous infusions.
- If child is near panic (air gulping) and able to follow instructions, tell child to follow breathing pattern of nurse; start with a rapid rate, then slow down gradually; encourage child to breathe in through nose, then exhale slowly through mouth.
- Provide cool, moist environment (mist tent or venti mask).
- Administer aerosol or nebulizer treatments as ordered.
- Perform percussion, vibration, postural drainage as indicated once airways have begun to open satisfactorily.
- Plan nursing tasks to allow for maximum rest.
- Administer sedatives as ordered.
- Encourage anxious parents to take small amounts of time away from child to see if child relaxes.
- Discuss with parents sensitivity testing and elimination diet.
- Teach parents and child early signs and symptoms of an attack.
- Teach parents and child to avoid: contact with allergens, extremes of temperature, overexcitement, and overexertion.
- Instruct parents and child in proper administration of medication. Stress that medications should be taken even when child is feeling well.
- Demonstrate correct use of inhaler and ask for return demonstration.
- Instruct parents and child in proper use and side effects of prophylactic medications. Alert them to dangers of overuse.
- Encourage parents to be alert to possibility of child's using his symptoms to manipulate his environment, and to avoid parental rejection or overprotection.
- Encourage exercise using stop-start activity not requiring endurance.
- Discuss use of bronchodilators 20–30 minutes before exercise.

d. **Evaluation**
   - Child's respiratory rate is within normal range for age
   - Child is not anxious and is able to interact with family, staff, and other patients.
   - Medications are within therapeutic range; child exhibits minimal side effects.

- Child/parents
  - describe signs of an impending attack, and what they would do to help alleviate it.
  - describe factors that precipitate attacks and measures they will take to avoid them.
  - use inhalers properly.
  - verbalize correct administration of medications, their benefits, and side effects.
  - discuss their feelings about the disease.
  - realistically describe child's limitations.
- Parents discuss how an attack could be used to manipulate others (Whaley & Wong).

## Other Possible Nursing Diagnoses

Impaired gas exchange
Impaired home maintenance management
Knowledge deficit
Potential for injury

## 4.  Status Asthmaticus

a. **Discussion**
   - The most severe and life-threatening form of asthma.
   - Produces a cycle of hypoxemia and acidosis, wheezing (bronchospasm), psychologic degeneration, and $CO_2$ narcosis.
   - Fails to respond to normal therapies. As this condition continues, pulmonary hypertension (reflecting gas exchange impairment), cor pulmonale, right-sided heart failure and, eventually, death, occur.

b. **Multidisciplinary Approaches**
   - Relief of bronchospasm and hypoxemia
     - corticosteroids, IV Isuprel, bronchodilators
     - intubation
     - mechanical ventilation (extreme cases only)
   - Respiratory therapy

## Additional Nursing Care That Can Be Incorporated into the Generic Care Plan

a. **Assessment**
   - See *Asthma,* page 236
   - Presence of complicating condition such as an upper respiratory infection or pneumonia
   - Response to epinephrine

b. **Goal**
Child will breathe at a normal rate and depth and will be adequately oxygenated.

c. **Interventions**
- Monitor effects of medications; note effects of bronchodilators and epinephrine.
- Monitor child's condition and ABGs for presence of acidosis.
- Reassure child and parents in order to decrease apprehension.

d. **Evaluation**
- Child breathes easily and is adequately oxygenated
  - vital signs returning to normal parameters.
  - diminished wheezes heard on auscultation of breath sounds.
  - ABGs returning to normal.
  - anxiety decreases.

# Other Possible Nursing Diagnoses

Anxiety
Impaired Gas Exchange

# 5.  Acute Epiglottitis

a. **Discussion:** This inflammatory edema of the epiglottis and aryepiglottic folds most often develops in children 2–6 years of age, although it has been observed in patients from 5 months through early adulthood. Epiglottitis is characterized by swelling and rounding of the epiglottis, blunting of the vallecula, hypopharyngeal ballooning, and edematous aryepiglottic folds. The patient assumes a "tripod" position (sitting up, learning forward, mouth open and chin forward) (Whaley & Wong). This diagnosis is considered a medical emergency. The child may be taken straight to the operating room where a small nasotracheal tube is inserted under general anesthesia. The epiglottis is cultured *only* after the airway is controlled.

b. **Multidisciplinary Approaches**
- Establish an airway (intubate if necessary)
- Lateral soft tissue neck x-ray (if clinical condition permits)
- Antibiotics (racemic epinephrine is of no value)
- Lab studies, blood cultures, ABGs
- Humidified $O_2$
- Observation in an ICU
- Respiratory therapy

# Additional Nursing Care That Can Be Incorporated into the Generic Care Plan

**a. Assessment**
- Sore throat
- Dysphagia
- High fever and toxicity
- Hoarseness
- Drooling
- Respiratory distress
- Sitting in the "tripod" position
- Air hunger
- Anxiety

**b. Goal**
Child will maintain a patent airway.

**c. Interventions**
- Maintain the child in a sitting position.
- Do not attempt to visualize the epiglottis; *under no circumstances place a tongue blade or other object in child's mouth.*
- Monitor vital signs closely; be alert for indications of airway obstruction.
- Keep npo.
- Have intubation or tracheotomy set at the bedside.
- Monitor for side effects of antibiotics.

**d. Evaluation**
- Child is free from dyspnea or other signs of respiratory distress; vital signs returning to normal.

# Other Possible Nursing Diagnoses

Anxiety
Impaired gas exchange
Potential for injury

# 6. Laryngotracheobronchitis (Croup)

**a. Definition/Discussion**
- A viral ailment that occurs predominantly in male children aged 3 months to 3 years, particularly between October and May.
- Characterized by subglottic edema and variable tracheal/ bronchial inflammation (due to a desquamating tracheitis).

**b. Multidisciplinary Approaches**
- X-ray (shows subglottic narrowing but a normal epiglottis)
- High humidity oxygen tent

- IV hydration
- Racemic epinephrine, steroids, or antibiotics
- Tracheostomy, intubation if necessary

# Additional Nursing Care That Can Be Incorporated into the Generic Care Plan

a. **Assessment**
   - Coryza
   - Barking cough
   - Hoarseness
   - Low-grade fever
   - Stridor
   - Respiratory distress
   - See Clinical Croup Score, table 7.10

**Table 7.10**   Clinical Croup Score
(can be used as an upper airway obstruction score)

|  | 0 | 1 | 2 | Score |
|---|---|---|---|---|
| Inspiratory breath sounds | Normal | Harsh with rhonchi and/or wheezing | Delayed | |
| Stridor | None | Inspiratory | Inspiratory and expiratory | |
| Cough | None | Hoarse cry | Bark | |
| Retractions and flaring | None | Flaring and suprasternal retractions | Same as score 1, plus subcostal, intercostal retractions | |
| Cyanosis | None | Present in room air | Present in 40% $O_2$ | Total Score |

A total score of 4–7 indicates moderately severe obstruction in which administration of racemic epinephrine may be beneficial.
A score of 7 or more with a $PCO_2 \geq 45$ mm Hg and a $pO_2 \leq 70$ mm Hg in room air (excluding chronic hypoxics) persisting for $> 30$ minutes, despite IV administration of fluid, use of mist, and recemic epinephrine, indicates need for an artificial airway.
(Downes & Raphaely, 1975; Anton, 1984)

b. **Goal**
   Child will remain oxygenated.

c. **Intervention**
   - Provide humid air to child (croup tent; humidifier, shower if at home).

   d.  **Evaluation**
- Child breathes easily; skin and fingernails are pink; cough and hoarseness decrease.

## 7. Foreign Body Aspiration

   a.  **Discussion**
- Suspect aspiration in any pediatric respiratory distress of unknown etiology.
- Most common in children aged 1–3 years.
- 85% of all aspirates are food (peanuts, popcorn, carrots, hot dogs) (Blazer, 1980).

   b.  **Multidisciplinary Approaches**
- If the child does not resume breathing after the foreign body is removed, begin assisted ventilation immediately; see *Cardiopulmonary Arrest*, page 205.
- If the obstruction cannot be removed, cricothyroidotomy may be done with a 14-gauge needle (frequently impossible in neonates, as the cricoid cannot be palpated).
- Bronchoscopy to remove foreign body

## Additional Nursing Care That Can Be Incorporated into the Generic Care Plan

   a.  **Assessment**
- See *Ineffective Airway Clearance,* page 229

   b.  **Goal**
Child will be able to breathe unobstructed.

   c.  **Interventions**
- If the child is cyanotic, unable to speak, or unconscious, the obstruction must be removed immediately; if a child can speak or cough, obstruction is not complete.
- Removal: Occasionally, an aspirated object can be removed with the fingers. Extreme caution is required to avoid pushing the object further down. When removal is not possible, utilize the following alternatives
  - *infants:* lay child face down over nurse's arm with head lower than trunk. Apply four quick blows to the area between the scapulae with the heel of hand; then turn to the supine position. (Keep the head lower than the trunk at all times; support the child with two hands.) Apply four upward chest compressions with two fingers or the heel of the hand. Repeat until the obstruction is relieved.
  - *children:* drape over nurse's thigh with head lower than the trunk. Administer four back blows, then place the child supine

on the floor. Administer chest thrusts with the heel of one or both hands, depending on the age of the child. Repeat if needed.
- *Heimlich maneuver* (controversial for use in children; there is risk of abdominal organ damage): attempt only if the above measures are ineffective, using the same basic technique as for adults; the one difference is the use of only two fingers of each hand for thrusts administered to infants.

**d. Evaluation**
- Child breathes easily; is free from respiratory obstruction or distress.

## Other Possible Nursing Diagnoses

Knowledge deficit
Potential for injury
Sensory-perceptual alteration

## 8. Tonsillectomy

**a. Discussion**
- Surgical removal of the tonsils
- Done for repeated occurrences of strep throat, when tonsils are chronically hypertrophied, or infected

**b. Multidisciplinary Approaches**
- PT/PTT preoperatively
- Play therapy

## Additional Nursing Care That Can Be Incorporated into the Generic Care Plan

**a. Assessment**
- Baseline vital signs
- Symptoms of upper respiratory infection
- History of bleeding tendencies
- Parental concerns, knowledge level about child's condition, and probability of compliance with medication regimen after discharge

**b. Goals**
Child will
- maintain patent airway clear of secretions.
- remain free of hemorrhage.
- have decrease in pain.
- be able to take clear liquids first day post-op, followed by soft diet.

Child/parents will be able to describe what to expect postoperatively. Parents will be able to describe care of child after discharge.

c.  **Interventions**
   – Before child is fully awake postoperatively, position on abdomen or side to facilitate drainage of secretions.
   – Inspect throat for bleeding, edema, accumulated secretions
     • inspect vomitus for blood (fresh or old)
     • observe for thirst, tolerance of liquids, rapid thready pulse, anxiety (indicate copious amounts of swallowed blood)
     • note continuous swallowing.
   – Observe for pharyngeal edema formation and signs of impending airway obstruction (e.g., difficulty breathing, swallowing).
   – Suction as needed; avoid operative site.
   – Administer sedatives as ordered if very irritable, crying.
   – Maintain bedrest during first post-op day.
   – Offer cool liquid diet 12–24 hours postoperatively, followed by soft diet; progress diet as tolerated; encourage eating to promote healing.
   – Provide discharge instruction to parents including
     • avoid highly seasoned or irritating foods
     • avoid gargling, rough tooth brushing
     • discourage child from coughing, clearing throat, or inserting objects into mouth
     • provide cool liquids, soft diet as tolerated; use mild analgesics, ice collar as needed
     • keep child quiet and indoors for first 3 days
     • call MD if there are signs of bleeding or persistent severe earache, fever, or cough
     • return to normal activities usually 1–2 weeks after surgery
     • instruct parents that wound area will have white membrane covering it, that throat may be sore for 7–10 days, and that if bleeding occurs, it will likely be on day of surgery or 5th to 10th day postoperatively, when membrane sloughs from operative site
     • provide cool mist vaporizer

d.  **Evaluation**
   – Child's vital signs are stable, operative site is intact, bleeding is minimal.
   – Child swallows food and fluid with minimum discomfort.
   – Parents verbalize understanding of medication administration and importance of compliance with regimen after discharge.

# Other Possible Nursing Diagnoses

Alteration in comfort: pain
Alteration in nutrition: less than body requirements

Anxiety
Knowledge deficit

## 9. Chest Trauma

a. **Discussion**
   - The most common cause of thoracic trauma in children is pedestrian/automobile accidents.
     - intrathoracic injury should be suspected if any of the following are reported
       * appropriate history (e.g., pedestrian hit by car, bicycle rider thrown across handlebars), especially with lacerations, contusions, or rib fracture
       * pain in thorax or upper abdomen
       * respiratory distress, cyanosis, signs of hypoxia
       * hypotension, tachycardia
       * tracheal deviation
       * crepitus of chest, neck, back, upper abdomen (Reece & Chamberlain, 1974)

b. **Multidisciplinary Approaches**
   - Restoration of chest wall integrity, re-expansion of the lungs, and optimal ventilation (Brunner & Suddarth, 1982); resuscitation measures if necessary
   - Treatments vary with the type of injury and include chest tube insertion, water-seal drainage of the chest, thoracotomy
   - Careful evaluation of all chest trauma victims for internal abdominal injury since the two conditions are often associated
   - Narcotic and/or non-narcotic analgesics

## Additional Nursing Care That Can Be Incorporated into the Generic Care Plan

a. **Assessment**
   - Vital signs
   - Level of consciousness
   - Integrity of water-seal drainage unit
   - Anxiety level of parents/child

b. **Goal**
   Child's lungs will return to full expansion and child will breathe without distress.

c. **Interventions**
   - See *Ineffective Airway Clearance*, page 231.
   - Monitor vital signs carefully for signs of shock.
   - Monitor chest tube and water-seal drainage system for patency every 2 hours.

- Measure chest tube output every 4 hours.
- Position child for comfort.
- Turn, cough, and deep breathe every 2 hours.
- Provide quiet diversional activity.
- Monitor effects of analgesics.
- Monitor for signs of renal and/or bladder trauma.
- Monitor neurologic status.

d. **Evaluation**
- Child regains full lung expansion and is adequately oxygenated as evidenced by
  - breath sounds clear and equal bilaterally
  - no cyanosis or other signs of hypoxia
  - pulse, respiration, and blood pressure within normal limits for age
  - no tracheal deviation
  - lack of crepitus in neck, back, upper abdomen
  - Child is alert and oriented.

## Other Possible Nursing Diagnoses

Alteration in cardiac output: decreased
Alteration in comfort: pain
Alteration in patterns of urinary elimination
Anxiety
Fluid volume deficit
Impaired gas exchange

## 10. Near Drowning

a. **Discussion**
- Death from drowning results from hypoxemia, which leads to cardiac arrest. Near drowning victims require vigorous therapy to increase the oxygen/carbon dioxide exchange in the lungs and correct acidosis (Reece & Chamberlain).
- It must be emphasized that drowning victims, especially those pulled from cold water, have been successfully revived after periods of oxygen deprivation that would cause brain damage in nondrowning arrest victims, probably due to the metabolic depression related to hypothermia.
- Resuscitation should be vigorous and prolonged.

b. **Multidisciplinary Approaches**
- Intubation if necessary (cuffed tube may be used to avoid aspiration of the almost inevitable vomitus)
- 100% $O_2$
- Correct acidosis; give $NaHCO_3$ 1 mEq/kg initially, then according to ABGs

- Give aminophylline for bronchospasm
- Hypothermia

# Additional Nursing Care That Can Be Incorporated into the Generic Care Plan

a. **Assessment**
   - Note type and temperature of water (salt or fresh), length of time submerged to determine physiologic response (hypervolemia vs pulmonary edema)
   - Respiratory status
     • ABGs, vital signs
     • bronchospasms
   - Neurologic status

b. **Goal**
   Child's pulmonary ventilation will be adequate to oxygenate vital organs

c. **Interventions**
   - Establish airway.
   - Perform CPR if child is in cardiac arrest (see *Cardiopulmonary Arrest,* page 205).
   - Provide care for comatose child (see page 271).
   - Monitor effects of $O_2$ therapy.
   - Monitor respiratory status for signs of pneumonia.
   - Monitor mechanical ventilation.
   - Control fever with cooling mattress.

d. **Evaluation**
   - Child regains adequate oxygenation as evidenced by
     • ABGs and vital signs return to normal
     • no signs or symptoms of pneumonia
     • temperature within normal limits
   - Child's level of consciousness is appropriate.

e. **Other Possible Nursing Diagnoses**
   Alteration in cardiac output: decreased
   Anxiety (parental)
   Impaired gas exchange
   Impaired physical mobility
   Impairment of skin integrity
   Ineffective airway clearance
   Sensory-perceptual alteration

**GENERIC CARE PLAN FOR THE NURSING DIAGNOSIS**
# ALTERATION IN TISSUE PERFUSION: PERIPHERAL

## 1. General Information

a. **Etiology**
   - Arterial or venous obstruction, sickle cell disease, anemia, thallasemia, erythroblastosis fetalis, transfusion reaction
   - Hypo/hypervolemia (congestive heart failure, hemorrhage)
   - Rh incompatibility
   - Trauma to an extremity
   - Fractures

b. **Clinical Manifestations**
   - Tachycardia
   - Diminished or absent arterial pulses
   - Decreased urinary output
   - Slow healing of lesions
   - Cool, pale extremities

c. **Multidisciplinary Approaches**
   - Correction of underlying problem
   - Reattachment of severed part
   - IV, appropriate medications

## 2. Nursing Process

a. **Assessment**
   - Cause and/or contributing factors
   - Cardiac function
   - Peripheral pulses
   - Hydration
   - Skin (temperature and integrity)

b. **Goal**
   Child will have adequate oxygenation of peripheral tissues.

c. **Interventions**
   - Relieve pressure from extremities.
   - Check capillary refill and temperature of extremities.
   - Provide adequate hydration (oral and/or IV).
   - Weigh daily.
   - Encourage limited activity.

d. **Evaluation**
   - Child's extremities are warm and pink.
   - Intake and output are balanced.
   - Weight is returning to normal.

# Selected Health Problem Frequently Associated with the Nursing Diagnosis ALTERATION IN TISSUE PERFUSION: PERIPHERAL

## Sickle Cell Anemia

a. **Discussion**
   - Sickle cell anemia is a chronic disease characterized by production of abnormal hemoglobin S and periods of crisis; most common in blacks
   - Vaso-occlusive (thrombocytic): malformed RBCs occlude small and peripheral blood vessels, leading to infarction of a given area
   - Sequestration: blood pools in the liver or spleen, producing circulatory collapse (more common in infants and frequently fatal)
   - Aplastic: lack of production of RBCs
   - Hyperhemolytic: increased destruction of RBCs
   - Crisis periods can be precipitated by dehydration, trauma, infection, extreme fatigue, exposure to cold, respiratory distress, or unusual physical exertion (Hazinski)

b. **Multidisciplinary Approaches**
   - IV or oral fluids
   - Temperature and pain control: narcotics are most effective in relieving visceral pain; non-narcotics are most effective for musculoskeletal pain
   - Treatment of precipitating factor (if known)
   - Blood transfusions
   - $O_2$ therapy

## Additional Nursing Care That Can Be Incorporated into the Generic Care Plan

a. **Assessment**
   - Joints (range of motion)
   - Pain and swelling: location, character, duration
   - Painful episode: frequency, whether "typical" or unusual
     - severe form: painful episodes 11–15 times/year requiring hospitalization and narcotic analgesia

- moderate form: 2 times/year
- mild form: 1 time/year or less
- Complications; presence of another disease or condition
- Precipitating factors: dehydration, infections, overexertion, weather changes, emotional stress

b. **Goals**
Child will
- experience decreased discomfort.
- be adequately hydrated.
Parents/child will
- be able to describe the etiology and course of sickle cell anemia and crisis-prevention measures.
- describe when necessary to seek medical attention.

c. **Interventions**
- Record I&O.
- Encourage child to drink 1½–2 times maintenance fluids.
- Observe lab values for hemoglobin, hematocrit, electrolyte imbalance.
- Note presence of anorexia, irritability, weakness, fever, and pallor.
- Help parents/child identify precipitating factors; plan to prevent further attacks.
- Maintain bedrest.
- Provide $O_2$ as ordered.
- Provide passive range-of-motion exercises when not in crisis.
- Apply warmth to painful areas, avoiding use of cold (exacerbates crisis).
- Monitor effectiveness of analgesics.
- Discuss home management with parents and child
  - prevent tissue deoxygenation by avoidance of strenuous physical activity, contact sports, emotional stress, low $O_2$ environments, infections (even mild ones)
  - when to seek medical help
    * temperature (greater than 38.5°C)
    * pain uncontrolled by oral medication.
    * inability to drink sufficient fluids.
- Refer to genetic counseling if parents so desire.

d. **Evaluation**
- Child
  - interacts with family, friends, and staff and verbalizes decreased discomfort from pain.
  - participates in age-appropriate play.
  - ingests 100–125 ml/kg/day; has urine output of at least 2–4 ml/kg/hour, with specific gravity of 1.005–1.010 or lower.
  - has moist mucous membranes, stable vital signs.

- Parents
  - describe sickle cell anemia, measures to prevent sickling.
  - identify conditions necessitating hospitalization.

## Other Possible Nursing Diagnoses

Alteration in comfort: pain
Alteration in family process
Impaired physical mobility
Knowledge deficit

## Problems of Mobility

The activity-exercise functional health pattern also includes problems of physical mobility and a number of conditions. For example, a child may sustain burn wound contractures or have a progressive neuromuscular disease. Both conditions result in impaired physical mobility. Since most children develop problems related to injuries or congenital skeletal anomalies, the focus in this section will be on orthopedic conditions. Some of the most common orthopedic problems and their associated nursing care are included.

### GENERIC CARE PLAN FOR THE NURSING DIAGNOSIS
## IMPAIRED PHYSICAL MOBILITY

### 1. General Information

a. **Etiology**
   - Neuromuscular problems (spinal cord injury, myelomeningocele, CNS tumor)
   - Musculoskeletal impairment (fracture, cerebral palsy, arthritis)

b. **Clinical Manifestation**
   - Inability to initiate movement
   - Imposed restriction of movement (cast, traction, bedrest)
   - Limited range of motion (ROM)
   - Impaired coordination

c. **Multidisciplinary Approaches**
   - Immobilization (casts, traction)
   - Medications: muscle relaxants, analgesics
   - Physical therapy
   - Occupational therapy

## 2.  Nursing Process

### a.  Assessment
- History of systemic disease, mobility problems, recent surgery or traumatic injury
- ROM of all joints
- Ability to bear weight
- Medical restrictions on mobility

### b.  Goals
Child will
- experience the maximum potential level of mobility.
- be free from complications of decreased mobility.

### c.  Interventions
- Ensure that child's body is in good alignment especially when traction, casts, braces, etc., are in use
- Ensure that child's position in bed is changed frequently (every 15 minutes to every 2 hours).
- Provide active and passive ROM activities at least 3–4 times a day.
- Encourage child to do as many activities as possible; assist when necessary.
- Provide age-appropriate diversion, school work.
- Inspect and massage body prominences regularly; be alert to signs of potential skin impairment.
- Encourage increased fluid and roughage intake to prevent constipation.
- Evaluate effectiveness of analgesics.
- Promote safe use of mobility aids, e.g., crutches, wheel chairs.
- Teach child/parents methods for increasing mobility.

### d.  Evaluation
- Child is
  - able to move as much as possible within the limits of own physical ability and mobility restrictions.
  - free from contractures or limited joint mobility.

### e.  Other Possible Nursing Diagnoses
Alteration in bowel elimination
Alteration in comfort: pain
Alteration in tissue perfusion: peripheral
Disturbance in self-concept: body image
Diversional activity deficit
Fear
Impairment of skin integrity
Knowledge deficit
Potential for injury

## Selected Health Problems Frequently Associated with the Nursing Diagnosis IMPAIRED PHYSICAL MOBILITY

### 1. Orthopedic Trauma

a. **Discussion**
- Orthopedic trauma includes fractures, sprains, strains, dislocations, and associated injuries.
- Two types of fractures are unique to children
  - greenstick fractures: bone, most commonly the radius, ulna, or clavicle, curves from impact and breaks on only one side of the curve; no associated loss of bone continuity
  - epiphyseal plate injuries: may cause growth disturbance
- Fractures in children usually cause rapid swelling that tends to recede in a short time.
- Pelvic fractures are often overlooked in children since they involve minimal deformity and little appreciable crepitus, but do cause pain. Pelvic fractures can lead to significant blood loss and shock, and often indicate associated injuries of the abdomen and bladder.
- Casts are usually made of plaster of Paris, fiberglass (lightweight), or resin-impregnated plaster of Paris bandages. Purposes of casting
  - immobilize affected limb
  - prevent or correct deformities
  - maintain, support, and protect realigned bone fragments
  - provide uniform pressure to soft tissue around fracture, thereby preventing edema
  - promote early weight bearing
- Common childhood fractures are summarized in table 7.11.

b. **Multidisciplinary Approaches**
- X-ray of injury; views of the opposite extremity may be a helpful standard for comparison
- Treat children's sprains, strains, and dislocations the same as adult injuries
- Treat fracture
  - closed reduction: bracing, casting, traction
  - open reduction: internal fixation

## Additional Nursing Care That Can Be Incorporated into the Generic Care Plan

a. **Assessment**
- See table 7.11

**Table 7.11**    Common Fractures in Children

| Location | Cause | Signs/Symptoms | Comment |
|---|---|---|---|
| Clavicle | Falls onto outstretched arm or shoulder | Tenderness, deformity; arm held against chest; pain with shoulder movement | Requires careful evaluation of distal pulses to assess for damage to subclavian and axillary arteries. Clavicle strap (splint) applied. |
| Humerus: Supracondylar | Fall onto outstreched arm or elbow | Deformity, swelling, tenderness, inability to move arm | Frequently associated with injury to brachial artery, median or radial nerves. Careful neurovascular assessment vital. |
| Humerus: Shaft | Fall or direct blow | Tenderness in upper $1/3$ of arm | |
| Elbow | Fall on outstretched arm or direct blow | Refusal to move arm, tenderness, deformity | Careful assessment of radial and brachial pulse, radial and median nerve function |
| Distal radius/ulna | Fall onto outstretched arm (frequently a greenstick fracture) | Pain, swelling, tenderness, deformity, shortening, angulation | Frequent radial epiphysis injuries. Colles fracture common in children |
| Fingers | Direct blow (common in contact sports) | Pain, tenderness, swelling, impaired range of motion | Distal joint most common |
| Femur | Motor vehicle accident, fall from height | Pain, crepitus, marked deformity, muscle spasm | Careful evaluation of distal pulses necessary; blood loss can cause shock. Frequently seen with other injuries. Often an open fracture |
| Tibia/fibula, ankle | Twisting injury, direct force | Pain, swelling, crepitus; degree of deformity varies greatly | Requires careful assessment of neurovascular status. Often seen as open fracture with soft tissue damage. |

- Developmental needs
- Pain
- Neurovascular status of affected extremity
- Vital signs

**b.  Goals**
   Child will
   - remain as active as possible during healing.
   - be free from further injury.

c.  **Interventions**
   - Monitor neurovascular status every 2–4 hours; check
     • pulses distal to cast or injury if possible
     • temperature and color of affected limb
     • sensation and capillary refill of extremity
     • range of motion (wiggling of fingers or toes)
   - Reposition child every 2 hours.
   - Maintain body and cast alignment.
   - Elevate casted extremity using pillows, or suspend the arm from an IV pole
     • elevate above level of the heart.
     • pillows should extend above and below the cast
   - Observe for drainage on cast; circle area, note date and time.
   - Handle cast carefully with palms of hands until dry.
   - Leave cast uncovered, open to air to dry.
   - Don't put cast on plastic (prevents drying).
   - Assess any complaints of pain.
   - Check for rough edges on cast; trim to prevent skin irritation petal edges with waterproof tape, then apply moleskin petals over tape.
   - Teach child and parent proper home care of cast
     • petaling of cast
     • activity restrictions
     • neurovascular checks
     • return to the hospital if child experiences pain, numbness; the cast breaks or smells purulent; extremity is red and swollen, cold and pale, temperature is elevated
     • keep extremity elevated
     • exercise fingers or toes
     • keep cast dry
     • protect cast during elimination
     • prevent child from putting anything inside the cast

d.  **Evaluation**
   - Child is
     • able to move within limitations of injury and orthopedic appliances.
     • free from neurologic or circulatory impairment, i.e., child's fingers/toes are warm, color is good and capillary refill is rapid.
   - Child's body is in good alignment.

## 2.  Congenital Hip Dysplasia

a.  **Discussion/Definition**
   - Presence of malformations of hip at birth
   - Etiology is unknown
   - Usually unilateral

**b. Multidisciplinary Approaches**
- X-ray
- Splints: double diaper, Frejka pillow splint
- Pavlik harness
- Hip spica cast
- Operative reduction in older children

# Additional Nursing Care That Can Be Incorporated into the Generic Nursing Plan

**a. Assessment**
- Ortolani's sign: audible click when hips flexed at right-angle and knees flexed when infant is supine
- ROM of hips
- Length of extremities (shortening on affected side), asymmetric thigh, gluteal folds

**b. Goal**
Child's hip joint will move normally.

**c. Interventions**
- Assess the parents' understanding as to purpose of a Pavlik harness and provide parental teaching
  - keep harness on at all times; removal may cause redislocation
  - adjust buckles if they become loose
  - do not remove harness for daily bathing; sponge bath is sufficient; give special skin care under straps and stirrups
  - do not use lotions, creams or powders
  - be alert for pressure points of harness
  - perineal care should not be a problem, as harness does not cover this area
  - promote normal development of infant (see page 264)
  - assess compliance in using harness
- Monitor hip spica cast
  - explain procedure to child and family
  - use palm of hand when lifting child to prevent indenting wet cast
  - use Bradford frame for infants and incontinent children to prevent soiling of cast by urine and feces
  - place child in supine position with buttocks over opening of frame and directly over bedpan
  - elevate the head of the frame slightly to prevent child from sliding, if necessary
  - restrain the child with a safety jacket

- place continent children on firm mattress with trapeze attached to overhead frame
- reposition every 2–4 hours during the day and every 4 hours at night (child may be placed on back, abdomen, or sides when cast is dry)
- place blanket roll under lower section of leg and pillow under chest
- place a pillow under each leg and one under head and shoulders when supine
- do not lift child by crossbar that maintains abduction
- check quality of respirations and aeration of lungs every 4 hours; encourage activities that promote lung expansion
- observe for irritation around and under cast edges regularly; ensure cast is not too tight (one finger should be easily inserted inside top of cast); check for any inconsistencies in cast itself
- observe for drainage on cast—circle area, noting date and time; note any foul odor coming from cast
- investigate verbal and nonverbal indications of pain
- provide age-appropriate play activities and socialization
- keep skin as clean and dry as possible
- toughen skin around cast edges by applying alcohol
- petal cast edges around the perineum with waterproof tape; apply moleskin petals over tape, place plastic wrap over the petals; replace petals as they become soiled
- increase the amount of roughage in the diet; encourage fresh fruits to avoid constipation
- provide child and parent education (see table 7.12)
  * petaling of cast
  * protecting cast with plastic
  * positioning
  * neurovascular checks

# Play

Play or diversional activity is an essential part of childhood. In order to develop increasing ability and skills, children practice in the form of play. Understanding of self begins in infancy as babies learn the boundaries and capabilities of their own bodies. As infants learn that they are separate from their caretakers, playful activities begin to develop into social awareness and interactive skills. Infants also develop fine and gross motor skills as they experiment with their bodies and their environment.

As children grow, the need for play grows also. The need for play continues while children are hospitalized and is a major area of nursing intervention. Diversional activity, while essential for all children who are hospitalized, is critical for children with chronic illnesses who are hospitalized repeatedly.

**Table 7.12**  Home Care of Child in a Hip Spica Cast

1. Call MD if
   - cast is broken
   - child experiences pain, numbness, tingling
   - cast has foul odor
   - child has constant pain in any one area.
2. Be sure to
   - keep cast dry
   - reapply waterproof tape and moleskin as necessary
   - *never* use the bar between the legs to lift or turn the child.
3. Provide good skin care
   - keep skin clean and dry
   - sponge bathe daily all areas not covered by cast
   - do not use powders, lotions, or oils around cast edges or down cast since they will soften the skin.
   - check frequently for skin irritation and breakdown
   - do not place objects down cast to "scratch"
   - turn every 2 hours
   - to turn, move child to side of bed, support the hip and leg and roll child over
   - place pillow under chest and blanket roll or small pillow under lower section of leg when child is prone
   - place pillow under each leg and one under head and shoulders when child is supine
   - place pillows snugly along the back of the cast for support, when child is in side-lying position.
4. Diet
   - resume regular diet
   - appetite might be diminished due to decrease in activity
   - offer food high in roughage and fresh fruits to avoid constipation.
5. Play
   - encourage activities that are age-appropriate
   - try to keep child as active as possible
   - include child in all activities of the family within limitations imposed by the cast.

(Sporing, 1984)


## GENERIC CARE PLAN FOR THE NURSING DIAGNOSIS
# DIVERSIONAL ACTIVITY DEFICIT


## 1. General Information

a. **Etiology**
   - Isolation
   - Long-term hospitalization
   - Bedrest
   - Physical immobility (casts, traction, etc.)

b. **Clinical Manifestations**
   - Verbal expressions of boredom or of feeling isolated, lonely
   - Statements that reflect a child's wishes for a specific activity or for a familiar toy or game
   - Excessive sleeping
   - Constant TV watching
   - Staring into space, lethargy, or restlessness
   - Few visitors (no one to spend time or to play with child)
   - Lack of interest in environment
   - Flat affect
   - Physical confinement

c. **Multidisciplinary Approaches**
   - Continued evaluation and updating of isolation and physical activity restrictions
   - Child-life therapist, physical therapist
   - Volunteers

## 2. Nursing Process

a. **Assessment**
   - Affect and activity level
   - Quality of activity
   - Number of visitors and frequency of visits

b. **Goals**
   Child will
   - select several appropriate diversional activities of interest.
   - engage in one or more age-appropriate activities.

c. **Interventions**
   - Include child in planning of daily activities.
   - Alter timing of nursing care to permit child to engage in selected activities.
   - Provide age- and development-appropriate games or playthings.
     *Infant (birth–12 months)*
     - feel and move own body
     - different textures and temperatures
     - solitary play
     - may be imitative
     - exploratory and manipulative
     - enjoys squeak toys, crumpled paper, mirror and water play, mobiles, body parts, blocks, push and pull toys, busy boxes, rattles, and noise toys
     - 4–10 months: repeats accidental activities, does not look for lost objects

- 5–7 months: picks up tiny objects, holds on to toys and resists having them taken away from grasp, plays peek-a-boo; works for toy out of reach
- 8–9 months: plays pat-a-cake, recognizes self in mirror
- 10–12 months: plays ball with examiner, object permanence achieved (i.e., searches for dropped objects)

*Toddler (1–3 years)*
- play is parallel (plays alongside but not with others)
- imitates adult roles, including housework
- 18 months: will help do simple tasks; removes garments
- 21–36 months: begins interactive games (e.g., hiding objects from another person); can wash and dry hands, dress (with supervision)
- enjoys water (supervised tub play), sandbox, clay/Play-Doh, crayons, puzzles, small wheeled vehicles, storybooks
- enjoys fantasy and "make-believe" play

*Preschool (3–6 years)*
- play is parallel—associated activity: plays with other children, engages in common activity
- defines own rules
- cooperative, play is organized, likes to join in games or activities of others
- plays interactive games
- content of play includes dramatic and socially affective, as well as imitative play
- enjoys water (with supervision), sandbox, clay/Play-Doh, small wheeled vehicles, tea sets, toy kitchens, dress-up clothes, story books, dolls of either sex, favorite toys of attachment, action games, guessing games, simple card or board games, make-believe
- "needle" play and using dolls or stuffed animals to demonstrate pre-op teaching is very useful in this group

*School Age (6–12 years)*
- cooperative "team" play
- skill play, testing, model-building, exploration.
- enjoys adventure—action figures are popular with young school-age children
- collects and classifies items, hobbies, sophisticated "dolls", board games (including chess and backgammon); reading for pleasure
- needs to be discouraged from long hours of television watching

*Adolescent (12–19 years)*
- group/peer activities (sports, academic teams, etc.)
- parental/adult "limit setting" continues to be sought, desired; independence testing continues
- avoid reinforcing thrill-seeking behaviors
- Encourage family/friends to visit and to engage child in play.

   – Encourage family to bring several favorite toys, games, and play-things from home.
   – Utilize play therapist, occupational therapist, or volunteers when family cannot visit.
   – Take child to playroom or teen center as often as possible.
   – Consider allowing a family pet to visit if properly supervised.

**d. Evaluation**
   – Child participates in play activities
     • interacts playfully with staff during daily routine.
     • plays with familiar toys and games from home.
   – Family visitors, therapist, or volunteers provide sufficient oppor-tunities for child to engage in diversional activities.

**e. Other Possible Nursing Diagnoses**
   Anxiety
   Impaired physical mobility
   Ineffective individual coping

# References

American Heart Association. (1980). Standards and guidelines for cardiopulmonary resuscitation and emergency cardiac care. *Journal of the American Medical Association, 244*, 476.

Anton, B. (1984). Pediatric respiratory therapy beyond the neonatal ICU. *Respiratory Therapy, 14*(4), 19–26.

Blazer, S., et al. (1980). Foreign body in the airway. *American Journal of Disabled Children, 134*, 67–81.

Brunner, L., & Suddarth, D. (1982). *Lippincott manual of nursing practice*. (3rd ed.). Philadelphia: Lippincott.

Castaneda, A., & Norwood, W. (1981). Repair of Fallot's tetralogy in infancy. *Modern Techniques of Surgery*, 42–47.

Chameides, L., Melker, R., Raye, J., Todres, I., & Viles, P. (1983). Resuscitation of infants and children (p. 264). In K. McIntyre & A. Lewis (Eds.). *Textbook of advanced cardiac life support*. American Heart Association.

Downes, J., & Raphaely, R. (1975). Pediatric intensive care. *Anesthesiology, 43*, 242.

Hazinski, M. (1984). *Nursing care of the critically ill child*. St. Louis: Mosby.

Johns Hopkins Hospital. *Pediatric intensive care unit protocols*. Baltimore: Author.

Kent, D. (1975). *Pulmonary diseases in childhood—clinical notes on respiratory diseases*. New York: American Lung Association.

Lough, M., & Doershuk, C. (1980). *Pediatric respiratory therapy*. Chicago: Year Book Medical Publishers.

Ng, L. (1983). Complete "D"—Transposition of the great arteries. *Cardiovascular disease in the young: nursing intervention series, 3*, 14–15.

Norwood, W., Lang, P., & Hansen D. (1983). Physiologic repair of aortic atresia—hypoplastic left heart syndrome. *New England Journal of Medicine, 308*, 23–26.

Reece, R., & Chamberlain, J. (1974). *Manual of emergency pediatrics*. Philadelphia: Saunders.

Shapiro, B. (1975). *Clinical applications of blood gases*. Chicago: Year Book Medical Publishers.

Waechter, E., & Blake, R. (1976). *Nursing of children*. Philadelphia: Lippincott.

Whaley, L. & Wong, D. (1983). *Nursing care of infants and children*. (2nd ed). St. Louis: Mosby.

# CHAPTER 8

# COGNITIVE-PERCEPTUAL
## FUNCTIONAL HEALTH PATTERN

T he cognitive-perceptual functional health pattern includes the concepts of sensation, perception, and cognition. During childhood these functions are developing and being refined, continually changing. Therefore this chapter contains many developmental concerns.

Development of the nervous system and the sensory modes of vision and hearing are addressed and specific alterations in perception and sensation such as seizures and increasing intracranial pressure are presented.

Principles of teaching and learning are addressed. The child's developing cognitive functional abilities are considered and the learning theories of Piaget and Skinner are presented. See tables 8.1 and 8.2. The importance of parent teaching is presented to emphasize the need for the practicing pediatric nurse to present ongoing anticipatory guidance related to growth and development as well as teaching specific health related topics to parents; see table 8.3. Pain perception and pain management are also discussed, with an emphasis on the need to address these issues in a developmentally appropriate manner.

## DEVELOPMENT OF THE NERVOUS SYSTEM

### Central Nervous System

Myelination of the central nervous system (CNS) begins in utero and continues in a cephalocaudal fashion for two years (longer in some nerve tracts such as spinothalamic). The neonate displays widely varied movement patterns characterized by "fetal movements" (outward swipes of the arms and legs). It is not clear how mature various parts of the CNS are at this time.

## Neurologic and Motor Development

### Infant (birth–12 months)

- Development is cephalocaudal in nature and direction (proximal to distal). Arm and hand skills develop prior to leg and feet.
- Gross Motor
  - birth: turns head when prone, but cannot support self unassisted; adjusts posture when held at shoulder; may squirm to corner or edge of crib when prone; reflexive arm and leg movements
  - 6 weeks–2 months: raises head to 45° (90° when prone); may hold head steady when in supported sitting position
  - 3 months: rolls over back to side
  - 4 months: may bear weight on legs when assisted; when pulled to sitting position, head lag disappears
  - 5 months: pulls to sitting position, rolls from back to stomach; sits alone momentarily; unilateral reaching
  - 6 months: sits without support; may creep an inch forward or backward; moves from place to place by rolling over
  - 7 months: stands (holding on); early stepping movements (prewalking progression); begins to crawl or hitch
  - 8 months: pulls self to standing position, raises self to sitting position
  - 9 months: walks (assisted); crawls or hitches when permitted; sits down
  - 10 months: continues, with help, to develop walking skills; stands alone; may climb up and down stairs
  - 11 months: may walk alone; begins to stoop and recover
  - 12 months: continues to refine walking skills
- Fine Adaptive
  - birth–2 months: follows to and slightly past midline
  - 2–3 months: hands predominantly open; reflex grasp replaced by voluntary action; grasps such objects as rattle in open hand; may bring hands together at midline
  - 3–4 months: ulnar-palmar prehension with a cube; reaches for objects
  - 5 months: attempts to "catch" dangling objects; begins use of forefinger and thumb in pincer grasp (opposable thumb—prehension); retains 2 cubes, recovers rattle, reaches and grasps objects
  - 6–7 months: can grasp at will; holds and manipulates objects, transfers from hand to hand; scoops pellets, demonstrates inferior pincer grasp
  - 8–9 months: combines spoons or cubes at the midline; retains 2 of 3 cubes offered; displays neat pincer grasp of a pellet
  - feeds self finger-foods
  - 10–11 months: plays pat-a-cake (a midline skill); puts several objects in a container; holds crayon adaptively; bangs 2 cubes together;

looks for hidden objects (object permanence); neat pincer grasp of tiny objects achieved

## Toddler (1–3 years)
- Gross Motor
  - 12–18 months: walks well, throws ball, stoops and recovers, walks up stairs with help, begins to run; walks sideways and backwards 10 feet; stands on one foot (with help)
  - 18–24 months: kicks ball forward, throws overhand, walks downstairs (with help) one at a time
  - 2–3 years: jumps and runs well; jumps from bottom step, jumps in place; balances on one foot for 1 second; pedals tricycle; walks on a straight line; tiptoes
  - 29–32 months: broad jumps a distance of 4–14 inches
- Fine Adaptive
  - 12–18 months: scribbles spontaneously; builds tower of 2, then 4 cubes; dumps raisin from container with demonstration, then spontaneously; may untie shoes; uses opposable thumb (prehension) well; favors one hand
  - 18–24 months: may remove articles of clothing; holds pencil well enough to scribble; builds tower of 4 cubes; imitates vertical line within 30°
  - 24–36 months: builds tower of 6–8 cubes; can use paint brush; imitates scribble; copies a circle

## Preschool (3–6 years)
- Gross Motor
  - 3 years: hops on 1 foot
  - 4 years: skips; balances on 1 foot for 5 seconds (2 of 3 attempts); heel to toe walk (2 of 3 attempts); catches bounced ball (2 of 3 attempts); dresses without supervision
  - 5 years: backward heel to toe (2 of 3 attempts); balances on 1 foot for 10 seconds (2 of 3 attempts)
- Fine Adaptive
  - 3–4 years: buttons large buttons; picks longer line (3 of 3)
  - 4–5 years: ties shoe laces; draws a man with 3–6 parts; copies a square
  - 5–6 years: draws a man with 6 parts; copies a triangle

## School Age (6–12 years)
- Gross Motor: by 6 years can walk a straight line; has mastered all skills on Denver Developmental Screening Test
- Fine Adaptive: continuously refining and improving previously learned skills

## Adolescent (12–19 years)
- Good posture hampered by rapid growth spurt that accompanies puberty. (Those active in sports tend to have fewer problems with posture.)

**Table 8.1**    Cognitive Development: Piaget

| Infant (birth–12 months) | Toddler (1–3 years) | Preschool (3–6 years) | School-age Child (6–12 years) | Adolescence (13–19 years) |
|---|---|---|---|---|
| Substage I (0–1 months): practice of reflexes, reflex-like actions | Sensorimotor (0–2 years) | Preoperational (2–7 years) | Concrete operations (7–11 years): Reasoning | Formal operations: Abstraction and hypothetical/deductive reasoning possible |
| Substage II (1–4 months): purposeful reproduction of reflex actions | Preoperational-preconceptual (2–7 years) | Egocentrism and "omnipotence" (inability to distinguish between own perception and someone else's) | Understands reversability (of actions or thinking) | Characterized by |
| Substage III (4–8 months): object orientation, imitative actions | Substage V (12–18 months): production of vowel behaviors and curiosity | | Classifies objects (e.g., leaf and rock collections) according to their characteristic (e.g., igneous vs sedimentary rocks) | • Adaptability/flexibility |
| | Substage VI (18–24 months): concept of object permanence fully achieved | Concrete, tangible thought, becoming intuitive toward the end of the stage | | • Abstract thought |
| | | | | • Use of abstract symbols |
| Accidents repeated | Reaches symbolic plane | "Transductive reasoning" from one event to another—e.g., if didn't like one food on table, won't like another | | • Drawing conclusions from observations |
| Substage IV (8–12 months): coordination, intentionality, goal direction, achievement | Still sensorimotor (18 months) | | Understands the concept of conservation; comprehends that amount, weight, physical properties, and volume of substances are not changed by physical movement (e.g., the volume of water poured from a cup to a glass is the same) | • Developing hypotheses |
| | Limited concept of time (no "tomorrow") | Animism/anthropomorphism (attributes human traits to inanimate objects or animals) | | • Considering abstract, theoretical, and philosophic matters |
| Experimentation and achievement of object-permanence (searches for a dropped object or person playing peek-a-boo) | Very egocentric | Magical thinking (imaginary playmates common) | | • Problem solving (there may be some confusion of the ideal with the practical) |
| | "Animistic" (e.g., talks to stuffed animals) | | | |
| | | | Grasps relativism that 2 or more aspects of a problem may be operated/manipulated simultaneously | Able to comprehend purely abstract or symbolic content and to solve advanced math and logic problems |
| Imitation, behavior modeling | Imaginary playmates | Artificialism (all things "made for a purpose") | | |
| | Parallel play | | | |
| | Premature sense of cause/effect | Irreversibility (can't backtrack steps in a thinking pattern) | Can place self in another's situation | |
| | Goal-directed behavior | | Serialization: masters the ordinal number line; can group and sort (place in logical order) | Can comprehend philosophic, moral, and political value and belief systems |
| | Deferred imitation | Centration (inability to consider several aspects of a situation simultaneously) | | |
| | "Transductive reasoning" from the particular to the particular, e.g., if didn't like one food won't like another | Trial vs error (prelogical thought processes) | | |
| | | Primitive concepts of space, time, causality | Develops fundamental skills of reading, writing and grammar | |
| | | Uses memory | Late school-age child (11 years) capable of abstraction, deductive reasoning | |

**Table 8.2**  Cognitive Development: Skinner

| Infant (birth–12 months) | Toddler (1–3 years) | Preschooler (3–6 years) |
|---|---|---|
| Learning takes place by operant conditioning, reinforcing the right response to a specific stimulus | Learning occurs with respondent or operant behavior | Unreinforced negative behaviors become extinct in normal individuals |
| Without reinforcement, response becomes extinct | | |

# COGNITIVE DEVELOPMENT: PIAGET, SKINNER

## Sensory Perception

Vision is central, not peripheral. At birth, infants can establish locked eye contact in the *en face* position or fix on objects 8–12 inches from their eyes. They prefer stark contrasts (e.g., black and white) and respond better to arrangements similar to the human face than to random, free-form shapes.

Infants respond slowly to all auditory stimuli, but are more receptive (and are comforted) by high-pitched tones, including female voices. They discriminate well, frowning and flinching at unpleasant noises.

Sweet tastes are preferred by most neonates, while bitter, salty, and sour tastes are rejected. When awake and offered noxious olfactory stimuli (e.g., an alcohol swab), the neonate will express displeasure. Further discrimination was reported by Klaus and Kennel (1976), who noted that breast-fed babies indicate preference for the breast pads of their own mothers over those of other women by day five of life.

**Table 8.3**  Topics for Parental Education

**Infant (birth–12 months)**
- Immunizations
  - 2 months: diphtheria, pertussis, tetanus (DPT); trivalent oral polio vaccine (TOPV)
  - 4 months: DPT, TOPV
  - 6 months: DPT, optional TOPV
  - 12 months: tuberculin testing
- Nutrition
  - Formula rule-of-thumb: use up to 1 year; do not introduce cow's milk until infant is tolerating 1½ jars of strained baby food/day to maintain nutritional balance.
  - Solid food introduction is controversial. Rice cereal, not mixed, may be given as early as 6 weeks but authorities see little or no need for supplementation prior to 4–6 months.
  - Introduce only one new food at a time. Use daily for several days. Observe for signs of allergy: rashes, diarrhea, vomiting, hives.
  - Start with single strained foods (e.g., applesauce), not "mixed fruit dessert."
  - after cereals have been introduced
    - 6 months: mashed egg yolk, strained or blenderized fruits, yellow vegetables, green vegetables, meats
    - 10–12 months: liquids in a cup

**Table 8.3**    Topics for Parental Education (continued)

- Prepared baby food is expensive and can contain large concentrations of sugar and sodium. Blenderized table food is more nutritious.
- Dental caries may become a problem if a child is permitted to sleep with a bottle of juice or formula. Prevent "bottle mouth" by putting only water in a child's bottle prior to bed. Allowing a child to go to sleep with a bottle also predisposes the child to otitis media from juice or formula that penetrates the child's short, wide eustachian tubes.
- Other Concerns
  - Each infant has own temperament and expresses needs through crying.
  - Accident and safety precautions: allow no unsupervised tub baths; "baby-proof" the environment.
  - Review normal infant development and provide anticipatory guidance when next developmental stage is approaching.

**Toddler (1–3 years)**
- Immunizations
  - 15 months: mumps, measles, and rubella (MMR)
  - 18 months: DPT, TOPV
- Nutrition
  - Wean gradually, as tolerated (child will indicate the appropriate pace)
  - Encourage drinking from a cup
- Other concerns
  - Accident prevention
    - Anticipate safety concerns, protect from falls, close/lock potentially dangerous areas (e.g., medications)
    - Remove tiny objects (peanuts, small candies/toys, etc.), sharp objects from environment
    - Keep cabinets locked (even those above high counters)
    - Use safety child car seats (now required by law in many states)
    - Minimize "attractive nuisances" (e.g., neighbor's pool, fountain, pond) that could lead to a near-drowning incident
    - Allow no unsupervised tub, wading pool, or water play
    - Do not leave stove tops unattended (burning/scalding accidents are common)
  - Schedule a dental checkup

**Preschooler (3–6 years)**
- Immunizations
  - 4–6 years: DPT, TOPV boosters
- Nutrition
  - Have parents do a premeasured dietary recall for 1 week if they are concerned that child eats too little. (Parents are usually impressed with amount consumed.)
- Other Concerns
  - Secure/lock up all poisons
  - Be aware of playing in the street (running after balls, riding tricycles, etc.)
  - Preschoolers respond well to safety education and limit setting. Use role modeling of good health and safety habits to produce careful children.

**School-age Child (6–12 years)**
- Immunizations
  - TB test usually every one to two years
- Nutrition
  - Counsel on proper dietary composition
- Other Concerns
  - Teach accident prevention related to sports, falls, etc.
  - Instruct in detecting behavior/socialization problems, learning disabilities.
  - Begin sex education.
  - Practice discretion in exposure to media production (TV, movies).

**Table 8.3**    Topics for Parental Education (continued)

- Describe communicable diseases related to school.
- Somatic complaints and fatigue not uncommon; most frequently seen at ages 6, 9, 11, and 12 years.
- Fears not uncommon, especially at ages 6, 7, 10, and 11 years.

**Adolescent (12–19 years)**
- Immunizations
  - 14–16 years: tetanus and diphtheria booster (repeat every 10 years during adulthood).
- Nutrition
  - Counsel about proper diet
- Other Concerns
  - Counsel about
    - Sex education/family planning (as indicated)
    - Poisoning, substance abuse (smoking, drugs, and alcohol) and consequences
    - Motor vehicle safety (both operator/passenger)
    - Skin care (acne vulgaris)
    - Sports injuries, drowning
    - Improper use of firearms

# Sensory-Perceptual Development

## Infant (birth–12 months)
- Vision
  - birth: fixes on human face; demonstrates preference
  - 2 months: follows to midline; produces tears
  - 4 months: follows objects 180°
  - 6 months: inspects hands; can fix on objects 3 feet away; strabismus is no longer within normal limits
  - 8 months: eye color permanent
  - 10 months: tilts head backwards to look up
  - 12 months: smooth visual pursuit of objects; 20/100 vision
- Sound, Language, and Learning
  - newborns prefer higher-pitched voices
  - all infants (including the deaf) coo and babble, especially at 6 months of age; newborns startle at loud noises
  - 2–3 months: laughing, squealing
  - 4 months: belly laughs
  - 4–5 months: turns toward voice (quiet listening)
  - 8–10 months: verbalizes "dada", "mama" (nonspecific); responds to own name (about 10 months); receptive language skills develop first; localizes sound above or below
  - 7–11 months: imitates speech sounds, understands name and "no," "bye," and "pat-a-cake"
  - 1 year: 1 word (or a few) in spoken vocabulary; comprehends "give" and stops when told "no"; receptive vocabulary of several dozen words

- 3–12 months: learned rather than reflex behavior—recognizes certain sounds, ignores others, attends to quiet sounds more than to loud ones; deaf infants lose vocal ability by 1 year

## Toddler (1–3 years)
- Vision
  - 18 months: interested in pictures
  - 2 years: identifies forms; 20/40 vision
  - 3 years: 20/30 vision
- Sound, Language, and Learning
  - begins spoken language (often around time of walking); concentration on one or the other may occur
  - 12–18 months: recognizes nouns that stand for objects; uses gestures to make needs known
  - 18–24 months: follows directions; points to nose, hair, eyes on command; comprehends "give me that" when accompanied by a gesture
  - 2–2½ years: 300 words, 2-word sentences; uses colors; understands action-oriented verbs and commands; understands size gradations and designates "me, I, mine;" uses plurals
  - 3 years: 3-word sentences; gives first and last names; progressive comprehension of speech; responds to musical sounds (pitch pipes)

## Preschool (3–6 years)
- Vision
  - 3 years: 20/30 vision
  - 4 years: cooperates with Snellen testing
  - 5 years: normal accommodation and refraction
  - clues to visual deficits
    * squinting
    * favoring one eye
    * tilting head
    * bumping into objects
- Sound, Language, and Learning
  - 4–5 word sentences, with adult syntax
  - vocabulary of around 2,100 words
  - can name body parts, recognize colors
  - talks frequently and listens; quiet sounds are more effective than loud ones
  - cooperates with systematic audiometric tests
  - 3–5 years: comprehends cold, tired, and hungry; understands prepositions
  - 4–5 years: knows opposite analogies (2 of 3 attempts, DDST)
  - 5–6 years: defines words (6 of 9 attempts, DDST); knows composition of objects (3 of 3 attempts, DDST)
  - clues to hearing deficits
    * high TV volume
    * poor/absent response to others

* results of formal audiometric testing
* unintelligible speech (age 5 + )

### School Age (6–12 years)
- Vision
  - 7 years: 20/20 vision
- Sound, Language, and Learning
  - continues to augment vocabulary and cognitive skills

### Adolescent (12–19 years)
- Vision
  - regular testing important
- Sound, Language, and Learning
  - adult verbal skills with ever-increasing vocabulary

## GENERIC CARE PLAN FOR THE NURSING DIAGNOSIS
## SENSORY-PERCEPTUAL ALTERATION (Specify)

## 1. General Information

### a. Etiology
- Sensory organ alterations
- Long-term neurologic sequelae after an insult to the CNS (encephalitis)
- Anesthetics
- Sensory deprivation (or overload)
- CNS hemorrhage
- CNS infection
- Impaired oxygenation
- Cerebral edema (Reye's syndrome, trauma)
- Musculoskeletal alterations (paralysis, amputation)
- Seizure activity
- Biochemical changes affecting CNS (hypoglycemia)

### b. Clinical Manifestations
- Disorientation
- Decreased cognitive ability
- Deterioration of developmental skills (language, locomotor, feeding, toileting, etc.)
- Lack of attention
- Restlessness
- Hearing, vision impairment
- Sleep disturbances

- Listlessness
- Auditory and/or visual hallucinations
- Immobility
- Unconsciousness
- Coma

c. **Multidisciplinary Approaches**
- Diagnostic tests (EEG, CAT scan, x-ray, brain scan, hearing and vision tests)
- Occupational, child-life, physical therapists
- Management of increasing intracranial pressure (diuresis, ventricular taps)
- Assistive devices: splints, braces
- Medications
  • diuretics
  • adrenocorticosteroids
  • antibiotics

## 2. Nursing Process

a. **Assessment**
- Cognitive abilities (language, reasoning)
- Sensory perception (vision, hearing, touch, taste, smell)
- Behavior
- Response to stimuli (pain, touch, warmth, etc.)

b. **Goal**
Child will function at optimal level of sensory ability.

c. **Interventions**
- Orient child with vision impairment to the environment.
- Provide (or enlist the help of parents in providing)
  • conversation with child during routine care
  • tape recordings of child's friends and family members
  • taped story readings
  • stories read in person
  • exposure to various textures
  • exposure to various smells
  • kinesthetic stimulation (massages, backrubs, touch)
  • visual stimuli if eye opening is present
  • passive range-of-motion exercises to all joints 4 times/day
- Provide routines and continuity of care with same nurse caring for child as much as possible.
- Ensure that no conversations regarding a child's grave prognosis take place at the bedside.
- Explain procedures before beginning.

**NURSING TIP: Hearing is the last sense to be lost with CNS injury. Even preverbal children may possibly sense the emotions of parents and caretakers. Children who "wake up" from a comatose state often remember the nurse who talked to them while administering care.**

- Provide only the stimulation that is minimally necessary to the child with a CNS infection, cerebral edema (trauma, Reye's syndrome), or intractable seizures.
- Monitor effects of drugs affecting the CNS.
- Maintain patency of airway (oral, endotracheal) by suctioning as often as needed to keep the child's airway open and free of secretions.
- Change child's position at least every 2 hours.
- Provide chest physical therapy.
- Monitor vital signs and neurologic status as often as necessary depending on stability of child's condition (every 15 minutes to every 2 hours); see *Seizure Assessment,* page 277, and table 8.4, *Glasgow Coma Scale.*

**Table 8.4**    Glasgow Coma Scale

| Eyes | Open | Spontaneously | 4 |
|---|---|---|---|
| | | To verbal command | 3 |
| | | To pain | 2 |
| | No response | | 1 |
| Best motor | To verbal | Obeys | 6 |
| response | command | Localizes pain | 5 |
| | To painful stimulus | Flexion, withdrawal | 4 |
| | | Flexion, abnormal (decorticate rigidity) | 3 |
| | | Extension (decerebrate rigidity) | 2 |
| | | No response | 1 |
| Best verbal | | Oriented and converses | 5 |
| response | | Disoriented and converses | 4 |
| | | Inappropriate words | 3 |
| | | Incomprehensible sounds | 2 |
| | | No response | 1 |
| TOTAL | | | 3–15 |

- Maintain skin integrity by placing child on egg-crate mattress or sheepskin.
- Brush teeth and rinse mouth with cleansing agent (mouthwash, hydrogen peroxide) at least twice a day.
- Monitor eyes for dryness and irritation and lubricate as needed (dressings, artificial tears).
- Monitor nutrition and hydration.

       – Check Foley drainage and give catheter care at least once/shift, according to hospital protocol.
       – Monitor bowel elimination and administer stool softeners or enemas as ordered.
       – Provide passive range of motion at least every 4 hours.
       – Prevent contractures by using hand rolls, footboards, high-top sneakers, braces, splints as needed.

**d. Evaluation**
       – Child regains sensory perceptual ability as evidenced by
         • improved level of consciousnesss
         • responding to stimuli
         • performing at previous developmental level.

**e. Possible Related Nursing Related Diagnoses**
Fluid volume deficit
Impaired physical mobility
Potential for injury

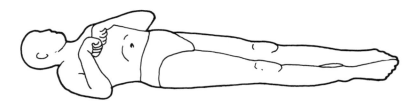

**Figure 8.1**  Decorticate Posturing
When there is loss of cerebral functioning, the child adducts the arms at the shoulders, flexes the arms on the chest, flexes the wrists and clenches the fist. The child's legs are extended and adducted.

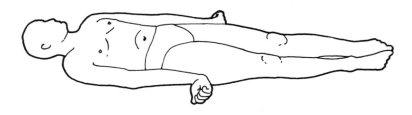

**Figure 8.2**  Decerebrate Posturing
When there is loss of midbrain functioning, the child extends his/her body, and pronates the arms and legs.

## Selected Health Problems Frequently Associated with the Nursing Diagnosis SENSORY-PERCEPTUAL ALTERATION

### 1. Seizures

#### a. Discussion

A seizure is a symptom of an underlying disorder of brain function. It characteristically consists of transient, involuntary alterations in consciousness or abnormalities in motor activity, behavior, sensation, or autonomic function. These changes result from a neuronal disturbance producing abnormal electrical discharges. The part of the brain affected and frequency of electrical aberrations may be indicated by clinical symptomatology.

"Epilepsy" traditionally refers to recurrent seizure activity, but has fallen out of common usage for the more acceptable "seizure disorder." Fortunately, most childhood seizure tendencies do not persist into adulthood, perhaps because of the brain's increasing functional maturity with age.

**Causes.**    It is estimated that 4%–6% of children will have one or more seizures during the first 16 years of life. Some known etiologies include infection (meningitis, sepsis), metabolic disturbance (hypoglycemia, hypocalcemia), trauma (child abuse, accidents), and intoxication (lead poisoning, drug ingestion). It is also known that fever may precipitate seizures in children with decreased neuronal thresholds.

Approximately 50% of children who experience recurrent seizures do so without any identifiable reason. This type of seizure activity is referred to as idiopathic (Chee, 1980).

**Diagnosis.**    Accurate diagnosis of seizure disorders requires consideration of many factors, from physical trauma to genetic heritage. The history and physical examination can offer invaluable clues to causal factors and seizure pattern. It is also imperative to describe all observable activity during an actual seizure (see *Seizure Assessment,* page 277). An electroencephalogram (EEG), the test most frequently used to establish seizure diagnosis, is a painless recording of electrical activity from the brain.

**Classification.**    Correct classification of seizure activity is crucial to proper management. It provides uniformity in diagnosis and evaluation and helps ensure better communication.

The International Classification of Epileptic Seizures was developed in 1964 and revised in 1981. This most common classification system draws upon clinical, pathophysiologic, and electroencephalographic prognostic and therapeutic considerations (Chee; Commission on Classification and Terminology of the International League Against Epilepsy, 1981) and is divided into three sections: generalized, partial, and unclassified.

Generalized seizures arise from neuronal hypersynchronized discharges from groups of cerebral neurons in both hemispheres. Three sub-types are

— *Tonic-clonic (grand mal):* onset is abrupt, and may be accompanied by an aura or prodrome. This aura may be described as a mood change, a visual or auditory disturbance, or a gastrointestinal upset; it is an integral part of the seizure and may be helpful in locating the focal origin in the brain.

Unconsciousness follows the prodrome, then a 10- to 20-second tonic (stiffening) phase. Cyanosis and upward deviation of the eyes may be observed. The clonic (jerking) phase follows, lasting 2–3 minutes; skeletal muscles rhythmically contract and relax, and the child may experience increased pharyngeal secretions, tongue biting, incontinence, or tachycardia. Postictal confusion, exhaustion, and headache are common.

Thirty minutes or more of uninterrupted seizure activity is termed status epilepticus. The cerebral anoxia and/or ischemic damage associated with this medical emergency may lead to permanent brain damage or death (Chee).
— *Absence (petit mal):* produce brief lapses of awareness and the child appears to be daydreaming. The child does not fall but ceases all verbal and motor activity. The seizure lasts 10 to 30 seconds and as many as 10 or more may occur daily. Postictal confusion is not evident (Chee).
— *Myoclonic:* characterized by brief involuntary muscular jerks of one or more muscles of the body. They may be localized or generalized (Chee).

Partial seizures arise from a localized area in the brain. Clinical signs depend on which brain segment experiences the hypersynchrony of discharges. Any portion of the body may be involved, depending on the site of origin. Usually the level of consciousness is not impaired. Partial seizures may evolve into generalized seizures. Three types are

— *Simple partial:* may have motor, sensory or autonomic components. Consciousness is not impaired. Tonic-clonic movements can be observed if the focus is near or in the motor region of the brain. If this type of activity continues and "marches" to include one entire side of the body it would be a Jacksonian seizure (Chee).
— *Complex partial* (psychomotor or temporal lobe): cause a wide variety of behaviors affecting cognitive, psychomotor, or psychosensory function. Level of consciousness is impaired. The child may appear to be daydreaming or staring. Activity lasts one to two minutes. Automatisms (repetition of inappropriate acts)

frequently accompany the above behavior. These might include lip smacking, picking at clothes, or walking in circles. Postictal confusion may be experienced (Chee).
- *Secondary generalized:* focal seizures that spread to both cerebral hemispheres (Chee).

   Unclassified seizures include all seizures that cannot be classified because of insufficient or incomplete data. Many neonatal seizures fall under this category (Chee).
   Febrile seizures are not usually associated with epilepsy. They usually consist of tonic-clonic movements and occur in children between 6 months and 3 years of age who are experiencing sudden temperature rise. Often fever is secondary to an upper respiratory infection (Chee).
   Many people still fear epilepsy and the seizure it causes. Children with seizure disorders are often treated differently from other children because of misconceptions about seizures. Children with seizure disorders can learn to manage their disease and minimize the occurrence of seizures.

b. **Multidisciplinary Approaches**
   - Diazepam or phenobarbital in the emergency room, if necessary, to control seizures
   - Respiratory and cardiac monitoring
   - Children suffering a first seizure will generally be referred for neurologic work-up

# Additional Nursing Care That Can Be Incorporated into the Generic Care Plan

a. **Assessment**
   - Activity preceding seizure(s)
     • fatigue, stress
     • presence/absence of aura (specific smell, noise, visual impression, headache, GI upset)
     • description of aura
   - Duration
   - Frequency
   - Behavior during seizure
   - Awareness of surroundings
     • conscious
     • semiconscious
     • unconscious
     • unaware that seizure activity has taken place
   - Continence/incontinence
     • urine
     • feces
   - Motor activity

- muscle tone
- eyes: staring, rolling back, movement to right, movement to left, rapid or slow blinking
- face: right twitches, left twitches
- mouth: right twitches, left twitches
- head: back, forward, right, left
- respirations: air movement, color
- right or left side: hand, arm, foot, leg twitching, other movements (describe)
- equality of sies: tonic-clonic movement or its absence
  - Postseizure (postictal) state
    - note degree of alertness, orientation to person, place, time, as well as weakness in extremities
    - postictal drowsiness
    - difficulty of arousal
  - History of prior seizure activity, anticonvulsant drugs (route, dose, frequency, patterns of compliance)
  - Parental feelings, knowledge, and concerns about management of seizures

b. **Goals**

Child will return to prior level of consciousness with no further injury.
Parents will verbalize care during and after seizures.
Parents/child will be able to realistically describe any necessary limitations in child's activity.

c. **Interventions**

- Remain calm.
- Maintain an adequate airway
  - do not place anything in the child's mouth
  - place the child in supine position and hyperextend the neck
  - turn the child's head to side if necessary to permit saliva and mucous to drain from mouth
  - have suction equipment available
- Protect the child from injury
  - do not restrain
  - pad siderails if needed
  - protect from falling; ease child to floor
- Observe and record progression of events.
- Observe postictal state; let child sleep until s/he awakens.
- Instruct parents in prompt treatment of fever and emergency management of seizures (a helpful "Parent Information Kit" is available from the Epilepsy Foundation of America) (Muehl, 1979).
- Instruct parents to observe time, and record seizure activity.
- Encourage age-appropriate self-care activities.
- Avoid unnecessary activity restrictions; discuss limitations in activity such as tree climbing or swimming.

- Teach about medication
  - benefits and side effects
  - how and when it is to be taken
  - possible consequences if medication is stopped abruptly
- Encourage parents to be honest and open about the disorder, and not to treat the child differently than they normally would.
- Refer parents to Epilepsy Foundation of America.

**d. Evaluation**
- Child is aware of surroundings, muscle tone is normal, pupils are equal and react to light and accommodation.
- Parents and child
  - verbalize an understanding of the seizure disorder, safety measures, medication administration, and notification of MD when complications arise.
  - maintain a positive attitude about the disorder.
- Parents maintain a written record of the child's seizure activity.
- Limitations (such as protective helmet) are discussed realistically and carried out in the home environment at time of discharge (Muehl).

## Other Possible Nursing Diagnoses

Alteration in bowel elimination: incontinence
Alteration in family process
Anxiety
Disturbance in self-concept
Fear
Impaired social interactions
Impaired verbal communication
Ineffective airway clearance
Knowledge deficit
Potential for injury
Powerlessness

## 2. Bacterial Meningitis

**a. Discussion**
- An inflammation of the meninges caused by bacterial infection of the CSF
- Etiology varies with age, geographical area, and from year to year
- Most common associated organisms are *E. coli, H. influenzae,* and *D. pneumoniae* (Chee).
- Antecedent factors can include upper respiratory infection, occasionally otitis media or mastoiditis, or a penetrating head wound

**b. Multidisciplinary Approaches**
- Lumbar puncture

    — Isolation
    — Antibiotic therapy

# Additional Nursing Care That Can Be Incorporated into the Generic Care Plan

   **a.**  **Assessment**  (age, causative agent, and stage of disease can all affect the presenting symptomatology)
      — *Neonates (to 1 month):* irritability, vomiting, anorexia, lethargy, seizures, fever unexplained by other symptoms
      — *Infants (to 2 years):* as above, also neck rigidity, tight fontanel, positive Kernig's or Brudzinski's sign
        • Kernig's: when child is lying prone and the thigh is passively flexed to a right angle, the leg is not able to extend completely
        • Brudzinski's: when one leg is flexed passively, the opposite leg also flexes
        • Brudzinski's neck sign: when the neck is flexed passively, both legs flex
      — *Children over 2 years:* vomiting, headache, decreased alertness followed by neck rigidity, seizures, positive Kernig's sign or Brudzinski's sign, markedly increased lethargy (Chee)

   **b.**  **Goals**
     Child
      — will return to pre-illness level of consciousness.
      — is free from further injury.

   **c.**  **Interventions**
      — Monitor airway and respiratory rate every 2 hours.
      — Monitor blood pressure, level of consciousness, neurologic status, I&O every 2 hours.
      — Assist with lumbar puncture.
      — Maintain seizure and isolation precautions.
      — Administer antibiotic therapy on time to ensure adequate blood levels.

   **d.**  **Evaluation**
      — Child can flex neck on command; has flat fontanel; has negative Kernigs' and Brudzinski's signs.

# Other Possible Nursing Diagnoses

Alteration in comfort: pain
Fluid volume deficit
Potential for injury

## 3. Hydrocephalus

a. **Definition/Discussion**
   – Hydrocephalus is a neurologic disorder involving an imbalance between the rate of cerebral spinal fluid (CSF) production and its absorption from the arachnoid villi. This results in an enlargement of the ventricles thereby causing an increase in the child's head circumference. Causes of this disorder include congenital malformations, infections, trauma, and neoplasms.
   – Two types
     • communicating (obstruction of CSF at the subarachnoid space)
     • noncommunicating (obstruction within the ventricular system)
   Symptomatology will be influenced by the age of the child, the acuteness of onset, and speed of progression. Signs of increased intracranial pressure will be evident in varied degrees.
   Ventriculoperitoneal or ventriculoatrial shunts are placed to decrease the intracranial pressure by diverting the CSF around the point of obstruction. The procedure consists of drilling a burrhole, inserting a ventricular catheter into the lateral ventricle, and bringing the tubing through the skull to the subcutaneous space of the scalp where a right angle is made. The catheter is then connected to a selected valve and placed subcutaneously into the abdominal cavity or right atrium (through a vein) where the CSF drains (see figure 8.3). Ventriculoperitoneal shunts are the procedure of choice for infants and young children; ventriculoatrial shunts are used most frequently in older children and adults.
   Some shunts are equipped with flushing valves that can aid in assessing function and patency of both proximal and distal ends of the drainage system. Flushing devices work under the principle that the CSF within the chamber can be forced out only if the distal catheter is patent and will refill only if the proximal catheter is patent. Once CSF drainage has stabilized the child may be placed on an "on/off" shunt schedule. This prevents slit-like ventricles from forming and promotes normal head configuration. Figure 8.4 shows one example of a flushing device.

b. **Multidisciplinary Approaches**
   – Computerized axial tomography (CAT scan)
   – Medicines
     • acetaminophen for headache and analgesia or fever; narcotics are contraindicated (may mask symptoms of deterioration)
     • IV antibiotics
     • dexamethasone/steroids to minimize intracranial inflammation
     • Diamox or other diuretics
     • anticonvulsants
   – Ventriculoperitoneal or ventriculoatrial shunt

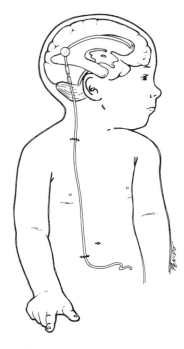 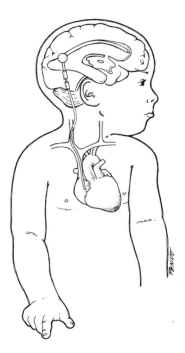

A. Ventriculoperitoneal Shunt
Cerebrospinal fluid drains from
ventricle into peritoneum.

B. Ventriculoatrial Shunt
Cerebrospinal fluid drains from
ventricle in right atrium.

**Figure 8.3**    Shunt Placement

        — Ventriculostomy: placement of a ventricular catheter, via a burrhole in the skull, into the lateral ventricle; catheter is attached to an external drainage system (placed to reduce intracranial pressure, as an alternative to standard shunt placement, and as a medication route).

## Additional Nursing Care That Can Be Incorporated into the Generic Care Plan

    a.  **Assessment**
        — Signs of infection: fever, subnormal temperature, lethargy, listlessness, "toxic look," seizures, anorexia
        — Vital signs, including blood pressure and neuro checks, for symptoms of increased ICP
           • elevated blood pressure and widening pulse pressure
           • respiratory depression (irregular and decreased respirations)
           • bradycardia
        — Feeding difficulty, sucking problems

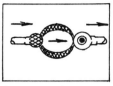 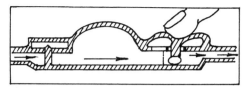

If valve cannot be compressed, there is an obstruction between the ventricle and the valve.

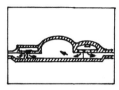 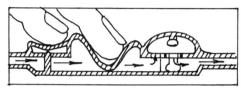

If valve does not refill, there is an obstruction between valve and anatomical reservoir.

**Figure 8.4**   Flushing Valve System for Shunt
Shunt valves control drainage of cerebrospinal fluid from ventricles or prevent reflux of cerebrospinal fluid back to ventricle. Some shunt valves may be flushed to insure patency.

— Occasional shrill, high-pitched cry
— Vomiting, especially projectile
— Opisthotonus
— Seizure activity
— Somnolence, irritability, photophobia
— Lower limb spasms, absence of normal lower limb reflexes
— Decreasing level of consciousness
— Variable responses to stimuli of different types
— Head circumference
   • fronto-occipital diameter above brows
   • same person measuring if possible
   • repeat measurements with a second opinion if they change
   • palpate separated sutures—observe for Macewen's sign (cracked-pot sound when the skull is percussed)
— Bulging, full, pulsating fontanels, depressed eyes where the sclera can be seen above the iris ("setting sun" sign), and dilated scalp veins
— Baseline behavior, sleep patterns, developmental level, achievements to date
— Child's and family's coping abilities and teaching needs
— Patency of shunt (observe for signs of increased ICP)

**b.   Goals**
Child will remain free from complications of increased ICP.
Family will
   — verbalize understanding of the mechanisms of hydrocephalus, prognosis, and reasons for interventions.

- list signs and symptoms of shunt infection and blockage prior to discharge.

c. **Interventions**
   - Feed small amounts frequently on a flexible schedule to accommodate diagnostic procedures (such as a CAT scan), which may induce an episode of vomiting.
   - Restrict fluids to $1/3$–$1/2$ of the daily maintenance level.
   - Shunt care
     - position head so that child will lie on unoperated side or will not lie prone if a VP shunt was inserted.
     - determine what type of shunt has been inserted and plan care accordingly. (Some shunts require elevating the head of the bed 30° to facilitate drainage; some require positioning flat in bed to avoid rapid loss of intracranial fluid.)
   - Assess neurologic status (level of consciousness, pupillary reaction, motor function, reflexes, vital signs) every hour.
   - Maintain hydration; assess daily weights, I&O.
   - Assess tissue perfusion (temperature of extremities, peripheral pulses, capillary refill) every 2 hours.
   - Prevent infection: observe wound sites for redness, drainage, edema, elevated temperature.
   - Provide comfort: medicate for pain.
   - Flush shunt as ordered.
   - Discuss signs of malfunction and infection with parents (medical emergencies)
     - infection: lethargy, nausea, vomiting, signs of meningeal irritation
     - obstruction: lethargy, vomiting, seizures, focal neurologic signs, swelling around the shunt site (signs of increased ICP)
   - Instruct parents how to flush shunt.
   - If ventriculostomy is used as an interim therapy
     - obtain specific written orders as to
       * degree of elevation of head of bed
       * height of inlet to collection bag
       * whether tubing is to be clamped, unclamped, or on an alternating schedule
       * the characteristics of expected drainage
       * need for IV fluids
     - continually assess the child for signs of increased intracranial pressure and amount of drainage from system
     - change the child's position carefully (positional changes can cause sudden changes in intraventricular pressure)
     - prevent infection by using aseptic technique when handling the drainage system
     - secure all tubing connections with tape to prevent unnecessary breaks in system

- note any changes in color, consistency, and amount of cerebrospinal fluid
- monitor vital signs frequently
- use protective isolation if indicated (Bonta & Blich-feldt, 1984)
- clamp ventriculostomy tubing if child is moved
- label ventriculostomy tubing with a special label so it is not mistaken for IV tubing (Sporing, Walton, & Cady, 1984; Masaorki & Piercy, 1984)

**d. Evaluation**
- Child's vital signs remain stable; pulse pressure does not change appreciably over time; no respiratory compromise.
- Parents verbalize and demonstrate knowledge and skills necessary to provide safe home care.

## Other Possible Nursing Diagnoses

Alteration in family process
Potential for injury

## 4. Cerebral Trauma/Edema

**a. Discussion**
- Children's proportionally large and heavy heads make them prime candidates for cerebrospinal trauma; most concussions are mild and do not require hospital admission.
- Common etiologies of head trauma are motor vehicle accidents, falls, and child abuse.
- The most common head injury from blunt trauma is concussion, see figure 8.5 for mechanism of a *coup contre coup* injury.
- Cerebral edema is a complication of every brain injury; the edema does not peak until 48–72 hours post-trauma, and the danger of complications from the edema lasts for days.

**b. Multidisciplinary Approaches**
- CAT scan, initial x-rays to distinguish diffuse edema from hematoma formation
- If no responsible person can care for the child, hospitalization or long term ER observation may be necessary.
- In severe injury
  - immediate transfer to a regional head trauma referral center
  - IV steroids (dexamethasone) to quell the inflammatory response.
- Intubation and mechanical ventilation to minimize $PCO_2$ even if patient is capable of respiratory effort
- $CO_2$ to decrease capillary permeability in the injured area and discourage fluid collection

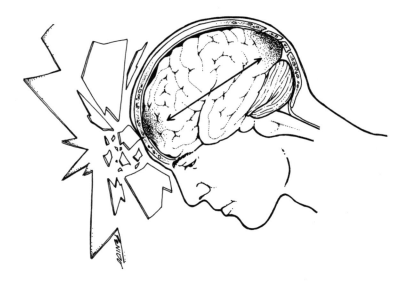

**Figure 8.5**  Mechanism of a Coup Contre Coup Injury
The coup contre coup injury occurs on the portion of the brain opposite the site of skull impact.

- Strict fluid restriction (to about ½ maintenance levels)
- Mannitol or similar osmotic diuretic when there is evidence of a dangerous increase in intracranial pressure
- Life-sustaining drugs (e.g., dopamine) as necessary
- Craniotomy to control bleeding, evacuate hematoma

## Additional Nursing Care That Can Be Incorporated into the Generic Care Plan

a.  **Assessment**
- Neurologic status (use table 8.4, Glasgow Coma Scale)
- Transient loss of consciousness
- Short-term amnesia regarding the accident
- Neurologic sequelae (e.g., weakness, tremors)
- Headache
- Lethargy and vomiting

b.  **Goal**
Child will maintain/regain previous level of consciousness.

c.  **Interventions**
- Monitor neurologic status and vital signs every 30 minutes to 1 hour (use Glasgow Coma Scale).
- Be alert to signs indicating a deterioration of status
  - altered mental status

- extreme lethargy
- increasingly severe headache (unrelieved by aspirin or acetaminophen)
- behavior/personality changes: somnolence or hyperactivity
- vomiting (more than 3 times), especially projectile
- unequal pupils/ocular changes, diminished response to light, blurred vision
- ataxia
- seizures
- involuntary motion of arms or legs.
  - Elevate the head of the bed at least 30° to promote jugular venous drainage from the head.
  - Do not administer narcotics or sedatives for pain (may mask symptoms of worsening of the injury).
  - Refer family members to the National Head Injury Foundation.

**d. Evaluation**
  - Child is arousable, free from head pain.

---

**NURSING TIP: If a serious injury is not suspected, the child may be sent home. Instruct parents to awaken the child every 1 to 2 hours to check level of consciousness. Provide a written list of symptoms that would indicate a worsening of the child's condition and necessitate immediate return to the hospital.**

---

## Other Possible Nursing Diagnoses

Fluid volume deficit or excess
Impaired physical mobility
Impaired skin integrity
Potential for injury

## 5. Reye's Syndrome

**a. Discussion**
  - An acute disease characterized by severe encephalopathy, increased intracranial pressure, hypoglycemia, and fatty degeneration of the viscera, primarily the liver, but also the kidneys, heart, lungs, pancreas, and skeletal muscle (Chee).
  - Etiology is unknown, although Reye's is often preceded by a viral infection. In younger children, chickenpox is the most common antecedent; in older children influenza B is most common.

- Clinical correlation has been shown between the use of aspirin in treatment of viral illness and Reye's syndrome.
- Symptoms vary with the child's age and stage of disease, but usually occur several hours to several days following recovery from a viral infection.
  - *infants:* hyperventilation or respiratory distress, high-pitched cry, mild twitching of extremities, irritability, and lethargy (Chee).
  - *older children:* persistent vomiting, altered sensorium (mild lethargy→stupor→seizures or coma), behavioral changes (irritability, irrational behavior), and hyperventilation (Chee)

---

**NURSING TIP: The same signs and symptoms occur in adolescents, but may be mistaken for drug or alcohol abuse (Chee).**

---

b. **Multidisciplinary Approaches**
   - Liver biopsy to provide a definitive diagnosis
   - SGOT, SGPT, ammonia, prothrombin time (all will be elevated)
   - Blood glucose (usually subnormal)
   - Drug screening (to rule out drug overdose)
   - Lumbar puncture (to rule out meningitis)
   - Specific treatment varies with the stage of the child's illness. Younger children, especially, may progress through the stages rapidly and require constant monitoring. In all cases, care is supportive.
     - IV therapy to correct dehydration and hypoglycemia, maintain adequate urine output
     - frequent neurologic assessment with invasive device (subarachnoid bolt) to monitor intracranial pressure
     - seizure control
     - adequate ventilation

# Additional Nursing Care That Can Be Incorporated into the Generic Care Plan

a. **Assessment**
   - Impaired blood coagulation
   - Glucose level
   - Vital signs
   - Hydration status
   - Neurologic status: intracranial pressure
   - Central venous pressure

**b. Goal**
Child will be free from residual effects.

**c. Interventions**
- Assist with lumbar puncture.
- Assist with ventilation if necessary; adjust respirator settings as ordered to maintain hypocapnia (hypocarbia).
- Monitor NG tube and Foley catheter for patency.
- Monitor vital signs including CVP frequently depending on child's condition.
- Monitor ABGs, serum electrolytes, BUN, and glucose levels.
- Check child for petechiae and signs of bleeding (e.g., hematest stool and urine).
- Adjust fluid volumes as ordered to prevent dehydration or cerebral edema depending upon cerebral perfusion pressures.
- Orient child (when conscious) to surroundings and to the events of the illness and hospitalization.

**d. Evaluation**
- Child is free from signs of complications as evidenced by
  - no emesis
  - no signs of bleeding
  - intracranial pressures within normal limits
  - respiratory rate within normal limits.

## Other Possible Nursing Diagnoses

Anxiety (child and parent)
Fluid volume deficit
Fluid volume excess (cerebral)
Impaired physical mobility
Impairment of skin integrity
Ineffective breathing pattern/impaired gas exchange
Knowledge deficit
Potential for injury

## 6. Plumbism (Lead Poisoning)

**a. Discussion:**  Sources of environmental lead include lead-containing gasoline, old peeling paint, pewter dishes (unglazed), some types of pottery.

**b. Multidisciplinary Approaches**
- Diagnostic tests: blood lead level, erythrocyte-protoporphyrin level, x-ray of long bones
- Calcium disodium edetate (EDTA) IM or IV every 4–6 hours, and British antilewisite (BAL) IM every 4 hours for 5 days

- Calcium gluconate
- Exchange transfusion if necessary
- Cleansing enema for acute lead ingestion
- IV if necessary
- Lumbar puncture to relieve CNS pressure if necessary
- Social service
  • home visit by visiting nurse for environmental assessment
  • child care services as needed

# Additional Nursing Care That Can Be Incorporated into the Generic Care Plan

a. **Assessment**
   - Early signs of poisoning from ingestion: hyperactivity, impulsiveness, aggression, no interest in play, irritability, lethargy, delay or loss of verbal ability, loss of recently acquired skills, clumsiness, sensory perception deficits, and shortening of attention span
   - Signs of toxicity from inhalation: tremor, irritability, confusion, hallucinations, ataxia, chorea, and sleep disturbances
   - History of pica, recent change in behavior, recent loss of acquired skills (particularly speech), or developmental delay
   - Environmental hazard profile

b. **Goals**
   Child will
   - remain free from injury from seizure.
   - be able to verbalize reason for treatment (if developmentally capable).
   Child's
   - serum and erythrocyte-protoporphyrin levels will decrease to normal levels.
   - environment will be free from sources of lead.

c. **Interventions**
   - Maintain seizure precautions and keep emergency equipment for respiratory arrest at bedside.
   - Provide child with explanations for treatments.
   - Forewarn parents of possible physical and psychologic reactions.
   - Keep detailed account of child's behavior to detect changes in personality and activity level (cerebral damage suggested if increased irritability or passivity, apathy, lethargy, a decrease in alertness, difficulty arousing from sleep, unconsciousness or coma).
   - If lumbar puncture is done to relieve pressure, observe for signs of respiratory arrest.
   - Observe for signs of hypocalcemia (e.g., tetany, convulsions, jittery behavior).

- Discuss with parents ways to decrease pica behavior; ways to remove sources of lead (Whaley & Wong, 1983).
- Refer family to community agency if follow-up on environmental lead screening is needed to remove sources of lead from child's environment.

**d. Evaluation**
- Child/parents describe reason for treatment.
- Child's serum lead and erythrocyte-protoporphyrin levels return to normal.
- Child decreases pica behavior.

## Other Possible Nursing Diagnoses

Activity intolerance
Alteration in nutrition: less than body requirements
Fluid volume deficit
Impaired physical mobility
Knowledge deficit

## 7. Eye Injuries

**a. Discussion**
- Eye injuries (chemical or toxic burns, foreign body or direct trauma) are the major cause of blindness in children over 2 years. Each type of injury carries its own specific risks. Blunt trauma, for instance, can cause hyphema, or hemorrhage into the anterior chamber of the eye.
  - Among the most often overlooked childhood ocular problems are intraocular foreign bodies. Although minimal pain may be involved, and the object may be visible only with x-ray assistance, immediate surgical removal is imperative.

**b. Multidisciplinary Approaches**
- Refer to ophthalmologist, if necessary, for examination (possibly under anesthesia) of the injured eye, removal of foreign body, or suturing laceration
- Antibiotics, steroids
- Bedrest

## Additional Nursing Care That Can Be Incorporated into the Generic Care Plan

**a. Assessment**
- Visual acuity before any other examination or treatment is done (if possible); check each eye separately and both together
- Presence of contact lenses

- Aqueous or vitreous leaks, pupil shape and equality, misshapen iris, pupil reaction, hyphema
- History for use of BB gun or other circumstances that suggest the possibility of foreign body intrusion

**b.  Goal**
Child will recover from injury free from visual impairment.

**c.  Interventions**
- Chemical or toxic burns
  - irrigate copiously with tap water or saline
    * for large amounts of solution, use IV bag of saline with regular IV tubing; for small amounts, a squeeze bottle may be used
    * have child lie supine with head tilted toward side of affected eye
    * place emesis basin or several towels to catch irrigant
    * retract lower lid with fingers
    * instruct child to look up
    * allow irrigant to flow at moderate rate; do not touch tubing to cornea
    * record any foreign material that drains from eye and child's response to irrigation
    * with young children, mummy restraints will probably be necessary, as well as at least one assistant
  - if causative agent is known, use specific neutralizing antidote as ordered
  - check pH if possible
- Foreign body
  - of conjunctiva: irrigate or remove with needle
  - of cornea: irrigate, remove with needle; check for rust ring if foreign body is metal
  - intraocular: patch eye, prevent child from rubbing
    * child should lie supine and close both eyes
    * patch the affected eye and tape securely (use several pieces of tape); be sure all edges are taped securely
- Blunt trauma
  - initiate/enforce emergency treatment: strict bedrest, bilateral patches, sedation
- Penetrating trauma
  - never remove an object impaled in the eye
  - patch both eyes
  - prepare for surgery

**d.  Evaluation**
- Child is able to see.
- Foreign body is removed; eye is not injured further.

## Other Possible Nursing Diagnoses

Alteration in comfort: pain
Guilt (parental/child)

## Child/Parent Education

In any nurse-patient relationship, the nurse is likely to identify gaps in the knowledge that patients and families have regarding their health care. There are many reasons why a child or the parents may be unable to take in information. The nurse should keep in mind that skills and information that she has internalized (and for which she has a scientific knowledge base) may not be "second nature" to patients or their families.

Assessment of the family's readiness to take in information is a key concept. There are many factors related to child/family readiness to acquire knowledge essential to health promotion. Low levels of readiness to take in information are usually related to anxiety, which may be immobilizing. There may be a lack of motivation to learn. For example, in some cultures, health belief patterns foster absolute dependence on providers. Cognitive limitations, such as illiteracy or retardation, may exist. A language barrier (either to foreign or medicotechnologic language) may be present. Inability to manipulate the health care system (e.g., providers) to divulge needed information is another possibility. Some families are more adept at meeting their information needs than other families who find themselves "in awe" of providers or the situation. Denial is a primitive defense mechanism that inhibits ability to learn as well. For example, denial of newly diagnosed cystic fibrosis will certainly preclude the family's ability to learn home IV administration of antibiotics. Finally, unfamiliarity with or inability to use information resources (electronic, human, educational or bureaucratic) may result in an inability to take in information.

## GENERIC CARE PLAN FOR THE NURSING DIAGNOSIS
## KNOWLEDGE DEFICIT

## 1.  General Information

a.  **Etiology**
    –  Lack of exposure
    –  Lack of recall
    –  Misinterpretation of health teaching
    –  Cognitive limitation
    –  Lack of interest
    –  Unfamiliarity with resources
    –  Anxiety

b.  **Clinical Manifestation**
    –  Inability to restate information concerning health care
    –  Inability to understand explanations about health care
    –  Misinterpreting instructions or explanations
    –  Lack of follow-through of previous teaching
    –  Inability to perform a necessary health care skill
    –  Inappropriate (hysterical, hostile, uninterested) behavior

## 2.  Nursing Process

a.  **Assessment**
    –  Level of growth and development in child
    –  Child's/parents' view of health problem
    –  Degree of denial and anger in child/parents
    –  Learning readiness of child/parents
    –  Health beliefs of the family
    –  Educational level of child/parents
    –  Intellectual capacity and learning style of parents/child
    –  Desire or perceived need of parents/child to learn
    –  Response to previous health teaching
    –  Level of knowledge about health problem
    –  Physical status and limitations
    –  Medical problems of child/parent
    –  Statements that reflect cultural, life-style, or ethnic impact on health practices
    –  Verbal acknowledgement of lack of information
    –  Impediments to learning
       •  anxiety
       •  stress
       •  illiteracy, retardation
       •  language barriers

b.  **Goals**
    Child/family will develop the necessary skills for immediate management of health problem.
    Family will identify necessary adjustments in the life-style to cope with health problem.

c.  **Interventions**
    –  Adjust teaching according to level of development of child and learning styles of parents and child; remember that children need shorter teaching sessions than adults.
    –  Plan teaching when child is rested and motivated.
    –  Keep environment free from noise, interruptions and distractions.
    –  Give content at three levels
       •  facts, knowledge, and understanding

- attitudes and feelings
- manual skills
  - Encourage child to assume responsibility for each aspect of self-management when capable.
  - Use written pamphlets and other learning aids to allow use of as many senses as possible and to provide another source of information; choose them carefully so that material is presented in a consistent manner.
  - Involve the learner actively in the learning process.
  - Use repetition and positive feedback to enhance retention.
  - Evaluate learner's progress; make appropriate follow-up referrals or reteach as needed.

**d. Evaluation**
  - Parents and child (if developmentally capable)
    - verbalize and demonstrate cognitive content and motor skills associated with the health promotion behaviors related to original knowledge deficit.
    - know where to obtain additional knowledge if needed.

# Pain

Like all humans, children experience pain. The perception of pain is a protective mechanism and involves the nerve endings, spinal cord, brain stem, and cerebral cortex. When perceived, pain is accompanied by emotional and/or physical reactions. Pain can be classified as

- *Superficial:* involves the cutaneous receptors, is localized, and has a sharp quality
- *Deep:* from muscles, viscera; more persistent and diffuse than superficial pain; usually dull in nature
- *Referred:* usually occurs at visceral level but actual point of focus of reaction or perception of pain is away from area of occurrence, e.g., pain in an ischemic heart is perceived in lower chest

Research indicates that children experience as much pain as adults, yet clinical studies show that physicians and nurses underestimate pain in children and tend not to offer pain medication or teach skills to cope with pain.

In children, nonverbal behaviors and changes in physiologic measures are present before verbal expression of pain, and are an important part of differential diagnosis. Children may deny pain in order to be "good" or to avoid a shot, or may fake pain in order to avoid school or unpleasant procedures. Table 8.5 details children's responses by age.

The dying child may be comfortable with little or no pain medication. This may be in contrast to a previous need for high doses of narcotics. If sedating drugs are administered only as required, most children are conscious until the very end (Whaley & Wong) and experience a period of peace and calm before death. A "period of restlessness," seen as a sign of approaching death, is frequently not altered by drugs or other physical comfort measures. Oversedation may prolong this restlessness and shorten the period of calm by diminishing internal controls. A description of the sensory-perceptual aspects of death is presented in table 8.6.

**Table 8.5**    Pain Responses in Children

| Pain Behaviors According to Age | Response Variables |
|---|---|
| *Infant and Toddler (1 month–1 year and 2–4 years)* | |
| Neonate reaction to pain is total body movement with brief, loud crying. In addition to the nonverbal and physiologic behaviors, the infant and toddler may also roll head from side to side, pull on ear for pain in ear or head, or flex knees to decrease pain in abdomen. Prior to 6 months of age no memory of painful experiences is evident; infant is easily distracted and comforted. After 6 months, infant may recall previous experience with pain from environmental cues (e.g., white uniforms or examining table), which can precipitate a response of intense physical resistance and emotional upset. | Separation from or presence of parents, emotional reactions of parents or siblings, memory of previous painful experience, physical restraints, differences in temperament and reactions. Intrusive procedures (e.g., rectal temperature, injections) are very threatening whether painless or painful. |
| Toddlers can verbally communicate their pain and are able to localize it (e.g., "owie on my knee"); rarely fake pain at this age. | Toddler may regress at threat of pain even without experiencing pain (might ask for bottle, blanket, or may wet pants even if potty trained). Response to medications will also vary because of individual differences, physiologic and emotional condition of child when drugs are given. |
| *Preschooler (3–5 years)* | |
| Respond with same physiologic and nonverbal behaviors as infant and toddler plus increased verbal expression (global response): "I don't feel good." "My tummy hurts." May respond with anger, aggression to pain or threat of pain ("Get out of here." "You're mean.") and may push nurse's hand away, kick, hide to escape. May act dependent, cling to parent, or regress. | Similar to those of the infant/toddler, but is more likely to have exaggerated fears about body injury (worries about bleeding, insides falling out, needle punctures, mutilation, and castration). "Magical thinking" (i.e., thoughts can cause events) lead to guilt, shame, and idea that pain is punishment for wrongdoing. |
| 4- to 5-year-old may be able to control self and not cry; if cannot, becomes upset and ashamed. May fake stomach ache, sore throat, or earache to get out of stressful situation. | |
| May prefer parent of opposite sex for comfort. Plea bargaining ("Don't give me a shot; I'll be good.") and denial of pain may occur. | |
| *School-age Child (6–11 years)* | |
| Physiologic behaviors same as toddler/preschool. | Examination and procedures in the genital area are especially threatening. |
| Increased ability to verbally describe location, intensity, and type of pain. Able to draw pictures, tell and read stories; | Has active imagination. Curious and wants to know rules and how things work. |

**Table 8.5**    Pain Responses in Children (continued)

| Pain Behaviors According to Age | Response Variables |
|---|---|
| increased cognitive abilities may lead to fear of death and disability. May be anxious and ask many questions or may withdraw and not ask any questions. May deny pain to avoid shot. May clench fists and teeth and try to act brave; if child cries or loses control, may become embarrassed about peers knowing and tend to deny this reaction later. May procrastinate and bargain. Older school-age child may be embarrassed and want privacy; may prefer parents to leave. | Likes to plan, boss, problem solve. Likes, humor, jokes, puns. |
| *Adolescent (12–19 years)* Uses self-control during pain episode; usually has some coping mechanisms to deal with pain. May withdraw or regress. May focus on body and have numerous psychosomatic-type complaints (e.g., headaches, chest pains, muscle tension, and anxiety-related disorders). May be impatient and want "instant relief." | Increased need for privacy. Worries about body being normal and able to function. Fears loss of control and body dysfunction; may act overconfident ("know it all," "cool") to compensate for extreme fear. Focuses on own body and may spend large amounts of time grooming self; may have increased somatic complaints. May criticize authority and parents and rebel against rules, persons. |

(Neal et al., 1986)

**Table 8.6**    Sensory-Perceptual Aspects of Death

| Physiologic Occurrence | Cause | Intervention |
|---|---|---|
| Tactile sensation decreases. Skin is cool to touch, particularly in extremities. | Blood is being shunted from the peripheral to the central circulation, causing a rise in child's internal temperature. | Touch the child if it is not annoying to the child. Keep excess covers off the child. |
| Vision decreases. | Blood supply to the occipital cortex diminishes. | Stand close to the child. |
| Hearing is last sense to decrease. | Less distance for neurotransmission of sound from ear to auditory center in the brain | Talk clearly and distinctly to the child even if the child appears to be comatose. |

## GENERIC CARE PLAN FOR THE NURSING DIAGNOSIS
# ALTERATION IN COMFORT: PAIN

## 1.  General Information

### a.  Etiology
- Biologic: infection
- Chemical: acid
- Thermal: burns
- Physical: surgery, fracture
- Psychologic: grief

### b.  Clinical Manifestations
- Behavioral cues: grimacing, crying, fist clenching, moaning, restlessness
- Diaphoresis, pallor, flushing, palpitations
- Decreased movement
- Anger, aggression, flat affect
- Alteration in vital signs: increased pulse, blood pressure, respirations
- Holding, supporting, or guarding involved body part
- Anorexia, nausea
- Sleep pattern disturbance
- Age-related variables (see table 8.5)

### c.  Multidisciplinary Approaches
- Analgesics
- Physical therapy

## 2.  Nursing Process

### a.  Assessment
- Clinical manifestations
- Verbal acknowledgement of pain
- Characteristics of pain
  - locate and describe type
  - determine time of onset and duration
  - describe how pain has an impact on activities of daily living
  - describe what treatment or activities improve or worsen pain
  - describe related events or circumstances (eating, movement, voiding)
- Cultural, life-style, or ethnic factors that have an impact on the expression of pain
- Severity of pain: if possible, ask child to rate the pain on a scale of 1–3 (or 5 or 10)

– Area of most severe discomfort
– Statements that reflect altered functional capacity as a result of pain

**b.  Goal**
Child will report an improvement in level of comfort or demonstrate relief of pain by reduction of pain behaviors.

**c.  Interventions**
– Demonstrate an acceptance of the child's report of pain.
– Work to develop a trusting nurse-child relationship by relating to and interacting with child in a developmentally appropriate manner.
– Determine physical factors that contribute to the onset of pain.
– Evaluate cultural, life-style, and ethnic factors that have an impact on the onset and expression of pain.
– Provide for adequate sleep, rest, and nap periods.
– Be alert to age related variables in table 8.5 and utilize growth and development principles to provide pain relief.
– Be truthful prior to a pain-producing procedure; schedule painful treatments after admininstration of pain medications.
– Administer and evaluate results of prescribed analgesics.
– Explore alterative modalities to reduce pain (e.g., positioning, backrest, deep breathing).
– Utilize distraction and environmental control as diversional strategies to reduce pain (e.g., pictures, music, story telling).
– Encourage child to verbalize what measures are the most helpful in pain reduction.
– Instruct child/parents in pain control as necessary.
– Teach parents alternative methods of dealing with child's pain (rocking, cuddling, stroking, distraction).

**d.  Evaluation**
– Child experiences pain relief as demonstrated by
  • resting quietly
  • participating in age-appropriate diversional activities.
– Child states what measures are most helpful in reducing pain.
– Family uses alternative measures to deal with child's pain.

# Other Possible Nursing Diagnoses

Anxiety
Noncompliance
Potential for injury

# References

Bonta, S., & Blichfeldt, M. (1984). What to watch for if your patient has a ventriculos-tomy. *RN, 47*(11), 63-73.

Chee, C. (1980). Seizure disorders. *Nursing Clinics of North America, 14*(1), 71–81.

Commission on Classification and Terminology of the International League Against Epilepsy. (1981). Proposal for revised clinical and electroencephalographic classification of epileptic seizures. *Epilepsia, 22,* 489–501.

Klaus, M., & Kennel, J. (1976). *Maternal-infant bonding.* St. Louis: Mosby.

Masaorki, S., & Piercy, S. (1984). A step-by-step guide to trouble free transfusions. *RN, 47*(5), 34-42.

Muehl, J. (1979). Seizure disorders in children: Prevention and care. *MCN, 4,* 154–160.

Neal, M. et al. (1986). *Nursing care planning guides, set 6: The child in pain.* Baltimore: Williams & Wilkins.

Sporing, E., Walton, M., & Cady, C. (1984). *The Children's Hospital of Philadelphia manual of pediatric nursing policy, procedures, and personnel.* Oradell, NJ: Medical Economics Books.

Whaley, L., & Wong, D. (1983). *Nursing care of infants and children.* (2nd ed.). St. Louis: Mosby.

# CHAPTER 9

# SELF-PERCEPTION
## FUNCTIONAL HEALTH PATTERN

C hildren's self-concept is shaped by their perception about themselves, their abilities, their bodies and the response of others to them. In order to develop self-esteem, children need to feel competent, worthy, and loved. Alterations in self-concept include a change in body image (loss of function or part), self-esteem (loss of confidence), role performance (inability to perform activities) and personal identity (confusion about "who am I").

## Self-Concept

The focus of a child's self-perception is developmentally determined. Infants are totally self-centered or egocentric. Infants are the center of their own universe and are dependent upon sensory and motor stimulation of their bodies for their self-perception. Toddlers, too, are very egocentric but, because of their increased physical capabilities are able to interact in a larger social sphere. They do not depend upon social approval of their competence for self-perception. Preschoolers and young school-age children, however, are very aware of their physical size and abilities. They observe the abilities of other children and compare themselves to the other children. Being tall or short, strong or weak, fast or slow is very important to the child's self-perception at this age. During the late school and early adolescent years the opinion of peers becomes extremely important to children's self-perception. Children are very concerned that their appearance and abilities are acceptable to their peers. In adolescence the focus of children's self-perception is the formation of a personal opinion of themselves and the formation and acceptance of their own identity—physical, social and spiritual.

**Table 9.1**    Physical Characteristics

**Infant (birth–12 months)**
- 10% loss of birthweight in first 3–4 days of life
- 73% of newborn's body weight is fluid ($H_2O$)
- 2–3 months: posterior fontanel closes
- 0–5 months (approximately): obligate (preferential) nose breathing
- 5–6 months: birth weight doubles by this time
- 6 months: teething begins (lower central incisors)
- 8 months: regular bowel and bladder patterns
- 12 months: head and chest circumference equal; average weight 20 lb

**Toddler (12–36 months)**
- 12–36 months: anterior fontanel closes; can "let go" and walk with a wide stance
- 2 years: average weight 30 lb
- 15–18 months: toilet training (possibly—don't rush)
- reduced need for food relative to size (permit acceptance/refusal)

**Preschooler (3–6 years)**
- First permanent tooth erupts at about 6 years; loss of deciduous teeth begins
- Walks erect, arms swing
- Rapid skeletal development

**School-age Child (6–12 years)**
- Adult height/weight comparison
    Females: 90%/50%
    Males: 80%/50%
- Most striking change (throughout developmental stage): long bone growth (proportional increase in leg length relative to height)
- Learns physical skills necessary for sophisticated games
- Begins Tanner stages of pubertal development; most children complete stages I-II (secondary sex characteristics), but striking individual differences occur (for instance, some females achieve menarche and are capable of child-bearing at 11 or 12)

**Adolescent (12–19 years)**
- Full height not attained until individual is 20–24 years, when epiphyseal plates close
- Adult cardiovascular rhythms by age 16
- Awesome nutritional needs. At peak of growth spurt, males may consume 3,600 calories and females 2,600 calories/day
- Menarche: 10–15 years; usually cannot reproduce for 1–2 years after menarche, due to anovulation. Usually, dysmenorrhea does not occur until ovulation begins
- Early use of oral contraceptives will limit potential height (elevated estrogen levels hasten closure of epiphyseal plates in the long bones)
- Males attain puberty between 12–16 years
- Marked increase in muscle mass in males related to androgen
- By age 17, muscle mass in males is 2 times greater than in females (overall strength is proportionally greater)
- At end of adolescence, male basal metabolic rate is about 10% greater than female
- Tanner stages I-V (complete development) usually attained between early and late adolescence

**Table 9.2**   Maslow's Hierarchy of Needs

| Infant | Toddler | Preschooler | School-age Child | Adolescent |
|---|---|---|---|---|
| Physiologic (survival) | Physiologic (survival) | Physiologic (survival) | Physiologic (survival) | Physiologic (survival) |
| Safety/security | Safety/security | Safety/security | Safety/security | Safety/security |
| Love/belonging | Love/belonging | Love/belonging | Love/belonging | Love/belonging |
| | Self-esteem | Self-esteem | Self-esteem | Self-esteem |
| | | Cognitive (knowledge, understanding) | Cognitive | Cognitive |
| | | | Beginning of self-actualization (recognizing and making maximum use of abilities | Self-actualization (some adolescents) |

**Table 9.3**   Psychosexual Development: Freud

| Infant | Toddler | Preschooler | School-age Child | Adolescent |
|---|---|---|---|---|
| Oral stage | Anal Stage | Phallic Stage | Latency Stage | Genital Stage |
| Oral gratification (sucking needs). Should promote feeling of security. If unsuccessful, produces oral dependent character. Egocentrism is complete. | Sensual pleasure shifts to anal and urethral areas. Toilet training as area of discipline and authority; if unsuccessful, personality may become possessive or child may refuse to release possessions, including waste materials. | Much genital manipulation and exploration (particularly with other children). Intense attraction and love for parent of opposite sex (Oedipal conflict in males, Electra conflict in females); rivalry with parent of same sex. Castration anxiety, mutilation fears: intrusive procedures threaten bodily integrity. Primitive sense of body image begins. Separates easily from mother. | Repressed impulses. Parents no longer viewed as omnipotent. Privacy becomes important (later school-age years: 10–12). | Personality and defense mechanisms become integrated into a character. Oral, anal, and phallic sensuality are incorporated into genitality. |

**Table 9.4**   Psychosocial Development: Erikson

| Infant (birth–12 months) | Toddler (1–3 years) | Preschooler (3–6 years) | School-age Child (6–12 years) | Adolescent (12–19 years) |
|---|---|---|---|---|
| Trust vs mistrust Quality of parental infant relationships important At birth: Notices faces, establishes eye contact 1–2 months: smiles responsively 2–3 months: smiles spontaneously 6 months: demonstrates fear, anger, and affection; can indicate desires without crying | Autonomy vs shame, doubt Doubt sense of self-control; personal behavior may be self-determined Overprotection, excessive criticism may be related to negative feelings Child is ritualistic; should be allowed to move at own pace Ambivalence, walking, toilet training, temper tantrums, and negative "oppositional" behaviors; dawdling without crying Magical thinking ("wishes make it so") Inconsistent limit-setting disrupts and upsets behavior patterns | Initiative vs guilt Locomotor—Genital Magical thinking: Much make-believe play activity, which, if stifled, is related to guilt Enhanced creativity Many fears (e.g., having one's head chopped off or being sucked down the drain) that become real and logical in the child's mind; everything understood literally | Industry vs inferiority Latency: When encouraged, the child enthusiastically makes, builds, constructs, sews various projects How things are made is a primary concern Sense of inferiority ensues when projects are not praised or creativity is squelched | Identity vs role confusion Puberty/adolescence Individual identity formulation (begins around age 12) characterized by • rapid, marked physical change • shattering of previous trust in one's body (especially if rapid growth is associated with poor physical coordination) • preoccupation with appearance • integration of personal values with those of society (role confusion may ensue) Later adolescence/young adulthood • intimacy vs isolation • capacity to share oneself with another/ foster an intimate relationship • inability to form intimate relationships may result in a sense of isolation |

**Table 9.5**    Adolescent Development: Elkind

**Adolescence (12–19 years)**

Pseudo-stupidity: asks "dumb" questions; has problems reconciling concrete and formal operations

The imaginary audience: super self-consciousness; belief that everybody is watching and evaluating

Personal fable: belief of being special, not subject to natural laws

Apparent hypocrisy: expressing an idea is tantamount to working for and attaining it

**Table 9.6**    Social Development: Sullivan

| Infant (birth–12 months) | Toddler (1–3 years) | Preschooler (3–6 years) | School-age Child (6–12 years) | Adolescent (12–19 years) |
|---|---|---|---|---|
| Two complex drives: satisfaction, security A self-system (self-esteem) develops in the context of parental approval and disapproval. Disapproval causes anxiety; if only disapproval is given, a negative self-system develops Infancy: Differentiation ("good mother/ bad mother") | Acculturation: Self-system continues to develop 0–18 months: "good mother/ bad mother" to "good me/bad me" or "not me" age 3: self-concept begins Two tasks • independence • individuation (differentiation from mother) Much testing of ability, self-control, disciplinary limits Oppositional behavior, mood swings (love to hate) Emptying and hoarding Frustration, saying "no" Ritualism (needs security of daily routine and familiar environment) | Competition, cooperation, compromise Increased acculturation: improved skill in playing with others Possessive, but able to "share" toys | Social participation (school, neighborhood, scouting groups) Independence within family "Compeer" relationships important Chumship: altruistic concern for others, particularly same sex or significant other Behavioral self-regulation Begins to manage cooperative, competitive relationships | Personal security, intimacy, lust Achieves intimate relationships, develops a personal philosophy, adjusts to bodily changes, becomes independent of adults |

Since physical and emotional development are interrelated in a child's self-concept, tables of standard physical and psychosocial growth and development are included with age ranges when specific developmental milestones are reached (tables 9.1–9.6). The nurse is also referred to the Denver Developmental Reference Chart (DDRC), which was developed as an aid to assist in follow-up discussion with the parents after a child has been evaluated by the DDST.

## GENERIC CARE PLAN FOR THE NURSING DIAGNOSIS
# DISTURBANCE IN SELF-CONCEPT: BODY IMAGE

## 1. General Information

Illness and hospitalization can affect children's perception of their bodies in several ways. Immobilization of children or their body parts decreases their ability to achieve mastery of their bodies and the environment. Changes in children's appearances from illness or treatment (e.g., cachexia, alopecia, edema, jaundice) may cause them to feel that they are not acceptable to others. Changes that mutilate children's bodies (e.g., amputation, tube placement) may disturb their sense of integrity or wholeness.

**a. Etiology**
- Physical illness or injury
- Treatments (e.g., radiation, chemotherapy, surgery)
- Perceptual distortions

**b. Clinical Manifestations**
- Refusal to look at or touch altered or missing body part
- Preoccupation with loss or change
- Feelings of shame, embarrassment, verbalized or demonstrated
- Distorted perception of normal body
- Fears of rejection or unwanted attention from others
- Overexposure or hiding of body part
- Actual or perceived change in structure and/or function of body or body part

**c. Multidisciplinary Approaches**
- Treatment is supportive, depending upon symptoms. The nurse makes referrals to appropriate professionals (e.g., counselors, dietary therapy, physical therapy, occupational therapy).
- When child's appearance and/or functioning have been drastically altered (such as with severe burns), nurse or other professional visits the child's school and/or church to talk with teachers and students before child returns to school or church.

- Peer groups of children with similar health problems in the hospital and/or in the community.

## 2. Nursing Process

### a. Assessment
- Change in life-style related to negative feelings or perceptions of body
- Verbalized fear of rejection or reaction by others
- Repetitious verbalizations focusing on loss or regarding equipment
- Verbalized negative feelings about body (e.g., dirty, big, small, unsightly)
- Giving a name to the body part or lost part
- Referring to body part by an impersonal pronoun ("she, he")
- Inability to acknowledge change in function or body part
- Unusual eating or drinking behaviors such as
  - drinking excessive quantities of fluid prior to weight checks
  - repetitious vomiting
  - preoccupation with food
  - anorexia

### b. Goals
Parent/child will
- verbalize areas where changes can be made to enhance level of functioning, adjustment to loss, or appearance.
- exhibit adaptive behavior and institute positive coping mechanisms.

### c. Interventions
- Provide ongoing support and encouragement to the family and child.
- Make referrals to appropriate professionals (e.g., psychotherapists, physical or occupational therapists).
- Point out and focus on positive aspects of child's body and functioning that compensate for loss.
- Monitor eating habits and stay with child during meal time to ensure proper nutrition.
- Use dolls and toys to demonstrate changes in body part; allow child to play with dolls to express their anxiety about altered body part.
- Encourage the child to play with other children with similar body changes and discuss feelings related to body image.
- Teach child new ways of handling situations to accommodate for loss of or change in body part such as use of mechanical aids and/or responses to comments from others regarding the change or loss.

- Talk with child about body differences and how to use camouflage when possible (e.g., wigs, scarves for baldness).
- Compliment child on behaviors indicating acceptance of altered body part.
- Offer diversional activities to lessen preoccupation with loss.

**d. Evaluation**
- Parents/child
  - indicate areas where they need assistance in adjusting to child's appearance.
  - begin to verbalize and/or demonstrate acceptance of child's appearance.
  - use positive coping behaviors (with regard to particular body image disturbance).

**e. Possible Related Nursing Diagnoses**
Anxiety
Disturbance in self-concept: self-esteem, role performance, personal identity
Dysfunctional grieving
Impaired physical mobility (specify level)
Ineffective family/individual coping
Knowledge deficit (specify)
Noncompliance (specify)
Potential alteration in parenting
Self-care deficit (specify level)

# GENERIC CARE PLAN FOR THE NURSING DIAGNOSIS ANXIETY

## 1. General Information

Anxiety is a vague uneasy feeling that arises when one faces a nonspecific threat to self or a significant other. It is different from fear in that the threat cannot be identified by the person. Changes and losses will raise one's anxiety level because there is usually an unknown aspect connected to the situation. Children will manifest anxiety in a variety of ways, and pediatric nurses need to stay aware of the ever-present phenomenon of anxiety in ill children.

**a. Etiology**
- Illness
- Treatments, diagnostic tests
- Hospitalization
- Disruption of familiar routine

- Unfamiliar people and environment
- Developmental: separation from parents, mutilation, peer relationships, sexual development

b. **Clinical Manifestations**
   - Statements that reflect inability to cope, isolation, rejection, apprehension, loneliness, suspiciousness, anger, aggression, being controlled by external forces
   - Verbal manifestations such as whining, moaning, uncooperativeness, hostility
   - Increase or decrease in motor activity pattern
   - Disruption in sleep and/or eating patterns
   - Alteration in communication/thought processes
   - Regressive behavior (e.g., thumb sucking, urinary and/or bowel incontinence)
   - Compulsiveness, acting out, retreating behaviors
   - Refusal to go for procedure
   - Crying, screaming
   - Asking same question repeatedly
   - Inability to recall information

c. **Multidisciplinary Approaches**
   - Counseling, e.g., psychologic, spiritual
   - Child-life therapist

## 2. Nursing Process

a. **Assessment**
   - Nursing admission history
   - Child's knowledge about illness and treatment, and its significance
   - Child's developmental level
   - Child's and parents' anxiety level
   - Child's response to separation
   - Behavior (e.g., fidgeting, squirming, following distractions, or running out of the room); regressive behavior
   - Usual coping strategies, particular fears, favorite toys

b. **Goals**
   The child will
   - demonstrate a reduction in anxiety evidenced by verbal and behavioral cues.
   - be able to describe treatments to be done, reason for them, and what to encounter with minimal/tolerable level of anxiety.

c. **Interventions**
   - Be aware of your own feelings when the child's speech and behavior reflects anxiety since anxiety is contagious.
   - Provide a secure, quiet, and threat-free environment.
   - Speak simply and quietly, using short phrases; repeat if necessary.

- Encourage child to verbalize concerns and feelings.
- Provide opportunity for child to physically express anger or fear.
- Encourage parents/family or friends to be involved in care or to visit and stay as long as possible.
- Provide opportunities for child to socialize with others.
- Give reassurance that child is not being punished (hug toddlers and infants after intrusive procedures).
- Be role model for parents in communicating to child.
- Inform child about the coming events in clear, simple, concrete ways, geared to actual developmental or regressed level of child.
  - use a drawing of a child of own age or a doll
  - show equipment to be used (e.g., syringes, tubes, ostomy bags, IV tubing)
  - encourage child to "play back" this information using doll, dressings, tubing
  - discuss injections, IV infusions, and other invasive procedures last
  - provide opportunity to practice procedures requiring child's cooperation

**d.  Evaluation**
- Child
  - shows evidence of resuming individualized patterns of daily living.
  - expresses understanding of procedures at his/her level of understanding.
  - is familiar with equipment to be used, and plays back information using dolls, dressings, syringes.
- Parents
  - verbalize that their questions have been answered satisfactorily.
  - have objective decrease in anxiety level, e.g., by intervening appropriately to comfort child, appearing comfortable and less anxious.
- Child/parent(s) show decreased anxiety as evidenced by talking calmly about forthcoming procedure, participating in treatment routines.

**e.  Possible Related Nursing Diagnoses**
Alteration in bowel elimination (specify)
Alteration in family process
Alteration in patterns of urinary elimination
Diversional activity deficit
Impaired verbal communication
Knowledge deficit
Noncompliance
Sleep pattern disturbance

# Selected Health Problem Frequently Associated with the Nursing Diagnosis ANXIETY

## Surgery

**a. Discussion**

Surgery represents a major disruption in a child's life, separating the child from familiar people and surroundings. Many hospitals have instituted prehospitalization visits for children who have elective or scheduled surgery. During these pre-op visits children see the hospital and the nurses and are involved in therapeutic play with medical equipment (e.g., mask, gown, gloves, surgical caps, stethoscopes) as a means of reducing their anxiety.

Many one-day or short-stay surgical units have been established to allow children to undergo minor surgical procedures and return home on the same day. Parents are with the child during the pre- and post-op periods and, under the direction of nurses, provide much of the child's care.

**b. Multidisciplinary Approaches**
   – Child-life therapists

# Additional Nursing Care That Can Be Incorporated into the Generic Care Plan

**a. Assessment**
   – Determine what child and parent know about the surgical procedure to be done and its significance to them

**b. Goals**

Child/parents will be able to describe the surgical procedure, reason for it, and what the child will encounter pre-op, in recovery, and post-op with minimal/tolerable level of anxiety.

**c. Interventions**
   – Explain what npo means to child and parents; place signs at bedside and tape on children under 6 years.
   – Explain nature and function of recovery room and allow child to visit prior to surgery.
   – Permit significant objects to accompany child (e.g., favorite toy marked with name).
   – Avoid leaving child unattended.
   – Involve child in therapeutic play with medical equipment, explaining purpose of each item.

- Reassure child someone (e.g., parents, nurse) will be there when it's over.
- Teach the child what to expect when surgery is over (e.g., bandages, IVs, cast).

**d. Evaluation**
- Child's anxiety is reduced to a manageable level.
- Child expresses feelings about procedures via puppet or doll play if age appropriate.

## Other Possible Nursing Diagnoses

Disturbance in self-concept
Fear
Ineffective individual coping
Social isolation

### GENERIC CARE PLAN FOR THE NURSING DIAGNOSIS FEAR

## 1. General Information

Fear is an emotional response to a specific perceived danger. It differs from anxiety, which does not necessarily identify the danger.

**a. Etiology**
- Pain, invasive procedures
- Loss of support system
- Unexpected occurrence
- Lack of knowledge
- Developmental, e.g., fear of dark, "bugs," strangers
- Environmental stimuli (loud noise)

**b. Clinical Manifestations**
- Statements that reflect loss of control, anticipation of unpleasant circumstances or procedures
- Statements that reflect physiologic changes (can't swallow, sweaty palms, palpitations)
- Verbal acknowledgement of fear, scared, jittery, frightened
- Changes in behavior when
  - child learns s/he is going to the hospital
  - procedures are pending
  - unknown personnel are present in child's environment
- Changes in vital signs: rapid pulse and respirations, increased blood pressure

- Fatigue, interrupted sleep patterns, nightmares
- Diaphoresis, pallor, flushing
- Dysphagia, nausea/vomiting, loose stools
- Rapid, loud speech or inability to speak
- Irritability
- Muscle tension or rigidity

c. **Multidisciplinary Approaches**
- Child-life or play therapists
- Counselor, psychologic or spiritual

## 2. Nursing Process

a. **Assessment**
- Prior knowledge and understanding of child's illness and treatment plan
- Verbal and nonverbal indicators of fear
- Signs of denial of real threats or dangers
- Vital signs
- Support systems of child and family

b. **Goals**
The child will
- verbalize specific fears to nurse.
- explore effective ways to cope with fears.
- utilize strategies to reduce fears.

c. **Interventions**
- Work to develop a trusting relationship with child.
- Provide a warm and supportive environment.
- Acknowledge the fears inherent in repeated hospitalizations and concerns for the unknown.
- Give permission for child to be afraid and to express fear.
- Encourage child to be specific about frightening circumstances.
- Allow child choices in deciding time and location for procedures.
- Introduce new personnel to child and provide ample time for them to become acquainted.
- Discuss with the child strategies useful in reducing fears (e.g., count to 10, relaxation).
- Explain all procedures well in advance.
- Use dolls, modified equipment, and tactile and visual involvement to reduce fears.

d. **Evaluation**
- Child
  - is able to verbalize fears.
  - sees new strategies to reduce fear during a frightening experience (e.g., counts out very loud, sings).

## Other Possible Nursing Diagnoses

Alteration in comfort: pain
Impaired physical mobility
Ineffective breathing pattern
Potential for injury

# CHAPTER 10

# ROLE-RELATIONSHIP
## FUNCTIONAL HEALTH PATTERN

T he role-relationship functional health pattern focuses on the relationships a child forms. As an egocentric being, the infant bonds with mother and with father to have his/her needs met. These attachments grow and the infant gives as well as takes. The infant then forms relationships with others in the family such as siblings and grandparents. The young child begins to expand horizons and relate to others in the environment, neighborhood, school, and finally, community. This chapter discusses the development of the growing individual's roles and responsibilities in life, family role development, and the loss of a relationship or grieving.

## The Development of Roles within the Family

According to Duvall, the family has developmental tasks to achieve at each stage of the child's growth (table 10.1).

## The Family in Crisis

Hospitalization and stressors related to this experience are perceived differently by each child's family. Some may take the experience in stride, others may perceive it as a crisis. Elements that define a crisis situation include the family's perception of the event, its meaning to them, availability (or lack) of support systems, and coping mechanisms.

**Table 10.1**    Family Developmental Tasks: Duvall

| Infant (birth–12 months) | Toddler (1–3 years) | Preschooler (3–6 years) | School-age Child (6–12 years) | Adolescent (13–19 years) |
|---|---|---|---|---|
| Marital—child-bearing family: Establishing a marriage and home, adjusting to parenthood | Child-bearing family: Further adjustment to parenting; stabilizing home | Preschool family: Nurturing children; socialization within the family environment | School-age family: Socialization and education of child in community | Teenage family: Balancing teenage freedom and responsibility; ends with launch (release of child) |

Nursing interventions can repattern the family's behaviors so that a more effective level of functioning occurs. Possible behavioral outcomes of a crisis situation include maintenance of pre-illness level of functioning, growth resulting in a higher level of functioning, or problem solving at a lower level. The nurse not only lends emotional support to children and their families, but also identifies additional resources for help and makes appropriate referrals.

The ability of children to function depends a great deal on the strength of their attachments. While preferential attachment begins in earnest in the 4- to 6-month-old infant, younger infants may be consoled more easily by familiar people and routines. Separation anxiety occurs in young children when they are removed from their usual environment and separated from their primary caretakers. Its stages include protest, despair, and detachment. Whaley and Wong (1983) explain that detachment (or denial) is a form of resignation. This form of depression may appear to be a form of adaptation to hospitalization.

Parents may become confused by the behavioral manifestations their children present. They may deal poorly with clinging behaviors when their children protest separation. Parents might decrease their visits or visiting time. They may lie to the child as well.

Another pattern may ensue. One parent may become completely absorbed in the ill child at the expense of spouse and siblings. The parent may become a sentry at the bedside, taking little time to meet his/her own needs or those of other family members.

# Family-centered Nursing.

It is easy for the nurse to prioritize patients' physiologic needs. A patent airway, for instance, is always of primary importance. Other needs, however, may not be so easily ranked, particularly when they are both very complex and difficult to fulfill.

Of particular concern are the needs of parents with ill children. Inpatient hospitalization, especially of very young children, constitutes a major family crisis and a substantial disruption of domestic routine and family roles. Some pediatric nurses have a natural talent for stepping into such situations and offering true support. "True support" is offered by knowing how to intervene in a psychologic crisis, i.e.

- Reduce anxiety (see Anxiety, page 308)
- Identify specific problem causing crisis (e.g., lack of money, travel, time, self-esteem, etc., creating additional stress related to child's illness).
- Identify meaning of event (sick child's hospitalization)
- Identify and support effective new coping.
- Encourage ventilation of feelings; offer empathy, validation, and comfort.
- Be physically present, act calm, explain procedures, use humor, offer coffee, snacks, etc.

Such intervention permits parents to parent, i.e., to fill roles for their children that are vitally important in maintaining as normal a parent-child relationship as possible, and is an essential part of family-centered care.

It is up to nurses to safeguard families' existing and potential supportive relationships. Many professional nurses find this concept difficult to understand, however, largely because medicine tends to either consciously or unconsciously blame pathologic processes on the family system. In cases of visible child abuse, it is easier to notice how health care reflects negative judgments about the abusers. The care giver's feelings might not be as clearly expressed in the case of a child with recurrent illnesses or accident-prone behaviors, but they are present nevertheless. In addition, many providers attach such importance to their own roles that they unwittingly place patients/families at the bottom of the hierarchy. The pediatric nurse may also alienate family members by refusing to interact with them on an adult-to-adult level. The nurses may take over all care of their pediatric patients. Such behavior is most often seen in infant intensive care units, where multiple lines, tubes, and wires are so intimidating to parents that some staff nurses can force parents into the role of "terrified incompetent."

Alienation of family members can occur in any setting, and it seems inveterately ingrained in today's health care system. Hospitalized children and their families may be depersonalized by health care providers. They may feel that they are not participants in the care of the hospitalized child. Family-centered practices, such as open visitation policies, are being used to allow and encourage family members to be part of the health care team.

Most in-patient pediatric settings have dramatically liberalized visiting policies in recent years. This significant movement began with Fagin's landmark research (1966). That study demonstrated that hospitalized children whose parents were permitted to stay with them had fewer post-hospitalization emotional sequelae, e.g., regression in toilet training, emotional dependence, and feeding disturbances, compared with children whose parents were not permitted to stay.

Maslow's hierarchy of needs is especially useful in identifying priorities for family-centered care. The nurse cannot be expected to meet all needs on all levels, but can be a facilitator for patient and family. Physiologic and safety needs are first priority, but the nurse must get past this minimal level and address needs on the levels of love, belonging, and esteem. It is probably beyond the scope of any provider to attempt to meet self-actualization needs, but it will certainly help the patient if the nurse encourages activities that are developmentally appropriate creatively and intellectually.

**Table 10.2**    Nursing Considerations to Promote Family-centered Care

1.  Encourage parental bonding with sick children, even those too ill to be held safely.
    • allow fingertip touching and talking to the child
    • comment on the child's positive features, e.g., pretty hair or eyes; parents of prema-
      ture or anomalous infants, who are probably mourning the loss of their anticipated
      "normal child", may particularly appreciate such compliments
2.  Delegate every possible aspect of the child's in-hospital care (feeding, bathing,
    cuddling) to the parents.
3.  Encourage parents to stay with their child overnight, if possible.
4.  Gently redirect negative parental behaviors as needed, since they can decrease the
    child's self-esteem and cause mistrust in future relationships with family members and
    health care providers.
5.  Gently discourage overly protective behavior. Giving the parent "permission" to take
    time away from the ill child is often an effective intervention. Offer to pay special atten-
    tion to the the child while the parent is away but do not make promises you cannot keep.

## GENERIC CARE PLAN FOR THE NURSING DIAGNOSIS
# ALTERATION IN FAMILY PROCESS

## 1.  General Information

### a.  Etiology
  – Pathophysiologic
    • illness of a family member
    • traumatic injury of a family member (e.g., surgery, accident)
  – Situational
    • loss or addition of a family member
    • financial insecurity
    • relocation
    • role change
    • family conflict

### b.  Clinical Manifestations
  – Inability of family members to meet own physical, financial, and/
    or emotional needs
  – Lack of knowledge and/or use of appropriate helping resources
  – Lack of communication among family members

c. **Multidisciplinary Approaches**
   - Counseling: family and/or individual
   - Social services
   - Support groups

## 2. Nursing Process

a. **Assessment**
   - Parental attitudes toward child
   - Family support systems (including extended family or friends willing to help), financial resources (including medical insurance coverage), family constellation (siblings)
   - Coping mechanisms (e.g., compliance with treatment regimen, denial, displacement).
   - Health and emotional status of family members
   - Family level of knowledge related to health problem, child care, nutrition, safety, etc.
   - Family structure and role performance of family members
   - Siblings for jealousy, lack of attention

b. **Goals**
   Parents/child will
   - verbalize areas where they will need assistance, changes to be made in life-style.
   - maximize use of available resources.

c. **Interventions**
   - Assist family to express feelings, problems, etc., about current situation.
   - Assist family to identify positive coping mechanisms that were successful in the past.
   - Help family to develop new ways to cope with current situation.
   - Refer to hospital and community resources as appropriate.
   - Reinforce all positive attempts to cope with current crisis.

d. **Evaluation**
   - Parents
     • verbalize areas where they need assistance.
     • have a list of available resources and verbalize plans to use them.
     • verbalize areas where changes are needed (e.g., seek people to stay with child for an evening out).

e. **Possible Related Nursing Diagnoses**
   Alteration in health maintenance
   Anxiety
   Disturbance in self-concept
   Fear
   Impaired home maintenance management

Impaired verbal communication
Knowledge deficit
Noncompliance
Potential for violence
Powerlessness

# GENERIC CARE PLAN FOR THE NURSING DIAGNOSIS
# ALTERATION IN PARENTING

## 1.  General Information

**a.  Etiology**
  - Poor parent role models
  - Inadequate financial resources
  - No available support systems
  - Multiple stressors (e.g., loss of a job, illness, disability)

**b.  Clinical Manifestations (Gordon, 1982)**
  - "Parentification" (role reversal) of child
  - Inappropriate developmental expectations
  - Pointing out "flaws" in child's characteristics
  - Disappointment with gender
  - Inappropriate visual, tactile, auditory stimulation
  - Inattentiveness to needs
  - Inappropriate care-giving behaviors (e.g., feeding, babysitting)
  - History of actual abuse/abandonment (in parents' history as well)
  - Evidence of physical/psychologic trauma
  - Child verbally uncontrollable
  - Verbalization of parental role inadequacy
  - Verbal disgust regarding child's bodily functions
  - Noncompliance with behaviors regarding child's health
  - Inconsistent or inappropriate discipline
  - Frequent accidents/illness
  - Developmental delay
  - Growth lag (failure to thrive)
  - Multiple care givers
  - Abandonment
  - Parental attention-seeking behaviors
  - Runaway

**c.  Multidisciplinary Approaches**
  - Family therapy
  - Social service

## 2. Nursing Process

### a. Assessment

- Developmental level of infant/child (with appropriate selected screening device)
  - newborn maturity rating and classification
  - Denver Developmental Screening Test
  - extensive developmental testing if appropriate
  - neurosensory capabilities (i.e., vision, hearing, taste, olfaction, touch)
  - sound, language, and learning skills
  - neuromotor development: gross vs fine motor skills
  - physical characteristics
- Developmental history (see Chapter 9)
  - age at which traditional milestones/capabilities reached
  - perinatal history (Apgar scores, infections, complications, type of birth)
  - parental attitudes toward pregnancy, their "life with this child"
- Stage of psychologic development using frameworks of major developmental theorists (see growth and development charts in Chapter 9)
  - Freud
  - Erickson
  - Piaget
  - Sullivan
  - Skinner
  - Havighurst
  - Kohlberg
  - level of needs met/unmet in Maslow's hierarchy
- Parental education/affective needs
  - Duvall's family development stage
  - knowledge of normal growth and development
  - readiness to engage in child-centered learning
  - appropriateness of developmental expectations
  - parental values for child's growth and development outcomes (active in sports, cognitive skills, physical beauty, good health)
  - parental education gaps concerning family health needs

### b. Goals

Parents will

- learn new behaviors/skills to strengthen their parental role.
- enlist the help of additional caretakers if needed (e.g., relatives).
- demonstrate developing awareness of helping systems available.
- contact and follow through on referrals to helping agencies, professionals, and other sources of support.
- display behaviors that indicate an investment in their child's care.

c. **Interventions**
  - Offer information to fill gaps in knowledge or skill deficits (e.g., parenting skills, developmental milestones).
  - Work with parents to identify effective role models for them.
  - Focus on fears of parents; help them to identify and articulate the fears.
  - Identify resources for parents to use to assist with social or legal stress.
  - Discuss how the parent will deal with developmental tasks of the child.
  - Avoid making parents dependent on professionals.
  - Facilitate bonding/reinvestment process
    • make personal comments about child's positive personality attributes, responses
    • role model appropriate parenting behaviors
    • reinforce positive normal parenting behaviors (e.g., diapering, feeding)
  - Determine age/ability-appropriate interventions by using various developmental "guides" to set individually determined goals
    • the Washington Guide to promoting development in the young child (includes expected tasks and suggested activities per age group); categories include motor, feeding, sleep, play, language, discipline, and toilet training (Whaley & Wong; Schraeder, 1980; Tudor, 1978).

d. **Evaluation**
  - Parents
    • discuss their feelings about current situations.
    • verbalize plans to follow through with referrals.
    • demonstrate incorporation of new, more effective coping behaviors (e.g., appropriate attention to child's needs).
  - Child and parents
    • display bonding behaviors to one another.
    • engage in developmental stimulation activities appropriate to the child's age.

# Possible Related Nursing Diagnoses

Anxiety
Depression
Disturbance in self-esteem
Diversional activity deficit
Fear
Impaired home maintenance management
Impaired thought processes
Ineffective family coping
Knowledge deficit (specify)
Potential cognitive impairment

## Selected Health Problem Frequently Associated with the Nursing Diagnosis ALTERATION IN PARENTING

### Lengthy Hospitalization

**a. Discussion**
- Children who are discharged from an extended stay in the newborn nursery or who are hospitalized frequently or for long periods of time are at risk for disturbed parenting.
- The bonding process occurs slowly over time and if the process is interrupted at a critical time by hospitalization it may be jeopardizied.
- Children with chronic health problems requiring frequent hospitalization may be seen by their parents as "imperfect" or inadequate.
- A catastrophe, accident, or illness may disturb a weak parent/child bond.

**b. Multidisciplinary Approaches**
- Visiting nurse
- Social service
- Community support groups (e.g., Cystic Fibrosis Foundation, Parents Anonymous)

### Additional Nursing Care That Can Be Incorporated into the Generic Care Plan

**a. Assessment**
- Stage of parental "binding in" to child (these behaviors will differ depending on nature of child's hospitalization)
  - what care-giving activities do the parents engage in? (e.g., diapering, feeding, cuddling, comforting, dressing)
  - what tasks can parents perform to meet child's specific health needs? (e.g., suctioning, changing equipment, doing treatments)
  - what behaviors do parents perform to indicate level of investment in their child? (e.g., regular visitation, focus of questions, i.e., are they on total child or on physiologic parameters?)
  - what parental affect is expressed in meeting the child's needs?
- What parents have been told
  - their actual understanding
  - acceptance/rejection of prognosis
  - denial of situation
  - unrealistic expectations for outcomes of therapy

   − Stage of crisis family members are in
      • capable of moving past grief/despair?

b. **Goals**
   Parents will
   − reinvest in parenting of the affected child.
   − provide age-appropriate developmental stimulation activities within the child's limitations.
   − assist their child in performing routine activities of daily living.
   − (and child if capable) collaborate with nurse and various appropriate therapists (e.g., occupational, physical, or speech) to set up developmentally appropriate goals for the child.

c. **Interventions**
   − Avoid making parents dependent on and "in awe" of the nurse (and other health professionals)
      • do not use medical terminology to intellectualize comments that might be emotionally painful for parents
      • focus parents on their child as a holistic being rather than many physiologic subsystems by commenting on the child rather than on vital signs or monitor readings
      • avoid the appearance of "taking over" the parenting role by purchasing toys and clothing, laundering clothes, or taking over routine care when parents are present
      • welcome parents' calls/visits around the clock
      • acknowledge family's stage in the grieving process/level of despair or sorrow
   − Facilitate the bonding/reinvestment process
      • give "permission" to undress, stroke, caress, hold, bond with their child
      • provide time for parental-child privacy
      • promote family holding child despite multiple tubes and wires
      • when ready, assist in performance of ongoing care activities necessary for physiologic survival (especially if eventual discharge is planned)
      • engage parents in discovering and carrying out comfort measures unique to their child
      • encourage "claiming behaviors" (e.g., taking home linens, bringing in or providing grooming aids)
      • accept, respect, and encourage advocacy behaviors (e.g., parental suggestions for changes in care routines)
      • suggest a visiting/teaching session contract if a positive pattern of care does not develop
      • reinforce that the child belongs to the parents, not to hospital personnel
      • arrange for regular sibling visitation
      • arrange for pets to visit if indicated
      • discuss parental rights and responsibilities in detail

- minimize number of care givers assigned to each child and provide staffing patterns so that care givers are consistent
- develop a developmental skills promotion "checklist" and document progress in nurses' notes
– Refer family to appropriate helping agencies (e.g., Cystic Fibrosis Foundation or Easter Seal Society.)

**d. Evaluation**
– Parents
- bring in toys, games; take photographs of child, note developmental milestones and work toward the achievement of next appropriate milestone.
- assist with activities of daily living and take responsibility to help with tasks such as child's laundry.
– Parents/child demonstrate a high level of investment by keeping appointments, administering medications/treatments skillfully, reporting that questions have been answered to their satisfaction.

**e. Other Possible Nursing Diagnoses**
Alteration in health maintenance
Anxiety
Disturbance in self-concept
Diversional activity deficit
Fear
Grieving
Impaired verbal communication
Ineffective coping
Knowledge deficit
Noncompliance
Potential for injury
Powerlessness

# Grief and Loss

Grief is a universal response to loss with a variety of manifestations. These manifestations depend upon the individual's situation and the family's coping skills. Its intensity varies with the child's and family's interpretation and the severity of the problem. Much more is known about adult grief reactions and patterns than about children's grief.

There are three stages of grief (AJN, 1986):

– Shock and disbelief, usually lasting 1–7 days
– Developing awareness of the loss, lasting from several weeks to several months
– Restitution, taking a year or more

Elizabeth Kübler-Ross (1969) notes five stages in the mourning process of the individual who is dying

- Denial: a method of mobilizing one's defenses and energy to cope with the terminal process
- Anger: occurs when death can no longer be denied
- Bargaining: used as a method of gaining more time
- Depression: resulting as a reaction to the anticipated loss
- Acceptance: a stage of passivity and withdrawal

Children react to loss differently, according to their stage of cognitive and emotional development. Toddlers and preschoolers cannot differentiate death from separation. Young school-age children accept the death of others as a fact, but feel that it is reversible. In the middle school-age years (6–9 years), children associate death with bodily injury and personify death (e.g., the "bogey man"). Older school-age children accept death as an inevitable occurrence for all and understand the physiologic changes associated with death (cessation of breathing and heartbeat). Adolescents begin to have a more abstract understanding of death. They realize the emotional impact of death on others, conceptualize their own death, and formulate a spiritual philosophy of death.

Grief reactions in children last varying amounts of time. No specific amount of time has been described as pathologic, however. Mott, Fazekas, and James (1985) suggest that "children also might rework grief reactions when they enter new developmental stages" (p. 824).

**Chronic Sorrow.**   The term *chronic sorrow* was coined by Olshansky in 1962 to describe an affect that stays with the family throughout the life of a defective child. Many families demonstrate admirable coping skills once they have mourned the loss of an imagined perfect child that was envisioned during the pregnancy. Young (1977) further explains the concept of chronic sorrow by stating that "only after the (actual) death of the constantly present, grief-producing child can parents move into the final stage of grief—resolution" (p. 39).

When the outcome of a pregnancy is not a healthy full-term infant, a process of grieving ensues within the family. In the face of major fetal damage, a minor defect that can be easily corrected with cosmetic surgery, or even no obvious physical abnormality at all, there is initial shock and disbelief. There may be a process of denial, prolonged by a detailed diagnostic work-up—the results of which may shatter what hopes the family continues to hold. Poor prognoses for the child, either in terms of life expectancy or function and development, can initiate the full grieving process.

Young describes a process of resolving chronic sorrow that includes the following phases

- Defective child lives and parents experience stages of acute grief over non-perfect child.
  - denial
  - developing awareness
  - restitution (two types of response)
    * adaptive
    * maladaptive (pathologic)

- Defective child dies and parents experience stages of acute grief over death of child
  - denial
  - developing awareness
  - restitution
  - resolution

Young states that "many defective children are fortunate in having easygoing, good-humored, accepting parents who love them and are supportive in helping them reach maximum potential" (p. 39). But she also identifies maladaptive extremes—parents who, out of guilt, dedicate themselves exclusively to their child or who feel such intolerance and revulsion that they deny the relationship completely.

Chronic sorrow is most poignantly seen in the family at the ages when a child should be reaching a developmental milestone and does not, an infant who should begin to sit unassisted around 6 months of age does not, or a child of parents who value education should be going off to college and is incapable of doing so.

Infants and children with defects are not the only ones who evoke grief responses in parents. The work of Benfield, Leib, and Reuter (1977) explores attitudes of parents whose critically ill newborns survived transfer from the hospitals where they were born to regional neonatal intensive care units. The findings are very compelling: "As measured by anticipatory grief score, most parents experienced grief reactions similar to those whose infants do not survive the newborn period" (p. 978). The impact of the transfer itself was so severe that it was like a death experience.

## GENERIC CARE PLAN FOR THE NURSING DIAGNOSIS
# GRIEVING

## 1. General Information

### a. Etiology
- Loss (e.g., relationship, health, loved one)
- Change in life-style or developmental stage

### b. Clinical Manifestations
- Normal grief
  - sensations of somatic distress
  - guilt
  - preoccupation or idealization with image of the loss (body part, person, level of functioning)
  - sadness, crying, painful feelings
  - anger, hostility
  - loss of usual patterns of daily living

- appetite decrease
- sleep-rest disturbance
- loss of concentration
- Unresolved grief
  - extended length of time or severity of grieving
  - grief from previous losses
  - continued verbal expression of loss
  - denial
  - eating disturbances
  - sleep-rest disturbances
  - idealization of the loss (body part, person, level of functioning)
  - inability to love or work
  - labile affect
  - concentration difficulty
  - hostility
  - psychosomatic diseases
  - self-defeating behaviors
  - self-depreciation
  - lack of ability to develop and maintain support systems
  - agitated depression

## 2. Nursing Process

**a. Assessment**
- Individual's stage of grief and mourning
- Individual's previous experience with and reaction to loss
- Value of the lost person or thing
- Developmental level of the grieving child
- Responses to loss: adaptive vs maladaptive

**b. Goal**

Parents/child will exhibit adaptive behavior to the potential or actual loss.

**c. Interventions**
- Allow grieving individual to express grief in own way as long as it is not physically destructive.
- Give positive feedback for adaptive methods of grieving.
- Tell child and family that grief is a normal reaction to loss and explain the various stages and responses.
- Encourage children to express grief symbolically through drawing, stories, therapeutic play, etc.
- Allow child to express feelings through anger, fear, withdrawal, and hostility as long as this behavior is not physically destructive.
- Refer suicidal individual for psychologic counseling.
- Recognize that, while parents are dealing with the shock of a baby that does not meet their idealized expectations, they must also face the demands of the unanticipated situation.

  - Give emotional support to parents when the infant's problem is potentially life-threatening or severely complicates meeting oxygenation or nutritional needs.
  - Understand that people can and do grieve for what they do not get from life, such as a perfect infant.

  **d. Evaluation**
  - The grieving individual is able to talk about the loss.
  - Parents/child express feelings in their own way (e.g., crying, drawing) and receive support from staff.

# Selected Health Problem Frequently Associated with the Nursing Diagnosis GRIEVING

## Sudden Infant Death Syndrome (SIDS)

  **a. Discussion**
  - SIDS, a specific entity of unknown etiology, is considered to be the cause of death in most cases when a previously healthy infant dies suddenly, during sleep, for no apparent reason.
  - It is the most common cause of documented death in children between the ages of 1 week and 1 year.
  - Peak age of occurrence is 2–4 months, with almost all cases occurring before 6 months.
  - Usually a rescue squad or police will be the first emergency personnel to see a SIDS child.
  - Frequently, no resuscitation attempts are made, and the child is transported to an ER for pronouncement of death.

  **b. Multidisciplinary Approach**
  - All parents of SIDS victims should be afforded the opportunity for follow-up counseling, preferably through the local SIDS foundation. This important step will help them deal with their grief and guilt, as well as with their uncertainty about future births (SIDS, 1982).

# Additional Nursing Care That Can Be Incorporated into the Generic Care Plan

  **a. Assessment**
  - Circumstances of the infant's health and activity prior to discovery
  - Reactions of the rescue squad, police, etc., to finding the infant
  - Family's knowledge of SIDS

b.  **Goals**
Family
- will see and be with infant (if desired) to express their grief before leaving hospital.
- will receive names of appropriate community or private resources.

c.  **Interventions**
- Interact sensitively with the bereaved parents; remember, they will be in a state of shock.
- Do not add to the parents' inevitable guilt by implying that abuse or neglect led to the child's death; emphasize instead that SIDS cannot be prevented.
- Quickly clean the child's body, remove any equipment.
- Allow parents to see/hold their child before they leave the hospital, if so desired.
- Provide parents undisturbed, private time and place in which to say goodbye.
- Provide informational literature about SIDS and SIDS Foundation.

d.  **Evaluation**
- Family
  - expresses grief in adaptive ways (e.g., crying).
  - is able to touch, hold, rock, or dress infant as they wish before leaving the hospital.
  - has information about SIDS and has the name of a SIDS support group.

## Other Possible Nursing Diagnoses

Alteration in family process
Alteration in parenting
Anxiety
Fear
Ineffective coping (individual or family)
Knowledge deficit
Sleep pattern disturbance
Spiritual distress
References

## References

American Journal of Nursing (1986). *1986 nursing boards review.* Baltimore: Williams & Wilkins.
Benfield, D., Leib, S., & Reuter, J. (1977). Grief response of parents after referral of the critically ill newborn to a regional center. *New England Journal of Medicine, 294,* 975-978.

Fagin, C. (1966). *The effects of maternal attendance during hospitalization on post hospital behavior of young children: A comparative study.* Philadelphia: Davis.

Gordon, M. (1982). *Manual of nursing diagnosis.* New York: McGraw-Hill.

Kübler-Ross, E. (1969). *On death and dying.* New York: Macmillan.

Mott, S., Fazekar, N., & James, S. (1985). *Nursing care of children and families.* Menlo Park, CA: Addison-Wesley.

National SIDS Foundation (1982). *Facts about sudden infant death syndrome.* Landover, MD: Author.

Olshansky, S. (1962). Chronic sorrow: A response to having a mentally defective child. *Social Casework, 43,* 190–193.

Whaley, L., & Wong, D. (1983). *Nursing care of infants and children.* (2nd ed.). St. Louis: Mosby.

Young, R. (1977). Chronic sorrow: Parents' response to the birth of a child with a defect. *American Journal of Maternal-Child Nursing, 1,* 39.

# CHAPTER 11

# COPING-STRESS TOLERANCE
## FUNCTIONAL HEALTH PATTERN

The coping-stress tolerance functional health pattern involves coping patterns and their use in the management of stress. How children handle stress, how the family system affects a child's ability to deal with stress, and how the family copes in general are important aspects of this functional health pattern.

Crisis and its effect on children is an important aspect of pediatric nursing. Knowing the psychologic phases of crises and a child's expected, "normal" responses are important concepts for every nurse caring for children. An overview of the family's response to hospitalization and related stressors is presented together with interventions to minimize stress in children and to promote effective coping.

This functional health pattern includes the nursing diagnosis *Ineffective Family Coping.* This refers to the family that copes ineffectively in general, and the coping level can decrease even further with the hospitalization of one of its members. When a family copes effectively most of the time but becomes stressed or in crisis because one of its family members is hospitalized, the nursing diagnosis is *Alteration in Family Process,* which is discussed in Chapter 10.

**Process.** Table 11.1 presents an overview of interventions to support the hospitalized child, thus promoting effective coping.

**Table 11.1** Nursing Interventions to Minimize Children's Stress and Promote Coping

| Age Group | Stressor | Interventions to Promote Coping |
|---|---|---|
| Infant | Separation | • Encourage parents to stay with their infant as much as possible.<br>• Provide consistent caretakers. |
| | Pain/intrusion | • Investigate the reason for an infant's crying.<br>• Initiate self-comforting behaviors, such as sucking, by bringing the infant's fingers toward the mouth.<br>• Decrease stimulation by holding the infant's arms close to the body or by swaddling.<br>• Talk quietly to the infant.<br>• Use touch to soothe the infant by stroking, patting, holding, or cuddling. |
| | Immobilization | • Provide changes in position by using an infant seat or by holding, rocking, or turning the infant.<br>• Remove restraints periodically to permit free movement under close supervision.<br>• Provide whatever exploration of the environment is possible in the crib or playpen or on the floor.<br>• Provide stimulation and opportunities for visual exploration with colorful mobiles, pictures, mirrors, and soft toys. |
| Toddler | Separation | • Encourage parents to stay with their toddler as much as possible.<br>• Provide consistent caretakers.<br>• Preserve ties to home by obtaining transitional objects, family photos, tape recordings of the family, objects from home, and by talking about home and family.<br>• Teach parents that withdrawal is a response to stress and helps the child to conserve energy. |
| | Pain/intrusion | • Accept that the toddler cannot differentiate pain from intrusion.<br>• Expect vigorous protest behavior and carry out painful procedures as quickly as safety permits with sufficient assistance and/or restraint.<br>• Teach parents that protest behavior is a healthy response.<br>• Comfort the child with holding and cuddling after painful procedures and assist parents to do the same.<br>• Provide "safe" times and places in which painful or intrusive procedures are prohibited.<br>• Provide rest periods between stressful procedures. |

**Table 11.1**    Nursing Interventions to Minimize Children's Stress and Promote Coping (continued)

| Age Group | Stressor | Interventions to Promote Coping |
|---|---|---|
| | Loss of self-control | • Continue rituals observed at home.<br>• Provide opportunities for autonomy by permitting choices.<br>• Provide as much physical activity as safety permits.<br>• Provide for exploration of the environment to whatever extent possible.<br>• Accept regression and teach parents that this is a healthy response and that their toddler will remaster "lost" skills after recovery. |
| Preschooler | Separation | • (see Toddlers)<br>• Teach parents that their young child still needs the reassurance of their continuing presence, especially when ill, and that fear of being alone is common in this age group. |
| | Pain/intrusion | • Help the child cooperate with procedures by providing information about the procedure and about what is expected of the child.<br>• Set realistic limits on undesirable behavior.<br>• Provide the child with opportunities to practice for potentially stressful procedures.<br>• Reassure the child that procedures are necessary and are not punishment.<br>• Use touch to convey comforting, warmth, and caring.<br>• Reassure the child about body intactness. |
| | Loss of self-control | • Provide opportunities for self-expression.<br>• Encourage autonomy by permitting choices and participation in self-care.<br>• Make reality-oriented statements to the child.<br>• Use play as a vehicle for teaching the child and encouraging expression of feeling.<br>• Utilize the child's ability to fantasize constructively. |
| School-age child | Separation | • Encourage parents to visit regularly and reliably.<br>• Provide consistent caretakers.<br>• Respond to withdrawn behavior or verbalization of loneliness with increased attention and closeness.<br>• Encourage communication with siblings and schoolmates.<br>• Keep the child informed about events at home and school. |
| | Pain/intrusion | • Provide privacy during procedures.<br>• Encourage the child's ability to learn through repetition by teaching about upcoming events well in advance.<br>• Accept aggressive verbal protests while setting realistic limits on undesirable behavior.<br>• Provide activities for the release of aggression. |

**Table 11.1**   Nursing Interventions to Minimize Children's Stress and Promote Coping (continued)

| Age Group | Stressor | Interventions to Promote Coping |
|---|---|---|
| | Loss of self-control | • Encourage the child to explain what s/he knows about the situation.<br>• Teach by means of honest explanations, diagrams, models, and actual equipment.<br>• Encourage the child to participate in self-care.<br>• Permit the child to make decisions and direct care whenever possible.<br>• Provide the child with meaningful tasks to perform.<br>• Use positive reinforcement for helpful behaviors. |
| Adolescent | Separation | • Encourage parents to visit regularly and reliably.<br>• Provide consistent caretakers.<br>• Assist parents in understanding their adolescent's need to be in control while recovering.<br>• Support communication with peers by providing flexible visiting hours for peers whenever feasible.<br>• Respect the adolescent's need to conform to peer expectations.<br>• Encourage verbalization of feelings with regard to peers, peer pressure, etc. |
| | Pain/intrusion | • Provide secure privacy during procedures.<br>• Assist the adolescent to prepare for stressful procedures.<br>• Accept aggressive verbal behavior without retaliating.<br>• Encourage verbalization of fears related to death or disability. |
| | Loss of self-control | • Encourage the adolescent's active participation in care.<br>• Consult the adolescent about the plan of care.<br>• Be flexible about hospital routines whenever possible.<br>• Promote cognitive mastery by asking the adolescent to explain what s/he knows.<br>• Be aware of intellectualization.<br>• Clarify misconceptions.<br>• Accept temporary withdrawal.<br>• Encourage expression of emotion by reflecting the adolescent's feelings.<br>• Respect the adolescent's need for independence. |

Note. From *Pediatric Critical Care* (pp. 16–18) by J. Smith, 1983, New York: Wiley. Copyright 1983 by Wiley. Reprinted by permission.

## GENERIC CARE PLAN FOR THE NURSING DIAGNOSIS INEFFECTIVE FAMILY COPING

# 1.  General Information

a.  **Etiology**
   - High-risk family structure (e.g., single, adolescent, emotionally or physically ill parent [s])
   - Child at risk (e.g., unwanted, physically or mentally handicapped, behaviorally disturbed, chronically or terminally ill)
   - Stressful environment (e.g., dissolved family, inadequate financial resources, family role changes, marital difficulty, relocation)
   - Emotional inadequacy (e.g., poor development of parental role, lack of knowledge of growth and developmental norms)
   - lack of physical, emotional, and/or psychologic resources
   - Unrealistic expectations

b.  **Clinical Manifestations**
   - Neglect of physical and/or emotional needs of child
   - Neglect of family needs (housing, food, emotional support)
   - Denial of problem
   - Unresolved anger, guilt, hostility, aggression, and/or depression
   - Observed or verbalized abuse
   - Lack of attainment of expected tasks by child
   - Destructive behavioral responses

c.  **Multidisciplinary Approaches**
   - Counseling: psychologic, financial, spiritual
   - Family therapy

# 2.  Nursing Process

a.  **Assessment**
   - Review this section in *Alteration in Family Process*, page 319, and *Alteration in Parenting*, page 323
   - Home environment for heat, ventilation, cleanliness, water supply, number of residents, presence of hazards
   - Parental knowledge, developmental expectations, and perceptions of their child
   - Level of anxiety
   - Family history, including stressful events and how the family copes
   - Interactions among family members
   - Risk level for ineffective family coping

b.  **Goals**
   Family will
   - acknowledge difficulties.

    — seek assistance in resolving family problems.
    — return to same or higher level of functioning.

**c. Interventions**
    — Provide information as needed about child's hospitalization.
    — Provide opportunities for family members to verbalize and ventilate their feelings; listen to and acknowledge what they say.
    — Reduce anxiety to prevent panic reactions (see *Anxiety,*page 308).
    — Assist family to identify available resources and options for changing the current situation.
    — Suggest more effective coping mechanisms that can be tried.
    — Refer family to appropriate sources for long-term intervention.

**d. Evaluation**
    — Family
      • identifies the source of the coping difficulty.
      • acknowledges family strengths and weaknesses.
      • identifies positive coping strategies.
      • obtains and uses available resources.
      • returns to prehospitalization level or functioning improves.

# Selected Health Problem Frequently Associated with the Nursing Diagnosis INEFFECTIVE FAMILY COPING

## Suspected Child Abuse and Neglect (SCAN)

**a. Discussion:**  Sometimes families do not develop a pattern of mutually supportive roles. For various reasons some parents do not develop a nurturing parental role and the family becomes dysfunctional. One result of this disturbance in role development is child abuse and/or neglect.

**Historical Perspectives.**  Child abuse is not a new product of modern technology and economic hard times. DeMause (1975) states that:

> "A child's life prior to modern times was uniformly bleak. . . . The further back in history we went, the lower the level of child care we found, and the more likely children were to have been killed, abandoned, whipped, sexually abused, and terrorized by their caretakers" (p. 85).

Even the Bible offers telling insight into the harshness of childhood.

> "Chastise your son while there is hope for him but be careful not to flog him to death." *Proverbs 19:18*
> "Rod and reprimand impart wisdom." *Proverbs 29:15*

DeMause also writes that the sexual abuse of children was common in ancient times. "Tiberius taught children of the most tender years . . . to play beneath his legs while he was in his bath. Those which had not yet been weaned . . . he set at fellatio" (p. 86).

**Forms of Child Abuse.**    The many forms of child abuse range from benign neglect and inappropriate developmental expectations to rape and murder. Those who inflict abuse on children may be parents, relatives, babysitters, daycare workers, school personnel, siblings, strangers, kidnappers, and so on. Abusers were generally abused themselves as children, and may appear to be functioning well in all other aspects of their personalities.

Child abuse, be it the lack of a safe environment that prevents growth and development or sodomization of a toddler, is not pleasant to think about. Indeed, it is easy to selectively tune out such things. Some types of abuse are not even within the frames of reference of many people; it does not occur to them that such things exist.

Physical abuse can be detected by a knowledgeable health care provider. It should be considered when *some* of the behaviors listed in table 11.2 are present.

**Table 11.2**    Indicators of Physical Abuse

When the Parent
1.  Shows evidence of loss of control, or fear of losing control
2.  Presents contradictory history
3.  Projects cause of injury onto a sibling or third party
4.  Has delayed unduly in bringing child in for care
5.  Shows detachment
6.  Reveals inappropriate awareness of seriousness of situation (either overreaction or underreaction)
7.  Continues to complain about irrelevant problems unrelated to the injury
8.  Personally is misusing drugs or alcohol
9.  Is disliked for unknown reasons by the physician
10. Presents a history that cannot or does not explain the injury
11. Gives specific "eye witness" history of abuse
12. Gives a history of repeated injury
13. Has no one to "bail" her/him out when "up tight" with the child
14. Is reluctant to give information
15. Refuses consent for further diagnostic studies
16. Hospital "shops"
17. Cannot be located
18. Is psychotic or psychopathic
19. Has been reared in a "motherless" atmosphere
20. Has unrealistic expectations of the child

When the Child
1.  Has an unexplained injury
2.  Shows evidence of dehydration and/or malnutrition without obvious cause
3.  Has been given inappropriate food, drink, and/or drugs
4.  Shows evidence of overall poor care
5.  Is unusually fearful
6.  Shows evidence of repeated injury
7.  "Takes over" and begins to care for parents' needs
8.  Is seen as "different" or "bad" by the parents

9.   Is indeed different in physical or emotional makeup
10.  Is dressed inappropriately for degree or type of injury
11.  Shows evidence of sexual abuse
12.  Shows evidence of repeated skin injuries
13.  Shows evidence of repeated fractures
14.  Shows evidence of "characteristic" x-ray changes to long bones
15.  Has injuries that are not mentioned in history

Note. From *Helping the battered child and his family* (p. 73) by C. Kempe and R. Helfer, 1972, Philadelphia: Lippincott. Copyright 1972 by Lippincott. Reprinted by permission.

Verbal abuse is particularly insidious because there is no physical evidence of foul play to betray it. Hallmarks of the verbally abused child are a sense of inadequacy, social isolation, and self-effacing behavior.

Neglect of a child can range from the well-meaning parent's inability to set limits for safe behavior to deliberate denial of adequate nutrition, clothing, shelter, or social interaction resulting in nonorganic failure to thrive (FTT). Medically, the neglected child can be difficult to identify, unless the child falls dramatically below accepted growth standards. As in all cases of abuse, diagnosis is all-important when neglect is suspected, and a full work-up is indicated, particularly in cases of FTT. Table 11.3 lists more specific indications of parent-child attachment deprivation syndrome, but even those conditions are not foolproof diagnostic clues. The most telling factor is much more elusive: the "degree of fit" between the temperaments of parents and child (e.g., the greater the variation between child and parental temperament, the greater the potential for abuse). Prognosis for such children is uncertain.

**Constellation of Abusive Behaviors in Familial Abuse.**    Kempe and Helfer (1972) identify four factors in the parental situation that are generally present before abuse occurs

- History of abuse
- Social isolation
- Spouse unavailable/unable to give support
- Inappropriate developmental expectations.

Being aware of inappropriate developmental expectations may help the nurse identify clues to potential abuse. These damaging parental attitudes may be directed toward any age child, and may revolve around cognitive, physical, or emotional growth. Most children will give clues as to their receptivity to training as well as physical evidence of development. The nurse should be particularly alert to parental boasts of or demands for accomplishment clearly beyond demonstrated levels, e.g.

- A couple brags that their child was toilet trained before the age of one year. In this case, it is more likely that the parents were trained to a child's patterns and placed the child on the potty at the proper times.
- Parents zealously use flashcards to teach their baby or toddler to "read" and "do mathematics." This is common behavior among members of

the competitive upper middle class, although there is little current evidence that this enhances later cognitive ability.

Kempe and Helfer stipulate that the abused child must be "seen differently by his parents; one who fails to respond in the expected manner; or possibly one who really is different (retarded, too smart, hyperactive, or has a birth defect)" (p. XIV-XV).

They emphasize that it "takes a very special kind of child for battering to occur" (p. 63). Unless the abusive potential is unusually strong, not every child in a family will be beaten. It is important to recognize that parents do not love and care for each child equally. If a child born into a family with the potential to abuse is an "easy" baby—that is, does not fuss for hours, does not have colic, eats and grows well, and does not get sick much—chances are the child will escape battering. If things aren't going well this infant can be in serious trouble.

The highest incidence of battering is inflicted on the toddler, the second on the pubertal adolescent. The awake toddler cannot safely be unsupervised for any amount of time, which can be very difficult for a parent. Sexuality in the budding teen causes its own unique trials for the parent. The true incidence of abuse is really not known, although in the past 10–12 years, increased public sensitivity has resulted in a greater willingness to report child abuse cases. Such action has improved the lives of many where the potential for tragedy exists.

**Table 11.3**   Family Characteristics Indicating Parent-Child Attachment Deprivation Syndrome

| *Parent(s)* | *Child* |
|---|---|
| • Isolation and inadequate support systems | Characteristic posture |
| • Poor parenting as a child | • Does not "mold" to caretaker's body when picked up or comforted |
| • Lack of education | • Remains rigid or floppy |
| • Physical and/or mental health problems (retardation, drug dependence, depression) | • Does not maintain eye contact |
| | • Inconsolable even when comfort measures are provided |
| • Lack of commitment to parenting | • "Difficult" to feed—vomits, ruminates, thrusts tongue, or sticks fingers down throat; poor appetite or suck; spits food; hoards food in mouth; appetite depression owing to chronic reduction in calories |
| • Immature, possibly adolescent parents | |
| • Multiple and chronic emotional, social, and financial crises | |
| • Father unsupportive | |
| • Little or no paternal support of child-rearing efforts | • "Difficult child pattern" |
| • No help or relief from child-rearing responsibilities during stressful periods | • Colicky |
| | • Irritable |
| • Inability to perceive or distinguish infant's needs | • Sleepy |
| | • Passive |
| • Inappropriate developmental expectations | • Lethargic |
| • Ambivalence toward pregnancy | |
| • Unwanted pregnancy | |

(Whaley & Wong, 1983)

The crisis situation that provokes an abusive incident varies greatly. Anything from an irritating behavior on the part of the child to an unexpected financial loss can precipitate an abusive incident. Stress that others may perceive as minor is enough to drive the abusing adult's existing anxiety level out of control.

**b.  Multidiciplinary Approaches**

Available Services: Most large, urban medical centers have networks in place to help abused and neglected children and their families. Beyond the diagnostic meaning, the SCAN acronym may also stand for "Supportive Child-Adult Network." Be aware of available services in the practice locality and utilize them when needed. Be aware, also, of the importance of intensive follow-up to determine whether or not the home is safe for a child to return to. A family's act of presenting an abused child to the health care system is an act of seeking help—a partial acknowledgement of an inability to cope. To merely treat physical injuries and release may place the child in greater danger than before, perhaps even jeopardizing the child's life. Table 11.4 summarizes the kind of support services that may be available in a SCAN network.

**Table 11.4**   Services in a Child Abuse Network

*Personnel*
  Department of Public Welfare social worker
  Emergency departments
  Physicians, RNs
  Nonemergency workers (specially trained)
  • psychiatrists/physicians/pediatricians
  • psychologists
  • family therapists
  • professional nurses
  • social workers/counselors
  • occupational/physical therapists

*Supervision and Care Options*
  Special placements for the handicapped such as residences, county homes, or centers
  • Long-term care/foster care for teenage parents as well as abused children
  • Educational or day care facilities
  • Homemakers with parenting skills
  • Trusted support people able to relieve parenting responsibilities
  • Emergency shelters (for abused wives as well as children)

*The Law*
  • Family Court—Child Protective Services
  • Legal Services attorneys (poverty law groups)

*Support Groups*
  Self-help groups (e.g., Parents Anonymous, Alcoholics Anonymous)
  • Methadone maintenance programs
  • Poly-drug abuse and substance abuse centers
  • Wife abuse programs
  • Centers for rape concern (e.g., Women Organized Against Rape [WOAR] or Women Against Rape [WAR])

# Additional Nursing Care That Can Be Incorporated into the Generic Care Plan

a. **Assessment**
   - Child's degree of willingness to be cared for by strangers
   - Presence of any cuts, bruises, welts, burns, or other signs of trauma
   - Wounds in different stages of healing
   - Basic hygiene, appropriateness of child's clothing
   - Height, weight, head circumference (if under two years of age), and plot on a growth chart
   - Disruptions in a consistent pattern or changes from previous measurements, if available
   - Previous hospital experience, seeking out of multiple medical caretakers
   - Favorite foods, eating, sleeping, play and toilet habits, siblings, security objects
   - 24-hour calorie count

b. **Goals**
   Parents will
   - visit as often as possible, and assist in child's care (e.g., helping bathe and feed).
   - increase own ability to nurture their child.
     - openly discuss their feelings and identify problems in their interactions with child and each other.
     - identify stressors in their lives and develop alternate ways of coping with them.
     - follow through on appropriate referrals.
   
   Child will
   - participate in age-appropriate play with peers, parents, and staff.
   - be safely returned home to his/her family or to a temporary caretaker.

c. **Interventions**
   - At least one person from every concerned discipline should make a point of collecting information about the three major predispositions for abuse
     - potential for abuse
     - the child
     - precipitating crisis
   - When conducting interview in suspected child abuse cases
     - find out whether the constellation of predisposing factors cited above is present; use great care not to alienate the parents or they will not provide the necessary information
     - resist the desire to find out what actually hurt the child (Kempe & Helfer)

- keep the conversation "parent-centered"—avoid discussing the child altogether
- choose a comfortable, relaxed setting; the child's bedside or a crowded emergency area is not appropriate
- keep the session brief
- interview each parent/guardian separately
- do not offer information to one parent and not the other
— Use a nonthreatening, nonjudgmental approach when interacting with parents in order to avoid alienating them from the health care system that could help them meet their children's—and their own—needs.
— Develop a thorough knowledge of growth and development in order to be able to identify inappropriate development expectations and the abuse that may arise from them.
— Establish a therapeutic relationship with the family; maintain a therapeutic rather than a punitive tone.
— Avoid assigning guilt or innocence, taking sides, or acting out anger toward parents.
— Orient child and parents to hospital routines and regulations.
— Encourage parents to visit as much as possible; provide opportunities for them to care for child, such as bathing and feeding.
— Provide explanation and reassurance to child and parents before and during all procedures.
— Be alert for superficial, indiscriminate affection from child and, instead of rejecting, provide appropriate affection.
— Set limits using planned responses to child's behavior.
— Use consistent caretakers, uniformity of approach.
— Establish a contract with the parents (e.g., for patting and stroking child, allow them to take child to lobby.)
— Convey to parents that abusive behavior is a serious problem and not merely "bad" behavior that can be excused.
— Recognize and praise parental strengths.
— Be available to parents to answer questions, to acknowledge difficulties/feelings, to listen, etc.
— Teach parents new ways to interact with child (e.g., speaking to child at eye level and making eye contact).
— Be a model for parents and child, using day-to-day care as an opportunity to demonstrate alternate ways of handling behaviors, feelings, and interactions with others.
— Share identified individual needs of parents and child with other staff members.
— Encourage group discussions among staff to help them work through their feelings.
— Explain age related behaviors to parents; reinforce with educational literature as appropriate.
— Be an advocate, counselor, educator, while at the same time monitoring the parent-child interactions.

- Be precise in documenting parent-child interactions and their expressed feelings; do not chart conjecture, etc.
- Refer family to community agencies and to community nurse (preferably a specialized team whose purpose is to deal with abused or neglected children).
- Prepare child and parents for separation after discharge, as necessary.
- If child is not discharged to own home, encourage family visit with new caretakers.
- Prepare parents/caretaker for possible posthospitilization problems with child (e.g., nightmares, sleep disturbances, and regressive behavior).
- Provide "hotline," etc., phone numbers for parents so they can call if they feel an inclination to injure child or a necessity to leave child.

d. **Evaluation**
   - Parents
     • agree that there is a family problem and identify behaviors they would like to change.
     • visit in the hospital every day and help to care for their child.
     • demonstrate a behavior not previously used (e.g., speaking to child at eye level).
     • take active steps to alleviate some of the stressors in their life (e.g., plan for some diversional activity outside the home).
     • seek outside help from community nurse and other agencies.
     • identify a constellation of individuals who may help or take over child's care if they "need a break".
   - Child/parents
     • use new coping mechanisms.
     • express their feelings.
     Child returns home or goes home with another caretaker.

# Other Possible Nursing Diagnoses

Alteration in nutrition: less than body requirements
Alteration in parenting
Alteration in thought processes
Anxiety
Diversional activity deficit
Fear
Impaired home maintenance management
Impairment of skin integrity
Ineffective individual coping
Knowledge deficit
Noncompliance
Potential for injury
Potential for violence

Powerlessness
Social isolation
Spiritual distress

# References

DeMause, L. (1975). Our forebears made childhood a nightmare. *Psychology Today, 8*(4), 85-88.

Kempe, C., & Helfer, R. (1972). *Helping the battered child and his family.* Philadelphia: Lippincott.

Whaley, L., & Wong, D. (1983). *Nursing care of infants and children.* (2nd ed.). St. Louis: Mosby.

# CHAPTER 12

# VALUE-BELIEF
## FUNCTIONAL HEALTH PATTERN

T he value-belief functional health pattern covers the areas of personal
values, beliefs, and philosophies. These beliefs and values differ among
people and may be acquired through cultural heritage, religious affiliation, or personal experience. Each individual and each family has unique values
and beliefs.

## Cultural Influences

Children are exposed to cultural beliefs and values about health care from the
moment they enter the family. A family will make decisions about health care
based, in part, on these beliefs and values. Understanding the influence of a
culture or subculture on the family can help the pediatric nurse provide care in
a more acceptable form. For example, making allowances in a necessary dietary
regimen for certain ethnic foods or rituals, or special foods considered
healthful by the family or child may make compliance more likely. The best way
to determine the beliefs and values of any family is through a careful assessment conducted in an accepting atmosphere.

## Spirituality

The development of spirituality is a life-long process that begins when the
infant learns to trust that s/he is safe in this world. During the ages of 4–6 the
child begins to internalize the religious values of the parents. This is a subtle

process based mostly on observation and nonverbal conveyance of attitudes. Adolescence is a time of major spiritual awakening. The individual begins to question "Who am I?" "How am I to express myself in this world?" This identity crisis encourages adolescents to reevalute parental values, and to begin to develop internal standards to guide their behavior. The moral development of a child as described by Kohlberg is outlined in table 12.1. This cognitive process leads the normal child to a level of adult moral reasoning.

**Table 12.1**   Moral Development: Kohlberg

| Infant (birth–12 months) | Toddler (1–3 years) | Preschooler (3–6 years) | School-age Child (6–12 years) | Adolescent (12–19 years) |
|---|---|---|---|---|
| Preconventional level (stage 1) Beginning of awareness of punishment (via deprivation or injury) but makes no cognitive connection No moral concepts or rules | Preconventional level (stage 2) Detects concepts of fairness, sharing "Instrumental-relativist" orientation Satisfies own needs Conventional level beginning ("good girl/ nice boy") Approval-seeking behavior coupled with desire to please | Preconventional level (stage 2) Conventional (stage 3) Child desires to please others, seeks approval/ attention through behaviors Social concern | Conventional (stage 3) resembling adult level of development Concern with authority figures, fixed rules in moral decisions (doesn't change own criteria with varying situations) Concern with obligation to duty Understands the concept of "bad act" that breaks a rule or does harm May interpret accidents or misfortunes as punishment Develops a conscience and sense of values | Conventional (stage 4) resembling adult Applies fixed rules in moral decisions; feels obligation to do no harm and to duty (many adults never advance beyond this stage of moral development) Postconventional (Stage 5) 16 + years, possible Social contracts understood and formulated Laws recognized as changeable Correct actions depend on standards and individual rights Postconventional (Stage 6) adult moral reasoning May occur in late adolescence, but only rarely Abstract moral principles govern behaviors Morality is easily separated from legality Orientation is based on universal, ethical orientation; situational ethics can be applied by |

**Table 12.1**   Moral Development: Kohlberg (continued)

| Infant (birth–12 months) | Toddler (1–3 years) | Preschooler (3–6 years) | School-age Child (6–12 years) | Adolescent (12–19 years) |
|---|---|---|---|---|
| | | | | those in this stage of moral reasoning Many individuals do not comprehend this level of development |

## GENERIC CARE PLAN FOR THE NURSING DIAGNOSIS
## SPIRITUAL DISTRESS

## 1.   General Information

Different hospitals meet the spiritual needs of patients in different ways, with varying degrees of success. Secular hospitals, particularly large teaching institutions, may overlook spiritual care. Therefore, it is especially important for nurses to find out whether these quieter, deeper needs are being met for children and their families. (See table 12.2 for a summary of spiritual concerns, cognitive conception of God, parental role, and possible nursing interventions for patients at each developmental stage.) Pay particular attention to children with chronic and/or life-threatening disease. They, or their families, may feel spiritually abandoned or a need to turn to religion at a time of crisis.

**Table 12.2**   Spiritual Concerns According to Developmental Stage

| Age Group | Cognitive Conception of God/ Religion | Spiritual Concerns | Parental Roles | Nursing Implications |
|---|---|---|---|---|
| Infancy (birth to 1 year) | None | Comfort and warmth Sense of trust | Ensure child is brought into the church • baptism • sacrament of the sick • annointing • circumcision | Contact priest, minister, rabbi or hospital chaplain, if necessary. Convey document of baptism to parents and chart it. Contact Mohel (for circumcision ceremony). Pray with parents if indicated; if uncomfortable, call hospital chaplain. |

**Table 12.2**    Spiritual Concerns According to Developmental Stage (continued)

| Age Group | Cognitive Conception of God/ Religion | Spiritual Concerns | Parental Roles | Nursing Implications |
|---|---|---|---|---|
| Toddler (1–3 years) | Representational thought: by 3 years, child can name God/Jesus in pictures | Sense of autonomy Rituals aid in mastering tasks • prayers at meals and bedtime • singing religious songs | Begin to develop a positive moral character in the child Provide positive and consistent role models in religious practice by attending church services and practicing the faith | Assess spiritual needs. Outline child's religious practices and determine if parents wish them to continue during hospitalization. Incorporate these practices in care plan. Provide religious readings and crafts for the child. Allow religious rituals to help decrease the psychologic threat of hospitalization. |
| Preschooler (3–6 years) | Preoperational thought • accepts fact of God as creative and loving Father • sometimes confuses names and persons of God, Jesus, Messiah • may worry that God sees everything child does | Sense of initiative Usually enjoys being in religious programs Likes to dramatize religious stories and events | Avoid swearing (can destroy child's beliefs) Avoid using good and bad labels | Continue to assist child in religious practices. Pray with child and family. Involve child in play activities, arts and crafts, for religious occasions (Passover, Christmas). Avoid expressions of bias regarding the religious practices of the child and family. |
| School-age Child (6–8 years) | Concrete thought • God is important • accepts that God sees him/her but cannot be seen • thinks carefully about God and heaven • begins to | Sense of accomplishment Begins to make religious decisions Reads from own religious books (Bible, catechism, scriptures) Attends Hebrew school, if | Know that religious ceremony (Communion, receiving ashes) can be performed in the hospital if desired Help the hospitalized child continue to prepare for the religious cere- | Allow child to verbalize feelings about illness. Foster child's ability to accomplish tasks in his/ her faith. Plan for child to receive sacraments during hospitalization (contact priest or minister). Allow child and |

**Table 12.2**    Spiritual Concerns According to Developmental Stage (continued)

| Age Group | Cognitive Conception of God/ Religion | Spiritual Concerns | Parental Roles | Nursing Implications |
|---|---|---|---|---|
| | question things that were previously accepted on faith | appropriate Begins to celebrate religious occasions | mony if s/he is capable | family to attend worship services within the hospital. |
| School-age Child (9–11 years) | Can grasp the history of his/ her faith through the use of religious readings and scripture Continues to learn about religious heritage and apply it to own life | Religious schools require religion as a major subject throughout school years and adolescence; tutoring may be necessary | Involvement in the child's religious studies May want to develop a diary of the child's experiences | Allow time for religious study during hospitalization. Encourage child to verbalize what s/he learns from religious studies. Determine if there are any dietary restrictions in the child's religious practices; document in care plan and notify dietician. |
| Adolescence (11 years to adulthood) | Formal operations, abstract thinking • discusses ethical issues • begins to ask questions about his/her faith • capable of deep emotional response to worship within his/her faith • debates questions about God, heaven, hell, immortality, and reason for living | Sense of identity Guidance and encouragement from a capable teacher of his/ her faith Help in understanding the problem of ethics Possibly contemplating a religious vocation Hebrew confirmation at 16 | Demonstrate patience, love, and understanding during the adolescent's struggle with faith Share doubts with the adolescent Foster the adolescent's self-esteem | Allow visitation by peers, clergy, religious teachers. Listen; pick up clues to spiritual distress. Reevaluate the adolescent's beliefs since this is an age of doubt and uncertainty. Do not evangelize; maintain the adolescent's integrity. Establish discussion groups. |

    **a.  Etiology**
- Separation from family, religion, or culture
- Challenge to belief and value system
- Response to a loss of health, body part, function
- Hospital barriers to practicing spiritual rituals
- Terminal illness and death of significant other

    **b.  Clinical Manifestations**
- Discouragement
- Asking "Why me?"
- Feeling sorry for oneself
- Anger toward God
- Nightmares or sleep disturbances
- Expresses concern about the meaning of life, illness
- Unable or unwilling to participate in religious rituals

    **c.  Multidisciplinary Approach**
- Pastoral counseling

## 2.  Nursing Process

    **a.  Assessment**
- Parents' and child's religious affiliation
- Religious commitments child has made to this point (e.g., baptism, confirmation, bar mitzvah)
- Current preparation for a religious event
- Attendance at a religious school
- Need for assistance in continuing religious education
- Child's spiritual rituals (e.g., prayer at meals, bedtime, religious songs or stories)
- How the family is involved in the spiritual growth of the child
- Name of clergy (rabbi, minister, priest)
- Wish of parents and/or child to receive spiritual support during this hospitalization (e.g., visits by clergy, hospital chaplain, receiving sacraments, attendance at worship services)
- Particular religious occasions the child will be observing during hospitalization (e.g., Passover, Good Friday, Yom Kippur); how it will be observed
- Dietary restrictions according to religious practices (within medical regimen)

    **b.  Goal**

    Parent/child will increase sense of hope and participate in spiritual activities as appropriate.

    **c.  Interventions**
- Integrate normal religious education and observance into hospital care whenever possible (this may also help distract the child from the discomfort of disease or treatment).

- Consult the hospital chaplain, parish priest, rabbi, or other member of the clergy if the patient's religious/spiritual needs are beyond the nurse's ability to help.
- Support the family religion in all dealings with young patients (for instance, it serves no purpose for a child of a nonchristian faith to be taught the gospel); be aware of the parents' desires.
- Baptize, if indicated, and record baptism on the child's chart and bed
  - notify the parents as quickly as possible
  - complete a baptismal certificate and present it to the parents as official documentation of the ritual
  - baptism may be performed by anyone when a clergyperson cannot be summoned quickly enough
  - the act may be accomplished by touching water to the child's scalp and saying, "I baptize you in the name of the Father, Son, and Holy Spirit."
- Construct an interdenominational religious calendar and post it for the staff.
- Do not display bias concerning the religious practices of patients or families.

d. **Evaluation**
   Parents and/or child
   - verbalize a feeling of hope.
   - carry out rituals regularly.
   - express a sense of comfort.

e. **Possible Related Nursing Diagnoses**
   Anxiety
   Disturbance in self-concept
   Fear
   Powerlessness

# Selected Health Problem Frequently Associated with the Nursing Diagnosis SPIRITUAL DISTRESS

## Terminal Illness

a. **Discussion**
   It is never easy for even the most seasoned professional to deal with the death of a child. It is difficult to accept that the hopes and dreams of the child and family will never be fulfilled. When death is imminent, it is usually the nurse who is there with the child and family. The nurse's anticipation of family needs, and subsequent interventions,

make a great deal of difference in how the family accepts the loss of a loved one.

Part of the caring role of nursing is to provide comfort to the dying. It is not uncommon for busy staff members to become very task oriented at this distressing time. Physical presence is not enough during a patient's declining moments. Emotional and spiritual support assist the individual to die with peace and dignity. One must be willing to listen nonjudgmentally and accept each person's unique way of grieving.

It is important that care be provided by a support person whom family members know, not a stranger called in as additional help. A part-time staff member who has a limited relationship with the family should not be responsible for care during such a critical time.

The family needs to spend time with their dying child. Many parents state that they feel relieved at having had the chance to hold their dying child and spend private time with the body after death. Some families express the desire to photograph or even wash the child's body, and there is no reason to prohibit such actions. Each family brings distinct personal and cultural values and beliefs to a death situation. Honor these needs regardless of your personal values and beliefs.

When death is sudden and unexpected, particularly as the result of an accident, the family does not have time to experience the anticipatory grief possible with expected deaths. They may feel extremely guilt ridden and think "if only" they had been more careful, brought the child to treatment sooner, or honored a specific request, the child would be alive. Some kind of follow up counseling or informal discussion of the events immediately preceding death may be necessary to help family members cope with their loss.

b. **Multidisciplinary Approach**
   – Psychologic counseling

# Additional Nursing Care That Can Be Incorporated into the Generic Care Plan

a. **Assessment**
   – Carefully assess personal reactions to death and dying, then use that knowledge to help assure that dying children and their families do not feel emotionally or spiritually abandoned.
   – Do not assume that ethnic families do or do not follow traditional faiths. Many Vietnamese immigrants, for example, have embraced the Christian faith. Conversely, some members of different ethnic groups continue to practice traditional beliefs in their homes.

b. **Goals**
   Child will die with physical, emotional, and spiritual support.

Parents will receive spiritual support and comfort during the final stages of the child's life.

c.  **Interventions**
    - Offer family members the option of sitting or not sitting with a dying child; most wish to do so, but some do not.
    - Know when a death should be reported, and to whom (see table 3.2).
    - Determine, as far in advance as possible, what clergy, if any, can provide comfort to the family. Even after death has occurred, the family might wish to have a priest, minister, or rabbi deliver parting prayers.
    - Notify parents, whenever possible, as soon as it is known that their child is dying. This is generally the physician's role, but if no physician is available, take the initiative to telephone family members and indicate that the child has taken a turn for the worse.
    - Plan assignments carefully so that familiar nurses will be available around the clock and on weekends.
    - Discuss the grieving process with the family and how the flux of feelings, different phases, etc. are normal and expected.
    - Meet siblings' needs according to the dictates of their developmental status.
    - Listen to child's/parents' expressions of anger with or alienation from God.
    - Ask how you can be most helpful.
    - Allow time during care to discuss spiritual and/or philosophical concerns.
    - Use therapeutic communication techniques such as reflection, clarification, etc. to help child or family resolve their distress.

d.  **Evaluation**
    - Child dies with dignity and peace.
    - Parents
        • carry out their personal wishes for the child's death.
        • are comforted and supported in their grieving.

e.  **Other Possible Nursing Diagnoses**
    Alteration in family processes
    Anxiety
    Fear
    Ineffective individual/family coping
    Powerlessness

# Reference

Mott, S., Fazekas, N., & James, S. (1985). *Nursing care of children and families: A holistic approach.* Menlo Park: Addison-Wesley.

# APPENDIX 1: NORMAL GROWTH AND DEVELOPMENT

## The Infant: Neonate through 12 months (wide ranges of normal for each task)

### Major Developmental Theorists

#### Duvall (Family Stages)
• Marital, childbearing family: establishing a marriage, adjusting to parenthood, and making a home for all

#### Maslow's Hierarchy of Needs
I. Physiologic needs for survival
II. Safety and security
III. Love and belonging

#### Sullivan (Interpersonal)
• Two complex drives
  - satisfaction
  - security
• A self-system (self-esteem) develops in the context of parental approval and disapproval; disapproval causes anxiety; if only disapproval is given, a negative self-system will develop.
• Infancy: differentiation of "good mother—bad mother‘

#### Skinner (Behavioral)
• Learning takes place by conditioning a child to give the right response when a stimulus is applied.
• Operant conditioning (by reinforcement); if no reinforcement, a response becomes extinct.

#### Freud (Psychosexual)
• Oral stage: oral gratification and sucking needs
  - If successful, feelings of security result.
  - If unsuccessful, an oral-dependent character results.
• Egocentrism is complete.

#### Erikson (Psychosocial)
• Trust versus mistrust
• Oral sensory
• Quality of parental-infant relationship important
• Birth: regards face and establishes eye contact.
• 1–2 months: smiles responsively.
• 2–3 months: smiles spontaneously.
• 6 months: exhibits stranger anxiety.
• Attachment to favorite objects (e.g., teddy bear or blanket)

- 12 months: demonstrates emotions of fear, anger, and affection; can indicate desires without crying.

## *Havighurst*
- Establishing self-awareness and self as a very dependent being
- Developing feelings for affection in a giving-receiving pattern
- Beginning awareness of animate versus inanimate and familiar versus unfamiliar
- Rudimentary social interaction
- Preverbal communication
- Adjusting to adult feeding and cleanliness demands
- Adjusting to adult attitudes toward genital manipulation
- Developing a physiologic equilibrium
- Establishment of a satisfactory sleep-activity pattern or rhythm
- Exploring the physical world
- Establishing eye-to-hand coordination
- Beginning of preverbal communication and rudimentary concept formation

## *Kohlberg (Moral)*
- Stage I: preconventional level
  - Beginning of punishment (via deprivation or injury, but makes no cognitive connection)
  - No moral concepts or rules exist.

## *Piaget (Cognitive)*
- Substage I (0–1 months): practice of reflexes and reflex-like actions
- Substage II (1–4 months): purposeful reproduction of reflex actions
- Substage III (4–8 months): object-oriented and imitative actions
- Accidental actions are repeated
- Substage IV (8–12 months): coordination, intentionality, goal direction, and achievement
- Experimentation and achievement of object-permanence (searches for a dropped object or person playing peek-a-boo)
- Imitates and models behavior.

## Developmental Timetable

### *Sound, Language, and Learning*
- Newborn prefers higher-pitched voices.
- All infants coo and babble, especially at 6 months of age including deaf infants; newborn startles to loud noises.
- 2–3 months: laughs and squeals.
- 4 months: produces belly laughs.
- 4–5 months: turns to voice (quiet listening).
- 8–10 months: uses "dada," "mama" (nonspecific); responds to own name at about 10 months (receptive language skills develop first); localizes sound from above or below.
- 7–11 months: imitates speech sounds; understands name and "no."

- 10 months: understands "bye" and "pat-a-cake."
- 1 year: has one word (or a few) in spoken vocabulary; comprehends "give" and stops when told "no"; has receptive vocabulary of several dozen words.
- 3–12 months: learned rather than reflex behavior; recognizes certain sounds, ignores others, attends to quiet sounds more than loud ones.
- Deaf infants lose ability to vocalize by age 1.

## Vision
- Birth: fixates on human face and demonstrates preference.
- 2 months: follows to midline; produces tears.
- 4 months: follows objects to 180°.
- 6 months: inspects hands, can fixate on objects 3 feet away; strabismus no longer within normal limits.
- 8 months: has permanent eye color.
- 10 months: tilts head backwards to see up.
- 12 months: shows smooth visual pursuit of objects with 20/100 vision.

## Neurologic and Motor Development
- Development is cephalocaudal and proximal to distal in nature and direction; arm and hand skills develop prior to leg and feet skills.
- *Gross motor*
  - Birth: turns head when prone, but cannot support head; adjusts posture when held at shoulder; may squirm to corner or edge of crib when prone; arm and leg movements reflexive.
  - 6 weeks–2 months: holds head up to 45°–90° when prone; may hold head steady when in supported sitting position.
  - 3 months: rolls over from back to side.
  - 4 months: may bear weight on legs when assisted to stand; head lag disappears when pulled to sitting position.
  - 5 months: pulls to sitting position; rolls from back to stomach; sits alone momentarily; shows unilateral reaching.
  - 6 months: sits without support; may creep an inch forward or backward; moves from place to place by rolling over.
  - 7 months: stands holding on; early stepping movements (prewalking progression); begins to crawl or hitch.
  - 8 months: pulls to standing position; raises self to sitting position.
  - 9 months: walks with help; crawls or hitches when permitted; sits down.
  - 10 months: continues walking skill development with help; stands alone; may climb up and down stairs.
  - 11 months: may walk alone; begins to stoop and recover.
  - 12 months: continues walking skills.
- *Fine motor (Adaptive)*
  - Birth–2 months: follows to and slightly past midline.
  - 2–3 months: keeps hands open predominantly; reflex grasp replaced by voluntary grasping; grasps objects such as rattle in open hand; may bring hands together at midline.

- 3–4 months: uses ulnar-palmar prehension with a cube; reaches for objects.
- 5 months: attempts to "catch" dangling objects; begins use of fore-finger and thumb in pincer grasp (opposable thumb—prehension); retains two cubes, recovers rattle, reaches and grasps objects.
- 6–7 months: can grasp at will; holds and manipulates objects; trans-fers from hand to hand; scoops pellet; demonstrates inferior pincer grasp.
- 8–9 months: combines spoons or cubes at the midline; retains two of three cubes offered; achieves neat pincer grasp of a pellet; feeds self finger foods.
- 10–11 months: plays pat-a-cake, a midline skill; puts several objects in a container; holds crayon adaptively; bangs two cubes together; looks for hidden objects (object permanence); achieves neat pincer grasp of tiny objects.

### Physical Characteristics
- 10% loss of birthweight in first 3–4 days of life
- 73% of body weight is fluid ($H_2O$) in the newborn
- 2–3 months: posterior fontanel closes; obligate (preferential) nose breathers until about 5 months.
- 5–6 months: doubles birth weight.
- 6 months: begins teething with lower central incisors.
- 8 months: develops regular bowel and bladder patterns.
- 1 year: average weight 20 lb; head and chest circumference equal.

### Play and Age-Appropriate Play Interventions
- Sensorimotor developmental ability controls movements, increases ability.
- Provide different textures and temperatures.
- Solitary play
- May be imitative
- Exploratory and manipulative
- Enjoys squeak toys, crumpled paper, mirror and water play, mobiles, body parts, blocks, push and pull toys, busy boxes, rattles, and noise toys.
- 5–7 months: resists toy pull; picks up tiny objects; plays peek-a-boo; works for toy out of reach.
- 8–9 months: plays pat-a-cake; recognizes self in mirror.
- 10–12 months: plays ball with examiner; achieves object permanence (searches for dropped objects).

### Parental Education, Nutrition, and Health Needs
- Immunizations
  - 2 months: DPT, TOPV
  - 4 months: DPT, TOPV
  - 6 months: DPT, optional TOPV
  - 1 year: tuberculin testing
- Solid food introduction (controversial)

- 6 weeks (optional): rice cereal (not mixed) (respected authorities see little or no need for supplementation prior to age 4–6 months)
- Formula rule of thumb: up to 1 year cow's milk should not be introduced until infant is tolerating 1½ jars of strained baby food/day to give nutritional balance.
- Introduce only one new food at a time, then use daily for several days; observe for rashes, diarrhea, vomiting, hives; start with simple strained foods (e.g., applesauce, not "mixed fruit dessert").
- Blenderized table food is more nutritious than commercially prepared baby foods. (*Note:* Commercial strained foods are expensive and may contain a lot of sugar and sodium.)
- Follow reasonable timetable after cereals have been introduced, e.g.
  * 6 months: mashed egg yolk, strained or blenderized fruits, yellow vegetables, green vegetables, meats.
  * 10–12 months: introduce liquids in a cup.
- Dental caries may become a problem if a child is permitted to sleep with a bottle of juice or formula; "bottle mouth" may be prevented by putting only water in a child's bottle prior to bed.
- Additional concerns/information
  - Accident and safety precautions: no unsupervised tub baths, baby-proof environment.
  - Encourage as much parental visiting as possible to minimize separation anxiety.
  - Review normal developmental behaviors for this age and provide anticipatory guidance around next developmental stage.
  - Each infant has own temperament; expresses needs through crying.

# The Toddler: 1–3 years

## Major Developmental Theorists

### Duvall (Family Stages)
- Childbearing family: adjusting to parenting and making a home for all

### Maslow's Hierarchy of Needs
  I. Physiologic
 II. Safety and security
III. Love and belonging
IV. Self-esteem

### Sullivan (Interpersonal)
- Acculturation: self-system forms in the context of approval and disapproval.
- 0–18 months: differentiation between "good mother—bad mother" to "good me—bad me" or "not me."
- Self–concept begins at age 3.
- Two tasks
  - independence

- individuation (differentiation from mother)
- Much testing of ability, self-control, limits discipline.
- Oppositional behavior
- Swings from love to hate.
- Emptying and hoarding
- Frustration: saying "no"
- Ritualistic: feels secure with daily routine and familiar environment.

### Skinner (Behavior)
- Learning occurs when respondent or operant behavior occurs.

### Freud (Psychosexual)
- Anal stage
  - Sensual pleasure shifts to anal and urethral areas.
  - Toilet training seen as area of discipline and authority; if unsuccessful, personality may become possessive or child may refuse to release possessions, including waste materials.

### Erikson (Psychosocial)
- Autonomy versus shame and doubt
- Doubts sense of self-control; personal behavior may be self-determined; overprotection and excessive criticism may be related to negative feelings; permit child to move at own pace; ritualistic.
- Ambivalence, walking, toilet training, temper tantrums, and negative "oppositional" behavior
- Dawdling
- Magical thinking: "wishes make it so"
- Inconsistent limit setting disrupts and upsets behavior patterns.

### Havighurst
1. Dependence: adjusting to less personal attention; physical independence/emotional dependence
2. Affection: developing ability to give/share affection
3. Beginning to develop ability to interact with age mates; adjusting to family expectations
4. Developing respect for authority and obedience in presence or absence of authority
5. Identification with male/female sex roles
6, 7. Improving coordination of large and small muscles; modesty
8–10. Improving use of symbol system; much improved elaboration of concept pattern

### Kohlberg (Moral)
- Stage 2: preconventional level
  - Detects concepts of fairness and sharing.
  - "Instrumental-relationistic" orientation
  - Satisfaction of own needs
  - Conventional level beginning: "good girl—nice boy'
  - Approval-seeking behavior coupled with desire to please

## *Piaget (Cognitive)*
- Sensorimotor (0–2 years)
- Preoperational-preconceptual (2–7 years)
- Substage V (12–18 months): production of vowel behaviors and curiosity
- Substage VI (18–24 months): concept of object permanence fully achieved
- Symbolic plane
- Limited concept of time (no "tomorrow')
- Very egocentric
- Animists (talk to stuffed animals)
- Imaginary playmates
- Parallel play
- Premature sense of cause/effect
- Goal-directed behavior

## Developmental Timetable

### *Sound, Language, and Learning*
- Beginning of spoken language.
- May occur at the same time as walking.
- Concentration on one or the other may occur.
- Has 300-word vocabulary and use of 2-word sentences by 2 years.
- Has 900-word vocabulary and use of 3-word sentences by 3 years.
- 12–18 months: recognizes nouns that stand for objects; uses gestures to make needs known.
- 18–24 months: follows directions; points to nose, hair, eyes on command; comprehends "give me that" when accompanied by a gesture.
- 2–2½ years: uses colors; understands action-oriented verbs and commands; understands size gradations and designates "me, I, mine"; uses plurals.
- 3 years: gives first and last names; progressive comprehension of speech response to musical sounds (pitch pipes).

### *Vision*
- 18 months: displays interest in pictures.
- 2 years: identifies forms (Snellen testing: 20/40 vision)
- 3 years: has 20/30 vision.

### *Neurologic and Motor Development*
- *Gross motor*
  - 12–18 months: walks well, throws ball, stoops and recovers, walks up stairs with help, begins to run; walks sideways and backwards 10 feet; stands on one foot with help.
  - 18–24 months: kicks ball forward, throws overhand, walks down stairs with help, one at a time.
  - 2–3 years: jumps and runs well; jumps from bottom step; jumps in place; balances on one foot for 1 second; pedals tricycle; walks on a straight line; tiptoes.

- – 29–32 months: broad jumps (distance) 4–14 inches.
- *Fine motor*
  - – 12–18 months: scribbles spontaneously; builds tower of two, then four cubes; dumps raisin from container after demonstration, then spontaneously; may untie shoes. Uses opposable thumb well (prehension); shows preference for hand.
  - – 18–24 months: may remove articles of clothing; holds pencil well enough for scribbling; builds tower of four cubes; imitates vertical line within 30°.
  - – 24–36 months: builds tower of 6–8 cubes; can use paint brush; imitates scribble; copies a circle; begins to wash and dry hands and dress with supervision.

### Physical Characteristics
- Can "let go" and walk with a wide stance.
- 1 year: triples birth weight to 20 lb.
- 2 years: average weight is 30 lb.
- 18–30 months: toilet training may be accomplished (do not rush).
- 18–24 months: anterior fontanel closes.
- Need for food relative to size not as great (permit to accept or refuse).

### Play and Age-appropriate Play Interventions
- Play is parallel: plays alongside, not with, others; imitates adult roles, including housework.
- 18 months: will help do simple tasks in household.
- 21–36 months: begins to play interactive games, such as tag.
- Play materials: water (supervised tub play), sand, clay, Play-Doh, crayons, puzzles, wheeled vehicles, story books
- Fantasy and "make-believe" play, action games (ritualistic, such as tag or hide and go seek).
- Verbal limits may not be sufficient in the toddler age group.

### Parental Education and Health Needs
- Immunizations
  - – 15 months: mumps, measles, and rubella vaccine (MMR)
  - – 18 months: DPT, TOPV
- Dental care: dental visits begin at 2½ years.
- Accident prevention
  - – anticipatory guidance concerning safety; protect from falls by keeping doors to rooms with dangers shut and locked (e.g., medication room).
  - – Avoid tiny objects in environment (e.g., peanuts, difficult-to-chew foods, small toys).
  - – Avoid sharp objects.
  - – Prevention of ingestion of toxic substances of paramount importance; particular concern should be taken in unfamiliar, non-child-proofed environments (e.g., homes of relatives).
  - – No unlocked cabinet (even above counters) can be considered safe.

- Car seat safety is now law in many states.
- Near-drowning accidents are common; "attractive nuisances" available (e.g., neighbor's pool, fountain, pond); no unsupervised tub, wading pool, or water play.
- Burning/scalding accidents common (unattended stove tops).
- Weaning
  - Encourage drinking from a cup.
  - Gradually wean as tolerated from breast or bottle; each child will indicate own pace.

# The Preschooler: 3–6 years

## Major Developmental Theorists

### Duvall (Family Stages)
- Preschool family, nurturing children
- Socialization within the family environment

### Maslow's Hierarchy of Needs
- I. Physiologic
- II. Safety and security
- III. Love and belonging
- IV. Self-esteem
- V. Cognitive needs

### Sullivan (Interpersonal)
- Competition, cooperation, compromise
- Skill in playing with others begins with increased acculturation.
- Able to "share" toys; still possessive

### Skinner (Behavior)
- If negative behaviors are not enforced, they will become extinct in normal individuals.

### Freud (Psychosexual)
- Phallic stage: much genital manipulation and exploration (particularly with other children).
- Shows intense attraction and love for parent of opposite sex (Oedipal conflict in males/Electra conflict in females).
- Rivalry with parent of opposite sex
- Castration anxiety, mutilation fears: intrusive procedures threaten body integrity.
- Primitive sense of body image begins.
- Separates easily from mother.

### Erikson (Psychosocial)
- Initiative versus guilt
- Locomotor, genital

- Magical thinking; much make-believe play activity, which, if stifled, is related to guilt.
- When permitted freedom, creativity is enhanced.
- Many fears, such as having head chopped off or being sucked down the drain.
- Fears become real and logical in the child's mind; takes things literally.

### Havighurst
- Similar to and evolving from tasks listed under the toddler age group:
  1. Adapting to less private attention
  2. Giving and receiving affection
  3. Interacting and sharing with age-mates
  4. Obedience to authority
  5. Identification with role models of same sex
  6, 7. Modesty; increasing motor coordination
  8–10. Concept pattern elaboration and relating oneself to the cosmos, in an uncritical fashion

### Kohlberg (Moral)
- Conventional stage in which child desires to please others; seeks approval (or attention) through behaviors.
- Social concern

### Piaget (Cognitive)
- Preoperational (2–7 years): egocentrism and "omnipotence" (inability to distinguish between own perception and that of someone else)
- Thinking is concrete and tangible, becoming intuitive toward the end of this stage
- "Transductive reasoning" from a particular event to another event
- Animism: anthropomorphism (attributes human traits to inanimate objects or animals)
- Magical thinking (imaginary playmates are common)
- Artificialism (all things are "made for a purpose")
- Irreversibility (cannot backtrack steps in a thinking pattern)
- Centration (inability to consider several aspects of the situation simultaneously)
- Trial versus error (prelogical thought processes)
- Primitive concepts of space, time, and causality
- Uses memory.

## Developmental Timetable

### Sound, Language, and Learning
- Uses 4- to 5-word sentences, with adult sense of syntax; has vocabulary of about 2,100 words.
- Can name body parts, recognize colors.
- Talks fluently and listens.
- Cooperates on systematic audiometric tests.

- 3–4 years: comprehends cold, tired, and hungry (2 of 3); comprehends prepositions.
- 4–5 years: knows opposite analogies (2 of 3); recognizes colors.
- 5–6 years: defines words (6 of 9); knows composition of objects (3 of 3).
- Clues to hearing deficits: volume of TV, whether child responds to you, formal audiometric testing, whether 5-year-old's speech is intelligible.

## Development: Vision, Neurologic, and Motor
- *Vision*
  - 3 years: has 20/30 vision, copies a circle.
  - 4 years: cooperates with Snellen testing; copies crosses.
  - 5 years: recognizes color; copies squares.
  - Clues to visual deficits: squints, favors one eye, tilts head, bumps into objects.
- *Gross motor*
  - 3 years: hops on one foot.
  - 4 years: skips; balances on 1 foot for 5 seconds (2 out of 3 tries); performs heel-to-toe walk (2 out of 3 tries); catches bounced ball (2 out of 3 tries); dresses without supervision.
  - 5 years: walks backward heel to toe (2 out of 3 tries); balances on 1 foot for 10 seconds (2 out of 3 tries).
- *Fine motor*
  - 3–4 years: buttons large buttons; picks longer line (3 out of 3 tries).
  - 4–5 years: ties shoe laces; draws a man with 3–6 parts; copies a square.
  - 5–6 years: draws a man with 6 parts; copies a triangle.

## Physical Characteristics
- First permanent tooth erupts at about 6 years; begins loss of deciduous teeth.
- Walks erect; swings arms.
- Rapid skeletal development taking place.

## Play and Age-appropriate Play Interventions
- Parallel/associative: child plays with other children and engages in common activity.
- Has no organization or group goals.
- Defines own rules.
- Cooperates.
- Play is organized in a group with other children.
- Joins in play of others.
- Plays interactive games.
- Content of play includes dramatic and socially affective as well as imitative play.
- Play materials: similar to those of the toddler (e.g., water with supervision, sand, clay, Play-Doh, wheeled vehicles, tea sets, toy kitchens, dress-up clothes, story books, dolls of either sex, favorite toys of attachment, action games, guessing games, simple card or board games, make believe). *Note:*

"Needle" play and using dolls or stuffed animals to demonstrate preoperative teaching is very useful in this group.

### Parental Education and Health Needs
- Immunization
  - 4–6 years: DPT, TOPV boosters
- Nutritional guidance
  - Common parental concern is that child of this age group eats little; have parents do a premeasured dietary recall for 1 week (they are usually impressed with amount consumed).
- Accident prevention
  - Poisoning is still a danger.
  - Playing in the street (running after balls, riding tricycles)
  - This age group responds to education for safety and limit setting; role modeling of good health and safety habits develops careful children.

# The School-age Child

## Major Developmental Theorists

### Duvall (Family Stages)
- School-age family: socializing and educating children

### Maslow's Hierarchy of Needs
- I. Physiologic
- II. Safety and security
- III. Love and belonging
- IV. Self-esteem
- V. Self-actualization (making maximum use of abilities)
- VI. Cognitive needs: seeking knowledge and understanding

### Sullivan (Interpersonal)
- Social participation: school, neighborhood, scouting groups
- Independence within family
- "Compeer" relationships important
- Chumships and altruistic concern for others, particularly one same-sex significant other
- Self-regulation of behavior
- Begins to manage cooperative and competitive relationships.

### Freud (Psychosexual)
- Latent stage
  - Sexual impulses are repressed.
  - Parents are no longer viewed as omnipotent.
  - Privacy becomes important in later school-age years.

### Erikson (Psychosocial)
- Industry versus inferiority
- Latency

- A sense of industry ensues when child is encouraged to make, build, construct, sew various projects; child displays keen sense of concern with how things are made; sense of inferiority ensues when projects are not praised or creativity is squelched.

## *Havighurst*
- Late childhood—early adolescence
  1. Freeing oneself from primary identification with adults
  2. Accepting oneself as really worthy of love
     - Peer friendships
     - Learning to give as much love as one receives
  3. Establishing peer groups, learning to belong, and behaving according to a shifting peer code
  4. Learning more rules and developing "true" morality
  5. Developing strong identification with social contemporaries of the same sex, and learning one's role in heterosexual relationships
  6, 7. Further refinement and development of small muscles and accepting oneself while controlling and using a new body
  8–10. Understanding of causal relationships
     - Thinking in a "scientific," problem-solving manner
     - Movement from concrete to abstract principles via use of language
     - Application of general principles to the particular

## *Kohlberg (Moral)*
- Stage IV: conventional (even adult-like) level of moral development
- Concern with authority figures, fixed rules in moral decisions (not changing criteria or varying with the situation)
- Concern with obligation to duty
- A "bad act" breaks a rule or does harm.
- Accidents or misfortunes may be interpreted as punishment.
- Develops a conscience and sense of values.

## *Piaget (Cognitive)*
- Concrete operations (7–11 years)
- Ability to reason
- Concept of reversibility: can reverse actions or thinking ($10 = 10$).
- Classifies objects (e.g., leaf and rock collections) according to their characteristics (e.g., igneous versus sedimentary rocks).
- Concept of conservation: comprehends that amount, weight, physical properties, and volume of substances are not changed by physical movement (e.g., the volume of water poured from a cup to a glass is the same).
- Concept of relativism: two or more aspects of a problem may be operated (manipulated) simultaneously.
- Can place self in another's situation.
- Serialization: masters the ordinal number line; can group and sort/place in logical order.

- Fundamental skills of reading, writing and grammar develop.
- Late school-age child (11 years) is capable of abstraction and deductive reasoning.

## Normal Growth and Development

### Sound, Language, and Learning
- Augments vocabulary and cognitive skills.

### Development: Vision, Neurologic, and Motor
- *Vision:* 20/20 at age 7.
- *Gross motor*
  - 6 years: walks a straight line; has mastered all skills on Denver Developmental Screening Test.
- *Fine motor*
  - Continually refines and improves previously learned skills.

### Physical Characteristics
- Preadolescence/pubescence.
- Females (at 11 years) have achieved 90% of adult height and 50% of adult weight.
- Males (at 12 years) have achieved 80% of adult height and 50% of adult weight.
- Throughout the whole age group (6–12 years) the most striking physical change is in growth of long bones (proportional increase in leg length in relation to height).
- Learns physical skills necessary for games.
- Begins Tanner stages of pubertal development: usually accomplishes stages I, II (secondary sex characteristics); however, some females are capable of menarche and child-bearing at ages 11 and 12; striking individual differences.

### Play and Age-appropriate Play Interventions
- Cooperative "team" play
- Skill play (e.g., jumping rope, skating)
- Testing, model building, exploration
- Enjoys camping.
- Collections (and classification of items collected), hobbies, sophisticated dolls, board games (including chess and backgammon)
- Reads for pleasure.
- Enjoys swimming and horseback riding.
- Needs to be distracted from long hours of idle TV watching.

### Parental Education and Health Needs
- Accident prevention related to sports, falls, etc.
- Recognizing behavior-socialization problems and learning disabilities.
- Sex education begins.
- Nutritional counseling
- Discretion in viewing media productions (TV, movies)

- Communicable diseases related to school
- If child is treated with antibiotics, stress importance of completing full course.
- Somatic complaints and fatigue not uncommon; more frequently seen at ages 6, 9, 11, and 12.
- Fears not uncommon; especially enhanced at ages 6, 7, 10, and 11.

## The Adolescent

### Major Developmental Theorists

#### Duvall (Family Stages)
- Teenage family: balancing teenage freedom and responsibility; ends with launching (releasing) of children.

#### Maslow's Hierarchy of Needs (all)
  I. Physiologic
 II. Safety and security
III. Love and belonging
IV. Self-esteem
 V. Self-actualization (some)
VI. Cognitive
VII. Aesthetic needs; desire for beauty

#### Sullivan (Interpersonal)
- Personal security, intimacy, lust
- Achieves intimate relationships, develops a personal philosophy, adjusts to body changes, becomes independent of adults

#### Elkind (1978)
1. Pseudo-stupidity: appears to ask "dumb" questions; difficulty reconciling concrete and formal operations.
2. The imaginary audience: super self-consciousness; believes that everybody is watching and evaluating.
3. Personal fable: belief of being special and not subject to natural laws
4. Apparent hypocrisy: the act of expressing an idea is tantamount to working for and attaining it.

#### Freud (Psychosexual)
- Genital
- Personality and defense mechanisms become integrated into a person's character.
- Oral, anal, and phallic sensuality are incorporated into genitality.

#### Erikson (Psychosocial)
- Identity versus role confusion
- Puberty and adolescence: sense of formulating an individual identity begins at age 12 characterized by
  - rapid and marked physical change.

- shattering of previous trust in own body (rapid growth may result in lack of physical coordination).
- preoccupation with appearance.
- integration of personal values with those of society; role confusion may ensue.
- Later adolescence and young adulthood
  - Intimacy versus isolation

## Havighurst
Early to late adolescence
1. Establishing independence from adults in all areas of behavior, in a mature manner
2. Accepting oneself as a worthwhile person, really worthy of love, and building a strong, mutual bond with possible marriage partner
3. Shifting peer codes should lead to adoption of adult-patterned set of social values by learning a new peer code
4. Verbalizes contradictions in moral codes, discrepancies between principle and practice, and striking a resolution.
5. Developing own role in heterosexual relationships, exploring possibilities for a future mate, and acquiring "desirability;" choosing an occupation; becoming a responsible citizen in the larger community
6, 7. Controlling and using a new body; learning appropriate outlets for sexual drives
8–10. Using language to clarify complex concepts
    - Moving from concrete to abstract principles, and from general to specific
    - Achieving level of reasoning of which one is capable
    - Formulating workable belief and value system
    - Adopting an ideology

## Kohlberg (Moral)
- Stage IV: conventional (12–16 years): fixed rules in moral decisions, with obligation to do no harm and to duty (many adults never get past this stage of moral development).
- Stage V: post-conventional: 16 years
  - Social contracts understood and formulated
  - Laws recognized as changeable
  - Correct actions depend on standards and individual rights
- Stage VI: adulthood: moral reasoning may occur in late adolescence, but probably will not; abstract moral principles govern behaviors.
  - Morality is easily separated from legality.
  - Orientation is based on universal, ethical orientation.
  - Situation ethics can be applied by those in this stage of moral reasoning (many individuals do not comprehend this level of development).

## Piaget (Cognitive)
- Formal operations (abstraction and hypothetical-deductive reasoning possible) characterized by

- Adaptability and flexibility
- Thinking in abstract terms
- Using abstract symbols
- Making conclusions drawn from a set of observations
- Developing hypotheses and testing them
- Considering abstract, theoretical and philosophical matters
- Problem solving (there may be some confusion of the ideal with the practical)
* The ability to comprehend purely abstract or symbolic content exists, as well as the ability to solve advanced math and logic problems
* Can comprehend value and belief systems in the philosophical, moral, and political realms.
* Capable of sharing self with another to foster an intimate relationship.
* Inability to form intimate relationships may result in a sense of isolation.

## Developmental Timetable

### Sound, Language, and Learning
* Has adult verbal skills, with ever-increasing vocabulary

### Development: Vision, Neurologic, and Motor
* Regular vision testing important
* Good posture impeded by rapid growth spurt that accompanies puberty.
* Those active in sports tend to have fewer problems with poor posture.

### Physical Characteristics
* Menarche: 10–15 years
* Usually cannot reproduce for 1–2 years after menarche because of anovulation; dysmenorrhea does not usually occur until ovulation begins.
* Early use of oral contraceptives will limit potential height (elevated estrogen levels hasten closure of epiphyseal plates in the long bones).
* Males attain puberty between 12–16 years.
* Tanner stages I-V (complete development) usually attained between early and late adolescence.
* Full height not attained until ages 20–24 when epiphyseal plates close.
* Marked increase in muscle mass in males related to androgen; by age 17, muscle mass in males is 2 times greater than in females, resulting in strength 2–4 times greater in males.
* Adult cardiovascular rhythms by age 16.
* Awesome nutritional needs; at peak of growth spurt, males may consume 3,600 calories and females 2,600 calories/day.
* At end of adolescence, male basal metabolic rate is about 10% greater than female.

### Entertainment
* Group/peer activities such as sports or academic teams
* Parental-adult "limit setting" continues to be sought and desired by the adolescent and should be given; testing of independence continues.
* Thrill-seeking behaviors should not be positively reinforced.

### *Parental-child Education and Health Needs*

- 14–16 years: tetanus and diphtheria booster (repeat every 10 years during adulthood)
- Sex education and family planning (as indicated)
- Poisoning and substance abuse and consequences (e.g., smoking, drugs, alcohol)
- Motor vehicle safety (both as operator and passenger)
- Skin care (acne vulgaris)
- Nutritional counseling
- Sports injuries, drowning
- Improper use of firearms

# Index

Page numbers followed by "t" denote tables; those followed by "f" denote figures.